# Seminars
# in the Psychiatry
# of Learning Disabilities

## Second edition

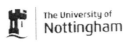
The University of
Nottingham

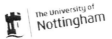

# College Seminars Series

## Series Editors

**Professor Anne Farmer**  Professor of Psychiatric Nosology, Institute of Psychiatry and Honorary Consultant Psychiatrist, South London and Maudsley NHS Trust, London

**Dr Louise Howard**  Research Fellow, Institute of Psychiatry, London

**Dr Elizabeth Walsh**  Clinical Senior Lecturer, Institute of Psychiatry, London

**Professor Greg Wilkinson**  Professor of Liaison Psychiatry, University of Liverpool and Honorary Consultant Psychiatrist, Royal Liverpool University Hospital

# Seminars in the Psychiatry of Learning Disabilities

## Second edition

Edited by William Fraser and Michael Kerr

Gaskell

Gaskell is an imprint of the Royal College of Psychiatrists, 17 Belgrave Square, London SW1X 8PG
http://www.rcpsych.ac.uk

British Library Cataloguing-in-Publication Data.
A catalogue record for this book is available from the British Library.
ISBN 1-901242-93-5

Distributed in North America by Balogh International Inc.

The Royal College of Psychiatrists is a registered charity (no. 228636).
Printed by Bell & Bain Limited, Glasgow, UK.

# Contents

# Tables, boxes and figures

*Figures*

# Contributors

**Zed Ahmed**, Consultant Psychiatrist, Welsh Centre for Learning Disabilities, Meridian Court, North Road, Cardiff CF14 3BL

**Helen Baxter**, Welsh Centre for Learning Disabilities, Meridian Court, North Road, Cardiff CF14 3BL

**Tom Berney**, Consultant Psychiatrist, Prudhoe Hospital, Prudhoe, Northumberland NE42 5NT

**Nick Bouras**, Professor and Consultant Psychiatrist, Estia Centre, York Clinic, 47 Weston Street, Guy's Hospital, London SE1 3RR

**John Cameron**, Consultant Clinical Psychologist, Gartnaval Royal Hospital, 1055 Great Western Road, Glasgow G12 OXH

**Sally-Ann Cooper**, Professor of Learning Disabilities, Section of Psychological Medicine, University of Glasgow, Academic Centre, Gartnavel Royal Hospital, 1055 Great Western Road, Glasgow G12 OXH

**Audrey Espie**, Chartered Clinical Psychologist, Old Johnstone Clinic, 1 Ludouic Square, Johnstone, Renfrewshire PA5 8EE

**William Fraser**, Emeritus Professor of Developmental Disabilities, Learning Disability Directorate, Tresender Way, Caeran, Cardiff CF5 5WF

**Tom Fryers**, Honorary Professor of Public Mental Health, Department of Psychiatry, University of Leicester, UK; Visiting Lecturer, New York Medical College, USA. Yan Yak, Old Hall Road, Troutbeck Bridge, Windermere, Cumbria LA23 1JA

**Anthony Holland**, Section of Developmental Psychiatry, University of Cambridge, Douglas House, 186 Trumpington Road, Cambridge CB2 2AH

**Sheila Hollins**, Department of Mental Health, St. George's Hospital Medical School, University of London, Cranmer Terrace, London SW17 ORE

**Geraldine Holt**, Senior Lecturer and Consultant Psychiatrist, Estia Centre, York Clinic, 47 Weston Street, Guy's Hospital, London SE1 3RR

**Andrew Jahoda**, University of Glasgow, Department of Psychological Medicine, Gartnaval Royal Hospital, 1055 Great Western Road, Glasgow G12 OXH

**Susan Johnston**, Consultant Psychiatrist, Nottinghamshire Healthcare NHS Trust, Rampton Hospital, Retford DN22 OPD

**Michael Kerr**, Professor of Learning Disability, Welsh Centre for Learning Disabilities, Meridian Court, North Road, Cardiff CF14 3BL

**Mary Lindsey**, Consultant Psychiatrist (Learning Disabilities), Cornwall Partnership NHS Trust, Kernow Building, Wilson Way, Pool, Cornwall TR15 3QE

**Craig Melville**, Specialist Registrar in the Psychiatry of Learning Disabilities, Section of Psychological Medicine, University of Glasgow, Academic Centre, Gartnaval Royal Hospital, 1055 Great Western Road, Glasgow G12 OXH

**Christopher Morgan**, Welsh Centre for Learning Disabilities, Meridian Court, North Road, Cardiff CF14 3BL

**Walter Muir**, Reader/Hon. Consultant Psychiatrist, University of Edinburgh, Kennedy Tower, Royal Edinburgh Hospital, Morningside Terrace, Edinburgh EH10 5HF

**Vee Prasher**, Associate Professor of Neurodevelopmental Psychiatry, c/o Monyhull, Monyhull Hall Road, Kings Norton, Birmingham B30 3QQ

**Oliver Russell**, Norah Fry Research Centre, 3 Priory Road, Bristol BS8 1TX

**Julia Scotland,** Specialist Speech and Language Therapist, Mid-Sussex Primary Healthcare Trust, Horsham Hospital, Hurst Road, Horsham, West Sussex RH12 2DR

**Bruce Tonge**, Head of Centre for Developmental Psychiatry, Monash University, Monash Medical Centre, Clayton, Victoria 3168, Australia

**Mike Vanstraelen**, Consultant Psychiatrist, Estia Centre, York Clinic, 47 Weston Street, Guy's Hospital, London SE1 3RR

# Foreword

## Series Editors

We are very pleased to introduce the second editions of *College Seminars*, now updated to reflect changes in the understanding, treatment and management of psychiatric illness and mental health, as well as changes in the MRCPsych examination and the need for continuing professional development. These titles represent a distillation of the collective wisdom of hundreds of individuals, but written in approachable, tutorial-style prose.

As the body responsible for maintaining professional standards and developing the MRCPsych curriculum, the Royal College of Psychiatrists has a duty to assist trainees in psychiatry as well as all practising psychiatrists throughout their careers. The first of the *College Seminars*, a series of textbooks covering the breadth of psychiatry, was published by the College in 1993. Widely acclaimed as essential and approachable texts, they were each written and edited to the brief of 'all the College requires the trainee to know about a sub-speciality, and a little bit more'.

*Anne Farmer*
*Louise Howard*
*Elizabeth Walsh*
*Greg Wilkinson*

# Preface

This volume – like the previous edition, edited by Oliver Russell – aims to provide an up-to-date account of current practice of psychiatry in the field of learning disabilities. The term 'learning disability', used in the United Kingdom and in this book, is equivalent to the term 'intellectual disability' as adopted in 1996 by the International Association for the Scientific Study of Intellectual Disability.

The book consists of 17 chapters that will meet the examination needs of young doctors specialising in the psychiatry of learning disability and inform their later practice. Most chapters are brief and further reading is advised, but we ensured that the key references to the topics are included and believe that this book will serve as a reference source. The topics cover knowledge required by the Joint Committee on Higher Psychiatric Training for those specialising in the field. In this edition, we have allowed some topics more space, such as the genetics of learning disability. Advances in molecular genetics have been rapid since the previous edition and a clear understanding of the genetic fundamentals of many conditions in learning disability is required. Advances in psychopharmacology in neurosciences and psychology have also been marked since the last edition and more space is also given to communicating with people with intellectual disability as a prerequisite to an understanding of their symptomatology and diagnosis. While this textbook is principally for psychiatrists in training, other professionals in the multi-disciplinary team will find the textbook relevant, reliable and stimulating.

*William Fraser*
*Michael Kerr*

# Acknowledgement

The editors are indebted to Joanne Wheeler, Academic Secretary, for her electronic meticulousness and mastery of coordinating authors and texts.

# CHAPTER 1

# New patterns of services

Mary Lindsey

The pattern of services developed for people with learning disabilities will reflect the culture, customs, history, values, beliefs, knowledge, resources and priorities of the society in which they live. In the Western world, in less than two centuries there has been a shift of policies from philanthropy in the 19th century to eugenics in the 20th century, and then to human rights and social inclusion in the past 30 years.

## The development of institutional care

In pre-industrial Britain, very few people with severe disabilities survived beyond infancy, and people with mild learning disabilities were cared for by their families and often occupied as unskilled labour. During the Industrial Revolution, people with learning disabilities (and those with mental illnesses) were frequently cared for in workhouses and prisons. An interest in people with learning disabilities, as a separate group, grew out of the work of the French physician Itard and his pupil Seguin. Their work led to considerable zeal in developing colonies and educational establishments across Europe and in the USA. The Idiots Act 1886 empowered local authorities to build special asylums and applied the same conditions for admission as for people with mental illness. The majority of mental deficiency colonies in Britain were constructed in the period between 1880 and 1910. Whereas the early institutions were concerned with training and rehabilitation, by the early 20th century there was a shift of emphasis to life-long segregation. The Mental Deficiency Act 1913 grew out of public concern about the control of a group of people who were seen as a threat to the physical, mental and moral well-being of the general population. It provided for both statutory institutional care and care in the community under guardianship or licence. By 1927, a survey by Dr E. O. Lewis for the Wood Committee found that 10% of 'defectives' were in mental deficiency institutions, 25% in mental hospitals, and 39% in Poor Law institutions. Professor Lionel Penrose, who in 1938 published a clinical and genetic study of 1280 cases known as the Colchester survey, undertook research into the biological basis of mental deficiency. This involvement of the medical profession led to the 'colonies' that had been established becoming designated as hospitals when the National Health Service was introduced.

# The demise of the institutions

With the Mental Health Act 1959, by which compulsory admission to hospital was possible on the basis of mental subnormality, care became polarised between hospital and the community. There was little change in services until the 1970s and the number of patients in hospitals continued to increase to over 60 000, with long waiting lists. Two Department of Health and Social Security hospital inquiries – Ely Hospital (Department of Health and Social Security, 1969) and Farleigh Hospital (Department of Health and Social Security, 1971) – and a large-scale survey, were to change this situation by revealing over-crowding, understaffing and serious ill-treatment. The Hospital Advisory Service was established in 1968 to inspect and advise, and influential publications by Goffman (1961) and Morris (1969) described the dehumanising effects of institutions.

As attitudes changed throughout the Western world, initiatives in community care consisted largely of building smaller institutions on less isolated sites but with very little real integration. Large hostels, often for 30 or more residents, were very similar to the wards of the hospitals that they replaced and the day centres were also large and institutional. They were exclusively for 'the mentally handicapped', who were in effect isolated from their non-disabled peers. This in itself restricted their opportunities for social learning and acquisition of independence (Zigler, 1969; Bjaanes & Butler, 1974). The Health Care Evaluation Research Centre in Wessex was established to carry out studies on epidemiology and deinstitutionalisation. Outcome studies were undertaken and showed that in community residential settings, the group care environment could be reorganised to increase the participation of residents and to enhance their competence (Kushlick, 1975). In the USA, the ideology of normalisation was promulgated by Wolfensberger (1972) and later described as 'social role valorization'. This was based on the belief that people with learning disabilities should be valued citizens with rights to dignity, growth and development, and should have accommodation and care that provided them with the same lifestyle and opportunities as the rest of the population. This led to rapid deinstitutionalisation in some states in the USA and in Sweden where people with learning disabilities were moved into ordinary houses within local communities, to be cared for by a non-professional staff team.

# The policy of community care

In the UK, the White Paper *Better Services for the Mentally Handicapped* (Department of Health and Social Security, 1971a) set the policy for the development of coordinated health and personal social services and a major shift in responsibility for residential care from health to local authorities. In 1974 it became evident that the implementation of the White Paper was not taking place as planned, and the National Development Group for the Mentally Handicapped was set up to provide advice on the development of community services. The Development Team for the Mentally Handicapped was established in 1976 to offer advice to individual authorities on how the White Paper could be translated into practical arrangements for the delivery of services. They produced a series of reports making recommendations for future community services.

As a result, a new service philosophy began to emerge, recognising that community care was based on different principles, as described by Towell (1988):

- people with learning disabilities have the same human value and rights as anyone else
- living with others in the community is both a right and a need
- services must recognise the individuality of people with learning disabilities.

A number of reports from the King's Fund introduced the term 'ordinary life' as the basis for future service delivery (King's Fund Centre, 1980). The implementation of the changes in community care also led to a much more personalised approach to care, based on individual need and choice, and to the concept of care management.

The National Health Service and Community Care Act 1990 that came into force in 1993 gave local authorities the lead role in the planning and coordination of social care for people with learning disabilities. Prior to this, there was clear policy guidance on community care (Department of Health and Social Security, 1989) which also introduced the separation of commissioning and providing functions, and encouraged the growth of the independent sector. Well before that, the All Wales Strategy aimed to 'correct the historic anomaly... which has left the bulk of service provision in large and, for many, remote hospitals whilst the great majority of mentally handicapped people and their families receive little or no support' and supported and funded a radical change in community services that included pilot projects offering intensive support in the community, even for those individuals with severe learning disabilities and very challenging behaviour (Welsh Office, 1983; Lowe & de Paiva, 1991).

Community care was initially regarded as a process of deinstitutionalisation with inherent benefits, but there has since been recognition that institutional practices can persist in many settings. Higher staffing ratios do not necessarily correlate with greater interaction with clients, or with reductions in maladaptive behaviours (Felce *et al*, 1991). However, overall research into service quality has shown better outcomes associated with ordinary housing compared with larger and more traditional provision (Felce, 1994). Whereas the early ordinary housing services usually provided staff teams supporting four or more people in one house, there has been recent emphasis on models of individual supported living whereby accommodation and staff support are provided from separate sources and the individual selects his or her own support workers. Such provision may be cost-effective for people with mild and moderate learning disabilities who are relatively independent but has not yet been widely adopted for more severely disabled people, except very high-cost provision for people with exceptionally challenging behaviour who put others at risk. While model projects demonstrate the viability of such care, the reality is that the majority of people in residential care are in much larger group settings.

The policy of deinstitutionalisation has also been applied to day care services and the large multi-function adult training centres, built in the 1970s and 1980s. These have gradually been replaced by employment schemes, more personalised day activities, support workers and smaller day centres. Colleges of further education have also become increasingly involved in provision, usually through the establishment of 'special needs' departments. The success of sheltered employment schemes is partly determined by the financial incentives, and the benefits system for people with disabilities is complex, with some perverse incentives.

Living in the community, while providing the opportunity for social integration, certainly does not guarantee it. There has been increasing emphasis on the many aspects of quality of life in which social integration plays an important part (Felce, 1996). Many people living in the community are very isolated socially and much of this is because, after an era of segregation, a large proportion of the general population is uncomfortable or embarrassed when meeting people with disabilities (McConkey *et al*, 1993). This can be reduced by personal contact in ordinary places, sharing activities together and by having channels of communication (McConkey, 1994). There has been increasing emphasis on the provision of appropriate support to enable people to access a range of leisure and social opportunities.

The importance of good-quality social care for people with learning disabilities cannot be overemphasised as it underpins physical and mental health promotion. Personal care plans are an important element of this, and should be delivered through a process over which the person has control.

# Services for children and families

Families have always been the major providers of care for people with learning disabilities, even at the peak of the institutional era. Families provide stable, consistent and personal care in a way that cannot be replicated in any residential setting. Emotional security and feelings of self-worth are primarily derived from being loved within a family. When this is not available from the natural family, then a substitute family through fostering or adoption should be available to the child. There is good evidence from the work of voluntary organisations such as Barnardos that, even if severely disabled, nearly all children can be found suitable foster or adoptive families with the right approach and with adequate levels of support (MacLachlan, 1986). The Children Act 1989, Volume 6, provides guidance and regulations for children with disabilities and reinforces their rights to family life. However, before the 1971 White Paper (Department of Health and Social Security, 1971) a large number of children were institutionalised from an early age without an understanding of the potential damage to their emotional and psychological development.

Families have to make many adjustments when they become aware that their child has a learning disability. Most go through a grieving process in relation to what they and their child have lost, and the importance of sensitive disclosure of diagnosis and appropriate support at this time is well recognised. At the same time as dealing with their bereavement reaction, parents also have to come to terms with a future containing many unknowns (Seligman & Darling, 1989). While facing many turbulent emotions, they also have to cope with the practicalities and demands of caring for a child who requires a higher than usual level of care or who may not respond to the more usual parenting strategies. In a minority of families, coping strategies may become dysfunctional. The impact of a persistently dependent child on the ordinary family life cycle can be considerable, with the transition to adulthood and independence being far more difficult to achieve (Goldberg *et al*, 1995). In adult life, ordinary people usually leave their family home and become independent, and this period of normal transition presents many more challenges for people with learning disabilities and their families. The tensions of adolescence are often exaggerated and the change of support systems from child to adult services exacerbates the problem and generates many anxieties. The shortage of suitable supports for independent living and of desirable residential resources results in parents being under pressure to continue to care well into adult life or until they are incapable of doing so. Also the natural protective instincts of parents, their awareness of the vulnerability of their child and their experience of service provision may result in them wanting to avoid the anxiety of their child leaving home and thus perpetuate the adolescent situation.

As the focus on family care has developed, and its importance has been recognised, so a number of service responses have been developed to address the issues that are raised. These include counselling, family therapy and also support through groups (often self-help groups), short breaks and practical help within the home. Community disability teams provided by paediatric or learning disability services can provide specialist therapy and advice. Financial assistance through disability and carer benefits is also available.

The changes in educational provision have had a considerable impact. Until the Education (Handicapped children) Act 1970, many children were deemed ineducable and excluded from school, leaving them totally in the care of their family or attending a 'junior training centre' with little opportunity for personal development, and with no financial support. This made it far more likely that families would seek institutional care for their child. In the 1970 Act, it was recognised that children who were 'educationally subnormal' had the right to education, and in 1981 the concept of assessment was introduced and a legal document, a Statement of Special Educational Needs, to identify and guarantee suitable provision. In recent years, the policy of inclusion in mainstream education has particularly applied to those children with mild and moderate learning disabilities.

Unfortunately, whereas education is now available to all, the availability of suitable counselling, respite and other support services is often poor, as shown by several surveys (Mental Health Foundation, 1996, 1997; Mencap, 1997; Department of Health, 1999). The legal framework for enforcing the provision of such services is not as robust as that for education. The service that families value most is that of short breaks, and such services have shifted from care in hostel and hospital settings to care with families that have been specially recruited and trained. There has also been a shift towards support services that offer care in the family home and those that support children in ordinary leisure activities or in special playschemes. The perpetuation of care from the family in adult life has led to a need for adult short-break services.

Most families also need to feel that they have control over their situation, and can make a positive contribution to the development of their child. Early pre-school intervention programmes such as Portage are available through the education system in most areas of the UK and have shown early benefits, particularly for children with Down's syndrome (Gibson & Harris, 1988). The evidence is that early gains may not be maintained, and there has recently been a shift of emphasis from just building on the specific strengths and weaknesses of the child to less academically oriented approaches that provide broader development of social competence (Marfo, 1991; Guralnick, 1997).

In the UK, most health services for children with learning disabilities are provided by the paediatric services. They may access the child and adolescent mental health services, but some of these services exclude them because they have insufficient resources and expertise. Some specialist learning disability services offer an age-span service, whereas others provide services only to adults. A survey carried out by the Royal College of Psychiatrists showed that in many areas of the UK there are no services available, despite the fact that it has been estimated that 50% of children and adolescents with learning disabilities are likely to need mental health services at some point during their childhood (Royal College of Psychiatrists, 1998).

## Specialist community teams for people with learning disabilities

As the hospitals closed from the 1970s onwards, so the professionals began to transfer their skills to working with families as well as with residential and day services within the community. Specialist community teams were developed that were multi-disciplinary and that could offer advice and support to families and carers as well as direct work with individuals with a learning disability. These teams vary in composition but usually include social workers, care managers, nurses trained in learning disability, speech and language therapists, occupational therapists, physiotherapists, clinical psychologists, learning disability psychiatrists and other therapists. Many also include less highly trained support workers.

As services and specialist teams have developed there has been increasing emphasis on the organisational aspects and management approaches that best underpin complex systems of service delivery (Barr, 1998). There are various models and memberships of teams across the UK and the importance of professionals working together effectively has been emphasised by the more recent development of care management and joint provision of services.

## Challenging behaviour

In the 1960s and 1970s, there was increasing interest and research into the effectiveness of behaviour modification in changing the behaviour of people with learning disabilities. This was targeted at both skill development and the reduction of challenging behaviour. The role of clinical psychologists became increasingly important in this area of expertise. Initially, both negative and positive reinforcements were used but there was growing concern about the use of aversive approaches and increasing emphasis on more positive and holistic approaches (Emerson, 1993; LaVigna & Willis, 1995). As well as being effective in behavioural terms, such interventions must also sustain and generalise the new behaviours. This requires considerable attention to carer training and behaviour. Challenging behaviour is a generic and descriptive term and the reasons for such behaviours are varied and complex. Thorough assessments should identify the key factors that may cause or maintain such behaviours and ensure that all of these are addressed, including developmental disorders, such as autism, and physical and mental health problems.

Initially it was assumed that behavioural and emotional problems were exacerbated by institutional care and that deinstitutionalisation would reduce them. However, it then became evident that this was not the case (Emerson & Hatton, 1994; Cullen *et al*, 1995; Nottestad & Linaker, 1999) and after deinstitutionalisation the frequency of behavioural problems often increased, while contact with psychiatric and psychology services decreased. As concern increased about community services for people with challenging behaviour, so providing for them was seen as a key aspect of community care. This led to a much better understanding of the use of behavioural approaches in such settings and the impact of the environment and staff attitudes and skills. The report of the Mansell Committee described a far more holistic approach to the care of people with learning disability and challenging behaviour (Mansell, 1992). It strongly recommended that competence in mainstream learning disability services should be increased and that specialist services should be provided locally to support good mainstream practice in learning disability services, as well as directly to serve a small number of people with the most challenging needs. In many areas this has been achieved through the development of multi-disciplinary teams that specialise in working intensively with people with challenging behaviour and their carers. The provision of such services is likely to reduce the frequently reported over-use of neuroleptic medication for behavioural control.

It is widely accepted that difficulties in communication underpin much challenging behaviour. Emphasis on communication skills in general has led to new approaches. These include the use of signing and symbols, sometimes known as augmentative communication systems, and interactive approaches based on developing a relationship with the individual through non-threatening and individually tailored approaches such as 'gentle teaching' (McGee & Gonzales, 1990). Art therapy, music therapy and drama therapy can facilitate communication and provide other therapeutic benefits.

Nevertheless, physical restraint or 'time out' is sometimes needed to prevent people from harming themselves and others. This has become increasingly regulated and training in its use has improved considerably. The emphasis has changed from control and restraint to care and responsibility, and any punitive element is seen as totally unacceptable.

# Health care

When people with learning disabilities were cared for in hospitals, it was assumed that all their health care needs could be met in that setting, whereas in reality many of the staff were not well trained in general medicine or psychiatry. The segregated nature of the hospitals and the prejudice against people with disabilities made access to mainstream health services difficult and inequitable, and as hospital care became discredited there was strong emphasis on avoidance of the medical approach. By the 1990s, there was greater acknowledgement of both the ordinary and special health care needs of people with learning disabilities and in 1992 the Department of Health published two important policy documents. One (Department of Health, 1992*a*) gave guidance to local authorities on planning services for adults with learning disabilities, particularly in relation to making arrangements to meet their social needs. The other (Department of Health, 1992*b*) provided guidelines on health services for people with learning disabilities. These guidelines stated that:

People with learning disabilities have the same rights of access to NHS services as everyone else but they may require assistance to use the services. Special care must be taken to ensure that they are not denied health care because of their disability, and that steps are taken to ensure that any barriers to access are minimised. Purchasing authorities should include in their contracts specific provision to enable people with learning disabilities to obtain NHS health care services and to ensure, where necessary, that special provision is made where the health care needs of people with learning disabilities cannot be met through the ordinary range of services.

In 1992, the Welsh Office also produced a report that identified specific health gain and service targets for people with learning disabilities (Welsh Health Planning Forum, 1992).

A survey of NHS trusts in England and Wales was undertaken in 1995 to ascertain the level of provision of specialist learning disability health services (Bailey & Cooper, 1997). Out of the 161 trusts that responded, 60.7% no longer had any long-stay beds in an institution but the majority (70.4%) had short-term assessment and treatment beds and also respite care beds (60.7%). The survey also showed considerable variation in the number of specialist professionals employed per 100 000 population. The trusts were also asked to indicate their priorities for service development and 61 were developing new services for people with challenging behavior, while 27 were further developing community services.

When the government of the day launched the 'Health of the Nation' initiative for England and Wales, a Health of the Nation Strategy for people with learning disabilities was also published (Department of Health, 1995) that drew attention to the ways of ensuring that the targets set for the general population in key areas of health were equally applicable. This was followed by good practice guidance on commissioning and providing health services for people with learning disabilities (Lindsey, 1998). This described the high level of health need in this population particularly in relation to mental health, physical disability, epilepsy and sensory impairments. The model was again that of accessing mainstream primary and specialist health services by overcoming barriers to access as much as possible, but also the provision of specialist services where these were needed both to support mainstream services and to provide services directly. Research had already shown the importance of access to primary health care and the value of health screening using health checks (Martin *et al*, 1996). The Department of Health has also produced good practice guidance to primary health care teams (Lindsey & Russell, 1999).

In the UK, the availability of specialist mental health services is very variable. A national survey of health and social care professionals' views about local services for adults with learning disabilities was carried out in 1994 (Gravestock & Bouras, 1996). This showed that most mental health services for adults with learning disabilities (66%) were within learning disability services rather than integrated within the general mental health services. More respondents (62%) had established specialised services (mainly assessment, treatment and community support services) than had not (36%). Respondents rated the general availability and accessibility of local learning disability services for adults with learning disabilities and mental health needs as significantly better than generic mental health services. Most respondents (94%) saw community learning disability teams as the major local service provider for this group, but only 48% thought that such teams offered adequate services to the group with mental health needs.

Another specialist area that has been much neglected is that of forensic psychiatry for people with learning disabilities, although the Reed Committee (Reed, 1994) reviewed the services. People with learning disabilities are over-represented at all levels in the criminal justice system, and are most likely to commit crimes against other people (Hayes, 1996). There is heavy demand on the small number of tertiary in-patient forensic units, particularly those offering secure facilities.

Demographic change has also affected the need for services, and it is estimated that since 1965 the number of people with severe learning disabilities has increased by 50% and will continue to grow by over 1% per year over the next 10 to 20 years (Scottish Executive, 2000; Department of Health, 2001). This is attributed to improved survival of children with more severe disabilities and also to a generally improved life expectancy. Despite this there has been very little development of health and social care to address the needs of people with learning disabilities in later life. Elderly people with learning disabilities have a higher rate of mental disorder compared with other elderly people and with younger adults with a learning disability (Cooper, 1997). Some of this is due to the high prevalence of dementia (Patel *et al*, 1993). Therefore, specialist learning disability services have had to develop their expertise in this area and work closely with psychiatric services for older people. The Royal College of Psychiatrists (1996/7) has produced a report that identifies the needs and required service responses for elderly people with learning disability.

# Self-advocacy, advocacy and human rights

There has been increasing emphasis on the participation of service users and their carers in decision-making in relation to service provision. This is both at an individual level and in service-planning. Gradually, the emphasis on service user involvement through self-advocacy or citizen advocacy has increased. The self-advocacy movement originated in Sweden in the 1960s and developed in the USA in the 1970s. The United Nations passed a resolution on the Declaration of Rights of Mentally Retarded Persons in 1971.

The first international self-advocacy conference was held in 1985. Many of the self-advocacy groups call themselves 'People First'. This movement has gradually increased throughout the UK and has had an increasing influence on service commissioners and providers. As the advantages of consultation with service users and carers have been recognised, so the methods of involving and consulting with them have improved. The introduction of advocates to speak on behalf of people who are unable to communicate sufficiently has also been developed in a fairly patchy way in some parts of the UK. Evans *et al* (1986) found that the involvement of parents led to a greater focus on people's needs rather than on service ideals. Voluntary sector involvement has increased and organisations that were initially parent-led, such as Mencap, now have people with learning disabilities closely involved in the running and management of the organisation and provide specific training to facilitate their involvement. Publications such as reports and policy documents now also have versions designed to be more easily understood by people with learning disabilities.

The European Convention on Human Rights was established by treaty in 1953. British citizens have been able to petition the European Court of Human Rights for some time, but until the Human Rights Act 1998 there was no direct remedy in the UK courts. The Act gives effect to the rights and fundamental freedoms set out in articles of the convention, making it unlawful for a public authority to act in a way that is incompatible with a convention right. There has also been legislation to ensure that the needs and rights of people with disabilities are protected. In addition, the Disability Discrimination Act 1995 is now fully in force, making it illegal for anyone providing services to discriminate against a disabled person in relation to access, including the way that information is provided and communication used.

Mental health and incapacity legislation is also very relevant in this context, and the Bournewood case (House of Lords, 1998) drew attention to the rights and autonomy of a person who cannot give valid consent to actions that affect health and well-being. The consultation document *Who Decides?* (Lord Chancellor's Department, 1997) describes the duty of care of society towards vulnerable people who cannot, for reasons of disability, express their wishes or make their own decisions, but incapacity legislation has not yet been enacted in England and Wales. The Adults with Incapacity (Scotland) Act 2000 has been passed by the Scottish Parliament.

# Current policy and service provision

Current policy on services for people with learning disabilities in the UK is very much based on their human rights and has been translated into practical recommendations through three important new policy initiatives. In 2000, the Scottish Executive published *The Same as You*. In 2001, a similar document *Valuing People* was published for England (Department of Health, 2001) and the Learning Disability Advisory Group in Wales has also made similar proposals to the National Assembly for Wales. Common themes include:

- the importance of person-centred life-planning (including health action plans in England) with the individual at the centre of decision-making and having control over his or her care
- availability of information through a Centre for Learning Disability that is to be established in Scotland and a National Information Centre in England
- strong support for advocacy services through the Scottish Centre for Learning Disability and through financial support to local self-advocacy groups and a National Citizen Advocacy Network in England
- the importance of ordinary housing and employment services to integrated community living
- appointment of care coordinators (local area coordinators in Scotland and health facilitators in England)
- more support to carers
- planning the transition from children's to adult services
- access to mainstream local social and health care services (including primary health care services) with support from specialist services as needed

- limited specialist provision
- better training and career structure for paid carers
- direct payment schemes
- multi-agency planning that involves service users and carers (through the establishment of Partnership Boards in England).

Therefore, the role of NHS specialist services for people with learning disabilities is now largely focused on the multi-disciplinary community teams. These offer support and advice to mainstream NHS services and to social services, as well as directly providing some services that are particularly specialist. For example, many provide neuropsychiatric and neuropsychology services particularly for people with learning disabilities and for developmental disorders such as autism. Likewise, people with learning disabilities should have access to the full range of mental health services, including in-patient services, but in addition there will continue to be a need for specialist learning disability assessment and treatment beds for adults. The Scottish Executive estimates that about 4 beds per 100 000 population will be required. The need for the NHS continuing care beds is not clear, but for the immediate future there is likely to be some residual provision for people with very high levels of physical or mental health care needs.

However, these and other reports (Department of Health, 1999) have also described considerable inequity of service provision. It is quite evident to all those who practice in the field that the service ideologies put forward in policy statements are very far from being implemented consistently across the UK. This is partly through lack of commitment and understanding of policy at a local level, but largely through under-investment in the major service developments that are needed if the reality is to match the rhetoric.

# References

Bailey, N. & Cooper, S-A. (1997) The provision of specialist health services to people with learning disabilities in England and Wales. *Journal of Intellectual Disability Research*, **41**, 52–59.

Barr, O. (1998) Community support teams. In *Hallas's The Care of People with Intellectual Disabilities* (9th edn) (eds W. Fraser, D. Sines & M. Kerr). Oxford: Butterworth Heinemann.

Bjaanes, A. & Butler, E. (1974) Environmental variations in community care facilities for mentally retarded persons. *American Journal of Mental Deficiency*, **78**, 429–439.

Cooper, S-A. (1997) Epidemiology of psychiatric disorders in elderly compared with younger adults with learning disabilities. *British Journal of Psychiatry*, **170**, 375–380.

Cullen, C., Whoriskey, M., Mackenzie, K., *et al* (1995) The effects of deinstitutionalization on adults with learning disabilities. *Journal of Intellectual Disability Research*, **39**, 484–494.

Department of Health and Social Security (1969) *Report of the Committee of Inquiry into Allegations of Ill Treatment and Other Irregularities at Ely Hospital, Cardiff* (Cmnd 3975). London: HMSO.

— (1989) *Caring for People: Community Care in the Next Decade and Beyond*. London: HMSO.

— (1971*a*) *Better Services for the Mentally Handicapped* (Cmnd 4683). London: HMSO.

— (1971*b*) *Report of the Farleigh Hospital Committee of Inquiry* (Cmnd 4557). London: HMSO.

Department of Health (1992*a*) *Social Care for Adults with Learning Disabilities (Mental Handicap)*. Local Authority Circular LAC(92)15. London: Department of Health.

— (1992*b*) *Health Services for People with Learning Disabilities (Mental Handicap)*. Health Service Guidelines HSG(92)42. London: Department of Health.

— (1995) *The Health of the Nation: A Strategy for People with Learning Disabilities*. London: Department of Health.

— (1999) *Facing the Facts: Services for People with Learning Disabilities: Policy Impact Study of Social Care and Health Services*. London: Stationery Office.

— (2001) *Valuing People* (Cm 5086). London: Department of Health.

Emerson, E. (1993) Challenging behaviours and severe learning disability: Recent developments in behavioural analysis and intervention. *Behavioural and Cognitive Psychotherapy*, **21**, 171–198.

— & Hatton, C. (1994) *The Impact of Relocation from Hospital to Community on the Quality of Life of People with Learning Disabilities*. London: HMSO.

Evans, G., Beyer, S., Todd, S., *et al* (1986) Planning for the all-Wales strategy. *Mental Handicap*, **14**, 108–110.

Felce, D. (1994) Costs, quality and staffing in services for people with severe learning disabilities. *Journal of Mental Health*, **3**, 495–506.

— (1996) Ways to measure quality of outcome – an essential ingredient in quality assurance. *Tizard Learning Disability Review*, **1**, 38–44.

—, Repp, A., Thomas, M., *et al* (1991) The relationship of staff : client ratios, interactions and residential placements. *Research in Developmental Disabilities*, **12**, 315–331.

Gibson, D. & Harris, A. (1988) Aggregated early intervention effects for Down's Syndrome persons: patterning and longevity of benefits. *Journal of Mental Deficiency Research*, **32**, 1–17.

Goffman, E. (1961) *Asylums*. New York: Doubleday.

Goldberg, D., Magrill, L. & Male, J. (1995) Protection and loss: working with learning disabled adults and their families. *Journal of Family Therapy*, **17**, 263–281.

Gravestock, S. & Bouras, N. (1996) Services for adults with learning disabilities and mental health needs. *Psychiatric Bulletin*, **19**, 288–290.

Guralnick, M. (ed.) (1997) *The Effectiveness of Early Intervention: Directions for Second Generation Research*. Baltimore: Paul H. Brookes.

Hayes, S. (1996) Recent research on offenders with learning disabilities. *Tizard Learning Disability Review*, **1**, 7–15.

House of Lords (1998) *Judgement in Re L* (by his next friend GE).

King's Fund Centre (1980) *Ordinary Life: Comprehensive Locally Based Services for Mentally Handicapped People*. London: King's Fund Centre.

Kushlick, A. (1975) The rehabilitation or habilitation of severely or profoundly retarded people. *Bulletin of the New York Academy of Medicine*, **51**, 143–161.

LaVigna, G. & Willis, T. (1995) Challenging behavior: a model for breaking the barriers to social and community integration. *Positive Practice*, **1**, 8–15.

Lindsey, M. (1998) *Signposts for Success in Commissioning and Providing Health Services for People with Learning Disabilities*. London: NHS Executive, Department of Health.

— & Russell, O. (1999) *Once A Day*. London: NHS Executive, Department of Health.

Lord Chancellor's Department (1997) *Who Decides? Making Decisions on Behalf of Mentally Incapacitated Adults*. London: Stationery Office.

Lowe, K. & de Paiva, S. (1991) *NIMROD: An Overview*. London: HMSO.

MacLachlan, R. (1986) Martin: a success story. *Community Care*, December, 1–6.

Mansell, J. (1992) *Services for People with Learning Disabilities and Challenging Behaviour or Mental Health Needs.* London: HMSO.

Marfo, K. (ed.) (1991) *Early Intervention in Transition: Current Perspectives on Programs for Handicapped Children.* New York: Praeger.

Martin, D., Roy, A. & Wells, M. (1996) Health gain through health checks. Improving access to primary health care for people with a learning disability. *Journal Intellectual Disability Research,* **41**, 401–408.

McConkey, R. (1994) *Innovations in Educating Communities About Learning Disabilities.* Chorley: Liseieux Hall Publications.

—, Walsh, P. & Conneally, S. (1993) Neighbour's reactions to community services: contrasts before and after services open in their locality. *Mental Handicap Research,* **6**, 131–141.

McGee, J. & Gonzales, L. (1990) Gentle teaching and the practice of human interdependence: a preliminary study of 15 persons with severe behaviour disorders and their caregivers. In *Perspectives on the Use of Nonaversive and Aversive Interventions for Persons with Developmental Disabilities* (eds A. C. Repp & N. N. Singh) Sycamore, IL: Sycamore Publishers.

Mencap (1997) *Prescription for Change.* London: Mencap.

Mental Health Foundation (1996) *Building Expectations.* London: Mental Health Foundation.

— (1997) *Don't Forget Us.* London: Mental Health Foundation.

Morris, P. (1969) *Put Away.* London: Routledge and Kegan Paul.

Nottestad, J. A. & Linaker, O. M. (1999) Psychiatric health needs and services before and after complete deinstitutionalization of people with intellectual disability. *Journal of Intellectual Disability Research,* **43**, 523–530.

Patel, P., Goldberg, D. & Moss, S. (1993) Psychiatric morbidity in older people with moderate and severe learning disability (mental retardation). Part II: The prevalence study. *British Journal of Psychiatry,* **163**, 481–491.

Reed, J. (1994) *Review of Health and Social Services for Mentally Disordered Offenders and Others Requiring Similar Services. Volume 7: People with Learning Disabilities or with Autism.* London: HMSO.

Royal College of Psychiatrists (1996/7) *Meeting the Mental Health Needs of People with Learning Disability.* Council Report CR56. London: Royal College of Psychiatrists.

— (1998) *Psychiatric Services for Children and Adolescents with a Learning Disability.* Council Report CR70. London: Royal College of Psychiatrists.

Scottish Executive (2000) *The Same as You – A review of services for people with learning disabilities.* Edinburgh: Stationary Office Bookshop.

Seligman, M. & Darling, R. (1989) *Ordinary Families, Special Children: A Systems Approach to Childhood Disability.* London: Guilford Press.

Towell, D, (ed.) (1988) *An Ordinary Life in Practice: Developing Community Based Services for People with Learning Disabilities.* London: King's Fund Centre.

Welsh Health Planning Forum (1992) *Protocol for Investment in Health Gain – Mental Handicap (Learning Disabilities).* Cardiff: Welsh Office.

Welsh Office (1983) *All Wales Strategy for the Development of Services for Mentally Handicapped People.* Cardiff: Welsh Office.

Wolfensburger, W. (ed.) (1972) *The Principle of Normalization in Human Services.* Toronto: National Institute on Mental Retardation.

Zigler, E. (1969) Developmental versus difference theories of mental retardation and the problems of motivation. *American Journal of Mental Deficiency,* **73**, 536–556.

# CHAPTER 2

# Applied epidemiology

Tom Fryers and Oliver Russell

Epidemiology is the study of health, disease and disorder, and factors affecting them, in human populations. Its methods are primarily statistical, but interpretations require knowledge of demographic, social, organisational and environmental sciences concerned with the collective experience and behaviour of human beings, and of clinical and pathological sciences. It is the foundation of public health practice, informing preventive programmes and the planning, organisation, development and evaluation of services.

Using epidemiological methods, we can validate taxonomies, discriminate categories, measure and compare the community dimensions and characteristics of health problems, search for causes and evaluate treatments and services. These methods need population data from well-designed studies or accurate and comprehensive information systems, both dependent upon high-quality clinical and personal data. For much of this work, we use the four classical designs of analytic study – cross-sectional, case–control, cohort and intervention studies. However, descriptive studies are important to generate hypotheses and are essential for planning, development and monitoring services. Definitions must be precise and consistent, measurements accurate and standardised, and analysis creative as well as statistically valid.

## Concepts and classifications

### History and conventions

The professional and scientific literature reveals a remarkable variety of incompatible terms, inconsistent categories and ambiguous concepts arising from diverse professional and scientific perspectives. Several equally important elements are difficult to reconcile in one taxonomy: genetic potential, aetiological diagnosis, brain damage and disorder, low measured intelligence and social maladaptation. Each alone poses serious problems of classification, standardisation and measurement; together the difficulties are insuperable. Most cultures use social labels, which are either stigmatising or promoted specifically because they are considered non-stigmatising, and these may change quite frequently. This should not affect professional and scientific terminology, although care professionals and researchers need to be aware of the differences between lay and professional language.

However, there has been little professional consensus on terminology. This has led to transient, culture-specific lay terms being used without discrimination or clear definition. The different needs of public acceptability, professional practice and scientific research cannot be accommodated in any one set of terms and categories. We require different taxonomies, categories and terms to serve different purposes, but always specified and defined.

The basic concepts of the first edition of the World Health Organization's *International Classification of Impairments, Disabilities and Handicaps* (World Health Organization, 1980) provided a coherent structure for this. Impairment was a fault in an organ or body system; disability was a loss of function normal for any human being; handicap was a social disadvantage accruing from the impairment and disability. These categories have been used to define mental retardation as a whole (global categories), or to define groups that have an important, but not exclusive, relationship with mental retardation (partial categories). See Fryers (1984, 1993, 2001) for the context of ICD–10 (World Health Organization, 1992), DSM–IV (American Psychiatric Association, 1995) and the American Association on Mental Retardation classification (Luckasson *et al*, 1992).

The World Health Organization classification has now been revised (World Health Organization, 2001). It has moved away from a model based on impairments as a consequence of disease towards a model based on the components of health. As a result, the boundaries and the terms used have changed. 'Impairment' is now subsumed under 'disability', which also encompasses 'activity limitation' (to which it was previously more or less restricted) and 'participation restriction', which more or less replaces 'handicap', a term considered prejudicial in some cultures. In the taxonomy of mental retardation, slight modification of previous terms will (avoiding 'handicap') acknowledge these changes, but some inconsistency remains. If the new terms and their conceptual boundaries are confirmed in practice over the next few years, it may become appropriate to make further modifications.

Discriminating multiple taxonomies within a common framework allows each to be researched or applied, both alone and in relation to others. Of course, no categories as such should determine the care individuals receive; that needs full individual assessment. Box 2.1 summarises the taxonomy described below.

**Box 2.1** Taxonomies in mental retardation

GLOBAL (OVERALL) CATEGORIES

*Intellectual impairment*
Criteria: intellectual
Measures: intelligence or developmental tests
Main categories: severe – IQ <50; mild – IQ 50–69

*Generalised learning disability*
Criteria: educational
Measures: mostly proxies of learning achievement (rather than learning process) such as memory recall, reading, number, problem solving, etc.
Main categories: in general, Severe, Moderate, and Mild are used but in non-standard ways; often ill-defined

*Generalised dependency (related to intellectual impairment)*
Criteria: social – highly variable in different societies
Measures: scales of dependency or maladaptation
Main categories:
   Severe – (or severe and profound combined) commonly limited to IQ <50,
      and therefore co-extensive with severe intellectual impairment
   Mild – used with very variable criteria of social selection

PARTIAL CATEGORIES

*Physical impairments, aetiological & pathological groups*
Criteria: commonly pathological or aetiological diagnosis
Measures: usually clinical and laboratory
Main categories: mostly neurological impairments providing 'medical' diagnostic groups

*Syndromes of impairments and/or disabilities*
Criteria: agreed (consensus) grouping of signs and symptoms with epidemiological validation
Measures: clinical, radiological, biochemical, etc.
Main categories: epilepsies; cerebral palsies; pervasive developmental disorders (mostly autism); challenging behaviours; psychiatric disorders

*Specific disabilities: losses of function*
Criteria: defined deficits in normal functions
Measures: standardised assessments where available
Main categories: specific motor, sensory, intellectual, emotional, and behavioural dysfunctions

*Specific social disadvantages; dependencies; restrictions of participation*
Criteria: social disadvantage
Measures: very few standard measures available

## Global categories

Retaining the internationally recognised term 'mental retardation' for the field of study and professional activity in general, three types of global category are useful: intellectual impairment, generalised learning disability and generalised dependency.

### Intellectual impairment

The fundamental global impairment is of the 'intellect', conceived as analogous to an organic body system in which lies the capacity to learn and reason. Intellectual impairment is measured, however inadequately, by intelligence tests, and summarised and simplified by the 'intelligence quotient' (IQ). There is no reason to assume that this capacity is immutable, and we know that its measurement is often prejudiced by other factors. Intelligence tests have often been discounted, but many (e.g. Berger & Yule, 1985) argue for their continued use in the absence of anything better. Epidemiologically, IQs have provided the sole basis for comparison between studies, and an IQ <50 is generally used to define the category of 'severe intellectual impairment' (Fryers, 1984). In human populations IQ approximates to a 'normal' distribution except for an excess at the lowest end, representing brain damage and disorder which mostly affects the prevalence of the severe group. 'Mild intellectual impairment', however, (IQ 50–69 by convention) is largely a product of the population distribution.

### Generalised learning disability

The primary function affected by intellectual impairment is learning, so 'learning disability' is the appropriate term (qualified by 'generalised' to avoid confusion with American usage in educational contexts). It should be measured by standard tests of the learning function, but these are not well developed per se, and tests generally measure performance of specific skills such as memorisation and recall, reading, writing and numeracy, which are outcomes of the learning process. It is not clear how these should be combined to describe generalised learning disability.

In recent years in the UK, 'learning disabled' has become the favoured lay term for all groups of people with mental retardation, but, as such, it has no scientific validity. School-based categories of learning disability have more validity for professional practice and administration of school systems, and are of little value for epidemiological research unless the criteria for selection are accurately described and measures are standardised and validated. If so, they can be studied in relation to various degrees of intellectual impairment. Of course, if a school category uses IQ<50 as the sole necessary criterion (given that all people in this category will undoubtedly have severe generalised learning disability and severe dependency), then we really have severe intellectual impairment in another guise.

In practice, categories of learning disability are likely to be determined by many more factors than IQ alone, such as the identification of educational special needs in schools (Department of Education, 1993), so they will not approximate to severe intellectual impairment or any other categories defined by IQ. This is important, as many children (and adults, such as those in prison) have learning disabilities not related to especially low intelligence. Nor do all persons with a similar IQ share the same degree of generalised learning disability, or types of specific learning disability. Current terms such as 'special needs' and 'learning difficulties', when used in an educational context, should probably be conceived as representing types of learning disability category. Outside educational contexts, they are likely to represent types of dependency category.

## Generalised dependency

The principal global, social disadvantage experienced by people with intellectual impairment is dependency (which may also be conceived as generalised restriction of participation, to apply the new World Health Organization terms). As with all social disadvantages, it is extremely variable in the experience of individuals but is a useful concept in populations. In this context, it is related to intellectual impairment and learning disability. Whatever term is applied to this group of people in a particular society – mentally retarded, mentally handicapped, learning disabled, developmentally disabled and so forth – without precise and standardised measures of intelligence or learning function, the group is in reality being conceived within 'generalised dependency' (related to intellectual impairment).

Many factors affect which groups of people are identified as 'learning disabled' (or whatever label is in fashion) in any community, but if the definition of a severe group specifies IQ <50 (whether adequately measured is another issue) as the sole essential criterion, this is again really severe intellectual impairment. Mild learning disability is never defined by IQ alone. Many other clinical, personal, social, cultural, legal and organisational criteria, some recognised and some not, determine who is selected. These factors operate differently in different communities and at different times, so that the number thus selected (usually called administrative prevalence) is immensely variable. There is no basis for comparing studies when the key data – the criteria by which people are selected in each community – are not presented and may not be known. However, they could be, and this would form the basis of very interesting and valuable comparative studies.

Discriminating in this way between global impairment, disability and social disadvantage in mental retardation encourages clarity of thinking, not least about causation. Causes of intellectual impairment are likely to be largely organic brain syndromes. Causes of learning disability may include these underlying processes, but also many other clinical conditions (e.g. cerebral palsy), especially those affecting communication, and social factors. Causes of generalised dependency (even when related to intellectual impairment) may include all these, but family and wider social and environmental factors will be equally prominent, and may be the most important in some cases. For example, society's demand for universal literacy may render dependent some who would otherwise fare well and live independently.

With the lack of precise definitions and measures in general use, 'generalised learning disability' and 'generalised dependency'(both related to intellectual impairment) can usually be considered together and, in recognition of the preferred term in the UK, will be referred to as 'learning disability'.

## Partial categories

Persons with intellectual impairment may, of course, experience any disease or disability, but here it is useful only to identify those 'partial categories' whose defining features are commonly related to learning disability, though not exclusively so. Serious investigation of causes in these groups requires studies of total human populations, not only those groups exhibiting intellectual impairment or selected as learning disabled. Five types are usefully described.

### Physical impairments: aetiological and pathological groups

These mostly relate to neurological impairments. They are rarely limited to specific degrees of intellectual impairment or learning disability, and many include people who would never be identified as such. Examples are phenylketonuria (including treated cases), Down's syndrome (including mosaics) and fragile X syndrome (including female carriers).

### Syndromes of impairments and/or disabilities

These include the epilepsies, cerebral palsies, psychiatric disorders, autistic disorders and 'challenging' behaviour. They are neither aetiological nor pathological entities, but are all important in the context of learning disability, showing higher frequencies than in the general population. They can pose serious problems for clinical and psychological assessment.

### Specific disabilities: losses of function

Motor and sensory disabilities are relatively common in people with intellectual impairment, and may represent additional factors in selecting a person as having learning disability. Disability categories do not correlate with IQ categories, organic impairments or aetiological entities. Studies of specific disabilities such as poor 'mobility' or 'inability to feed oneself' can guide habilitative practice. The 'learning disorders' of DSM–IV may be seen as specific learning disabilities, related partially to intellectual impairment.

### Specific social disadvantages; dependencies; restrictions of participation

Specific social disadvantages are even less well defined, and there has been little research, but there is great potential in such studies for improving the lives of people with learning disabilities. It is worth remembering that, for many individuals, it is the specific social disadvantages they experience in housing, employment, income, social networks, leisure opportunities and so on that give them their greatest frustrations and their greatest sense of alienation.

### Carers' concerns: parent and family disadvantages

Only recently have these concerns been widely acknowledged, though there is a small body of research. In practice, a large proportion of care is provided by families, and professionals need to recognise the partnership involved. But 'informal' carers also have their own needs and social disadvantages, which must be accommodated by professional services.

# Frequencies in populations

## Descriptive epidemiology of severe intellectual impairment (IQ <50)

Severe intellectual impairment is co-extensive with severe mental retardation/severe learning disabilities, etc., if these are defined by IQ <50. The main points are listed in Box 2.2 and described in more detail below.

### Factors affecting frequencies

The two basic measures of disease or disorder in populations are incidence and prevalence. Incidence is a measure of events in a period of time, commonly new cases in a year, but similarly admissions to hospital, births and deaths. Incidence rates relate the frequency of these events to a population (as $n/1000$). Point prevalence is the number of people with a particular condition at a point in time; prevalence ratios (or rates) relate these numbers to the population ($n/1000$, often age and gender specific). The point in time can be a point in lifetime rather than calendar time; we use prevalence at birth (or birth frequency, the number of babies with a particular condition in 1000 consecutive births), rather than incidence, to accommodate geographical and temporal variations in birth rate. (This is sometimes wrongly called incidence at birth). Variation in prevalence between successive birth cohorts will be masked, and comparative studies made difficult, unless data are restricted to small age-groups (e.g. 5 years).

Incidence and prevalence of a heterogeneous group such as 'people with learning disabilities' are highly dynamic. However categories are defined, their frequencies are determined by the frequencies of very many disorders of widely varying genesis. Some disorders arise at conception and their causes must be looked for before conception; others arise in early foetal life, around birth, and in early postnatal life. New cases become progressively less frequent with age, with very few after 4 or 5 years of age. Mortality of abnormal foetuses follows a similar dynamic, being concentrated in early foetal life, around birth and in

---

**Box 2.2** Basic epidemiology of severe intellectual impairment

There is geographical variation within similar birth cohorts: range at least 1.62–7.34/1000

There is temporal variation in successive birth cohorts in the same community, e.g. 1.98–5.54/1000 in Salford children aged 5–9, 1961–1971

There has been a similar pattern of temporal change in many developed countries:
Low prevalence for children born in the early to mid-1950s
High prevalence for children born in the early to mid-1960s

There is variation by age due to variations between birth cohorts in incidence and mortality.
Recently, the highest prevalence ratios have been in the age group 30–34 years. By 2005, it will be 35–39 years

There is increased survival at all ages and into old age; there are more clients aged >45 than aged <15

There are usually more males than females, but there are no consistent patterns in the gender ratio

There is probably a social class gradient in both incidence and mortality: there are excesses in lower socio-economic groups

There may be variation by ethnic group, or immigrant status

These features are typical of developed countries. They will be true to varying extents for communities in developing countries, depending upon development and economic status, demographic characteristics, vital statistics, and many other social indicators (see text)

---

early infancy, and then almost levelling off. Prevalence at any age is determined by both earlier inception rates and mortality rates; known prevalence also depends upon the identification rate. Prevalence ratios are also susceptible to differential migration – the epidemiologist must therefore attend to both denominators and numerators.

These processes give rise to substantial variation in prevalence, in different communities and at different times. The assertion common in the literature that prevalence ratios for severe learning disability are 'stable' or consistent is not true, even for clearly defined severe intellectual impairment. It would indeed be very strange if this were true, given the social determinants of population frequency of the causes of neurological impairment, which vary so much between cultures and communities. These social factors (e.g. diet in neural tube defects; patterns of fertility in Down's syndrome; alcohol price and supply in foetal alcohol syndrome; consanguinity in recessive genetic disorders) are most likely to offer scope for prevention.

## Geographical variation in prevalence

Point prevalence varies between similar birth cohorts (concurrent age groups) in different communities. Reliable studies (see Fryers, 1984) found 1.62/1000 children born 1951–1955 in Salford, UK, and 7.34/1000 children born in 1957 in Amsterdam. Greater variation is to be expected in developing countries. Prevalence varies with genetic, cultural, economic, environmental and service factors, largely by influencing the spectrum of biomedical causes and early mortality.

Sometimes there is one dominant cause, for example, iodine deficiency disease, where more than 10% of village populations may be affected by congenital hypothyroidism (Fryers, 1996). In other populations, Down's syndrome often shows the greatest frequency of any one aetiological group, and in communities with traditions of late marriage, large families and taboos against contraception and/or abortion, may dominate the scene unless early mortality is very high. Congenital anomalies may be relatively high in small, isolated communities with traditions of consanguineous marriage, but few are associated with intellectual impairment. Mortality and survival are extremely variable, and can be generally related to the 'development status' of the community.

## Temporal variation in prevalence

Age-specific prevalence varies over time in the same community, because the spectrum of causes and the extent of early mortality change. In Salford, prevalence for children aged 5–9 was 1.98/1000 in 1961, 5.54/1000 in 1971 and 3.86/1000 in 1980. The same factors affecting incidence and mortality that explain differences between communities may explain changes over time in the same community.

A similar pattern of temporal change is seen throughout the developed world, with a low range of values for age-specific prevalence (1.8–4.0/1000) for children born in the early 1950s, a high range (3.3–5.5/1000) for those born in the early to mid-1960s, and falling prevalence ratios since then (and into the early 1980s, when the last longitudinal data were collected). The increase was almost certainly due to a rapid decrease in early mortality associated with developments in neonatal care; this has no doubt continued since. Such increased survival is well documented for Down's syndrome by life-table studies from birth. Other aetiological groups are too rare or too inconsistent in case definition or diagnosis to be studied in a similar way, but we can assume similar processes have operated, and continue to operate to increase survival.

The progressive decrease in prevalence in young children, experienced in most developed communities since the late 1960s, reflects many different processes reducing inceptions; large-scale oral contraception led to both reduced mean maternal age and dramatic reductions in conceptions to women in the highest child-bearing age groups. This greatly reduced the incidence of Down's syndrome. Later, mostly in the 1980s, widespread amniocentesis and abortion programmes reduced Down's syndrome even more, although the impact was diminished by the lack of conceptions in older women. In recent years, the age of conception has begun to increase again, which will increase the number of Down's conceptions and the potential impact of abortion programmes (see McGrother et al, 2001).

All other contributions must each be very small because the number in each aetiological group is very small, but the cumulative effect may be significant. Postnatal screening programmes for inherited metabolic disorders and sporadic congenital hypothyroidism have been very successful. Perinatal factors, which probably increased the number of babies with neurological defects surviving in the 1970s, probably produced far less neurological impairment in the 1980s, although proof is extremely difficult to generate.

In the UK, the reduction of encephalitis, encephalopathy and rubella syndrome by effective immunisation (and other measures for tuberculosis and bacterial meningitis) may have had a small effect in the 1970s and 1980s, but the major impact will be revealed in figures from the 1990s since achieving immunisation rates of over 95%, which produces herd immunity, for pertussis, measles, mumps, haemophilus, influenza type B and rubella.

The widespread adoption of early stimulation and training programmes for severely intellectually impaired infants, especially those with Down's syndrome, might have removed a few individuals from the 'severe' group at later ages by improving their test performance, but the impact on prevalence rates must be extremely small and would be expected to be a 'one-off' effect in any one community. Overall, though many small contributions are possible, recent low prevalence figures do not seem to be fully explained. There are also exceptions, such as Northern Ireland, with equally unexplained continuing high rates (McDonald & McKay, 1996).

## Variation in prevalence by age

Prevalence varies by age because of cohort differences from birth and early infancy. In many developed countries, the highest age-specific prevalence is exhibited by those born in the early to mid-1960s, although this will not be 'in phase' everywhere. This means that in the UK, for example, around the year 2000, the largest age group was in their early 30s. Younger age groups, that is later birth cohorts, have had progressively lower prevalence ratios (e.g. from France; Rumeau-Roquette et al, 1997). In most UK communities, this has enhanced the effect of smaller total child cohorts on the numbers of children with learning disabilities in school-age groups. The larger cohorts will move progressively through the age groups in future decades.

Prevalence also varies by age and time because reduced mortality has increased survival at all ages. McGrother et al (2001) project a continuing 1% per annum increase in the adult prevalence in the UK. In developed countries, there are currently more adults over 45 than children under 15 in most communities, and there are now substantial numbers of elderly people with severe intellectual impairments since childhood. The orientation of professionals and service planners needs to adjust in order to accommodate this (Hogg & Moss, 1993).

From the prevalence and mortality data available, estimates can be made of age-specific prevalence ratios for severe intellectual impairment (IQ <50). They can only be a rough guide; they assume a stable population over the past half-century, and no unusual factors affecting particular important aetiological groups. The original estimates for a 'representative' UK district in January 1990 were probably fairly reliable, but few new data from precise studies have become available to confirm them or otherwise, and estimates for later dates are increasingly speculative. Projected figures for the youngest age group, and to a large extent those for the oldest age group, are necessarily little more than informed guesses to assist planning and resourcing services in a district. What data have been published are difficult to apply because of lax methodology, wide age groups or unknown details of the population and its history; individual communities will of course vary, because of the specificities of their populations.

In Table 2.1 below, estimates for 1990 and mortality expectations for 1990–1994 were derived from the literature available up to that time, but mortality data are now available from the Leicestershire Learning Disabilities Information System (Case Register) (McGrother and Thorp, personal communication; McGrother *et al*, 2001), and the estimates for 2000 were derived by applying these to the previous figures. The figures for the youngest and oldest age groups are necessarily speculative.

However speculative these projections are, they illustrate the dynamics of the population, which will inevitably move the statistics in the direction indicated. In 2000, the largest cohort in such a 'standard' district would be aged 30–34; by 2005 it would be aged 35–39, and it is likely that most UK districts will not vary significantly from that. Government departments depend on estimates of statistical trends in order to inform effective planning of future services (Scottish Executive, 2000; Department of Health, 2001; National Assembly for Wales, 2001).

## Variation between different groups

There are usually more males than females at all ages, the ratio varying between 1:1 and 2:1, but with no clear pattern. It most likely depends upon the particular spectrum of causes of central neurological damage and disorder in any population, but differential mortality may also affect it. Some biomedical causes favour males (e.g. fragile X syndrome), but males are also generally thought to be more vulnerable. Reduced mortality in recent years may, therefore, have increased the male excess.

Many early studies found severe intellectual impairment to be evenly distributed across socio-economic groups, a surprising finding given the social class differential of most measures of morbidity and mortality, and the social factors involved in the causes of severe intellectual impairment. More recent studies have tended to show the expected social class gradient. It therefore seems likely that a differential in

**Table 2.1** Estimated point prevalence of severe intellectual impairment (IQ <50) in the UK at different time points

| | Prevalence per 1000 at time point | | |
|---|---|---|---|
| Age | 1 January 1990 | 1 January 1995 | 1 January 2000 |
| 0–4 | 2.5? | 2.50? | 2.50? |
| 5–9 | 3.0 | 2.25 | 2.25 |
| 10–14 | 4.0 | 2.75 | 2.10 |
| 15–19 | 4.5 | 3.70 | 2.67 |
| 20–24 | 5.0 | 4.20 | 3.59 |
| 25–29 | 4.5 | 4.65 | 4.07 |
| 30–34 | 4.0 | 4.10 | 4.48 |
| 35–39 | 3.5 | 3.60 | 3.93 |
| 40–44 | 3.0 | 3.10 | 3.46 |
| 45–54 | 2.5 | 2.55 | 3.90 |
| 55–64 | 2.0 | 2.10 | 2.30 |
| 65–74 | 1.0 | 1.20 | 2.71 |
| 75+ | very few | very few | 0.80? |

inceptions, masked by a similar differential in early mortality, has been revealed by much lower mortality.

During the late 1990s, published studies often found higher frequencies for non-European sub-populations in European countries (e.g. in Sweden (Fernell, 1998) and in the UK (Emerson *et al*, 1997; Emerson & Hatton, 1999)). However, it is not clear whether explanations lie in increased risk factors for specific syndromes, disadvantageous social environments or inappropriate test characteristics, and to what degree these might vary in different cohorts, especially for those born before or after migration.

## Epidemiology of mild intellectual impairment

Prevalence of a group defined by IQ 50–69 reflects almost entirely the 'normal' statistical distribution of IQ in populations, that is, symmetrically distributed around the arithmetic mean. Standard intelligence tests must be validated for specific populations. Ideally, test means and standard deviations should be known from recent studies, because test means in particular populations change over time as a result of developments in education and other cultural changes. Although tests were originally designed with a mean of 100, the test mean for a particular population may now be substantially greater. This requires adjustment of IQ scores, which only relate to the mean. Unfortunately, current data are not available for most populations.

For a test of mean 100 (s.d.=15), 2.27% of the population will fall below IQ 70 (two standard deviations below the mean), plus a small effect mostly below IQ 50 from specific pathologies. The few populations providing data confirm this with figures of 25–30/1000. Because measured IQ in populations is a dynamic feature, studies of the effects on IQ of early exposure to hazards such as those associated with birth trauma or ingestion of lead must assess their outcome in relation to population norms in a related cohort of births (e.g. Smith *et al*, 1991).

## Mild learning disability (mild mental retardation)

However defined in practice, people with mild learning disability are never within the same groups as those with mild intellectual impairment, described in the previous section. Many individuals with mild intellectual impairment are identified at school as having a learning disability, but most are not regarded as such as adults. It is important to recognise that, as usually used for adults (and to a lesser extent for children), mild learning disability is always socially determined, although IQ (if known) and biomedical factors may be prominent among the overt criteria. The vast variation in prevalence recorded by studies of adults in the past 40 years (eg. 2.97/1000 in Wessex, UK, and

77.91/1000 in Rose County, USA, both published in 1968) illustrates the situation. These, and all other studies, use (or record service systems' use of) different criteria for selection; there is no standardisation. There are no standard or representative data for prevalence of mild learning disability.

To be fruitful, research must recognise that who is called 'learning disabled' in a particular community or culture is a phenomenon to be explored and explained. Local 'registers' are valid measures because they record precisely those for whom the label is perceived as appropriate in each community. We can only speak of 'underestimated' or 'hidden' mild learning disability in respect of those who fulfil local criteria but who have not been identified. In practice, this is seldom known because many criteria are not overt, are ambiguous or are variable in application. Studies identifying and explaining the criteria for selection that operate in different communities, and which determine prevalence, would help us to understand the social context of service provision, the variants and determinants of stigma and discrimination, the concomitants of labelling, and the advantages and disadvantages to vulnerable people of being excluded from the group. This might guide much community care planning.

We know many factors that commonly affect selection apart from perceived low intelligence (measured or not) and certain medical diagnoses (such as Down's syndrome) commonly assumed to dictate selection. Legislation relating to mental health, education and criminal offences may all determine selection, as may regulations, institutional traditions, conventions of practice, and professional attitudes in health, education and social services. For example, 'mild mental handicap' dramatically reduced in the UK as social services took over the lead from health, because social workers did not label people in that way as often as doctors had done. People with mild intellectual impairment are more likely to be selected if they also have communication problems, multiple physical disabilities, mental illness or, especially, challenging behaviour, and if they suffer unemployment, low socio-economic status, a poor home environment or inadequate parental care. There are also some people in long-stay institutions who would not now be labelled as having a learning disability but were inherited by current services. These many factors in selection are summarised in Box 2.3.

It is these selection criteria, recognised or unrecognised, that lead to the commonly observed characteristics of the groups described as having mild learning disability. There may be few precise aetiological diagnoses, but many neurological impairments and motor and sensory disabilities. Epilepsy, cerebral palsy, mental illness and challenging behaviour are more common than in the general population; so are social deprivation, educational failure and poor employment records. Since selection criteria change in all societies, prevalence of the group

---

**Box 2.3** Factors affecting selection as mentally retarded

Legislation: criminal, health, education, social welfare and employment law

Service structures and traditions: in education, health, social welfare, etc.

Professional cultures: concepts, perceptions, expectations, labelling, etc.

Patterns of employment and unemployment: work and training opportunities

Social class and social attitudes: cultural expectations, deprivation, discrimination, etc., especially in education.

Family support: structures and security of families

Historical service patterns: older clients inherited from former situations, e.g. in institutional care

Perceived low intelligence: with or without additional factors (e.g. antisocial behaviour; mental illness; motor, sensory or communication disabilities; multiple disabilities)

Certain medical diagnoses: especially Down's syndrome

---

and the balance of characteristics will change over time. However, most individuals have the basic capacity to be independent and to enjoy an essentially normal lifestyle. Successful rehabilitation, or simply maturing with age, may move people out of the category as they get older.

## Intellectual impairment in developing countries

There are few reliable sources for estimating prevalence in most countries, but the data suggest wide variations related to the varying spectrum of organic causes, mortality and social situations (see Fryers, 1996). Conceptual and methodological problems are also harder for researchers in developing countries to solve. Precise comparative statistics are not crucial in this context. However, descriptive epidemiological work identifying groups of people with particular needs, establishing the aetiological processes and factors that are locally preventable, and estimating the order of size of the group for resourcing service developments are all extremely important, for example in China (Tao, 1988), in Pakistan (Durkin *et al*, 1998) and in Bangladesh (Durkin *et al*, 2000).

Severe intellectual impairment (IQ <50), whatever it is called, will be recognised in all societies, but mild intellectual impairment may not be. A non-technological, non-literate society may impose no social disadvantage on many of those with limited learning and reasoning powers; they may have acceptable roles and adequate support in the family and community. But increasing technological demands, and universal education requiring literacy and numeracy, identifies those who function well below average as having problems and may disadvantage them in their prospects for employment and marriage. The rapid and universal urbanisation of society may also disadvantage the less able, as extended family networks are disrupted.

# Aetiology and prevention of neurological impairments

## Cause and outcome in individuals and populations

Whatever definitions are used for learning disability, causes of neurological impairment are of fundamental importance. Cause is a complex idea, which should be conceived in terms of causal processes, causal factors and a variety of precise outcomes. For example, the rubella virus can be said to cause rubella syndrome, but what determines maternal infection, foetal infection and foetal response to infection? In Down's syndrome, we know a great deal about the processes of causation, but nothing of the ultimate causal agents. Aetiological studies must try to relate specific causal factors to specific pathological outcomes; multiple exposure variables and multiple outcome variables almost always preclude clear conclusions, as illustrated by the many studies of perinatal factors.

Epidemiologically, cause encompasses a different concept: factors and processes, mostly social and environmental, that increase frequencies in populations. It is often these that offer most potential for prevention, that is, for decreasing prevalence (Fryers, 1990).

## Types and frequencies of organic syndromes

The main organic syndromes related to intellectual impairment are summarised systematically in Boxes 2.4, 2.5 and 2.6. Many of the hundreds of syndromes are so rare as to pose extreme difficulty in establishing frequency data; nevertheless, a few are major contributors (Gilbert, 1992). The genetic processes underlying many of these disorders are described more fully in Chapter 3.

### Pure primary disorders (Box 2.4)

These are present from conception, an autosome or sex chromosome aberration in one gamete producing an abnormal chromosome constitution. Trisomy 21 (Down's syndrome) is the archetype, but trisomies 13 (Patau's syndrome), 18 (Edward's syndrome) and others also occur. Sex chromosome disorders are seldom associated with significant intellectual impairment. X-linked disorders gained prominence with the elucidation of fragile X syndrome.

---

**Box 2.4** Aetiology of primary organic syndromes related to intellectual impairment (frequencies are approximate and sometimes insecure) (adapted from Fryers, 1984, with permission)

*Down's syndrome*
Trisomy 21 (94% of all Downs) – birth prevalence varies with maternal age:
    age 20: 0.5/1000    age 35: 2.5/1000    age 45: 40/1000
    age 30: 1.0/1000    age 40: 10/1000    age 50: 150/1000
Trisomy mosaics (1–3%): birth prevalence 0.03/1000
Translocation (3–5%): birth prevalence 0.03/1000
(All except a few mosaics show intellectual impairment, mostly severe; IQ range is generally 30–55.)

*Other autosomal anomalies*: birth prevalence 2–4/1000
Includes Patau's, Edward's & cri-du-chat syndromes (only occasionally severe or mild intellectual impairment)

*Sex chromosome disorders*: birth prevalence 2–3/1000 (only occasionally severe or mild intellectual impairment)

*Non-specific disorders associated with intellectual impairment*
Recessive: birth prevalence ?0.5/1000
X-linked: birth prevalence 1/1000 – most boys but few girls have intellectual impairment; see text

*Doubtful aetiology*
De Lange syndrome: always shows intellectual impairment
Hypercalcaemia syndrome: usually shows intellectual impairment by later childhood

---

## Pure primary disorders with secondary neurological damage (Box 2.5)

These do not affect the general constitution, but a genetically determined specific defect affects development, with or without environmental provocation. They are called the 'inborn errors of metabolism' or 'inherited disorders of metabolism'. Phenylketonuria (PKU) is the most common of several disorders, in which enzyme defects can prejudice normal metabolism. Sporadic congenital hypothyroidism leads to cretinism if not identified and treated from early infancy.

## Pure secondary disorders (Box 2.6)

Pure secondary disorders arise from environmental insults to a normal zygote after conception. Prenatal causes include neural tube defects, iodine deficiency disease, rhesus incompatibility, and the effects of communicable diseases and other agents such as alcohol, drugs and radiation. Perinatal processes are complex: the main factors are hypoxia, hypoglycaemia, cerebral thrombosis and haemorrhage, and gross trauma. Factors increasing vulnerability in the baby include large size, small

---

**Box 2.5** Aetiology of primary organic syndromes with secondary neurological damage related to intellectual impairment (frequencies are approximate and sometimes insecure) (adapted from Fryers, 1984, with permission)

*Defects of protein metabolism (all show severe intellectual impairment if untreated)*
Phenylketonuria (PKU): birth prevalence 0.05–0.2/1000
At least five others: aggregated birth prevalence 0.1/000

*Defects of carbohydrate metabolism (all show severe intellectual impairment and die young if untreated)*
Galactosaemia: birth prevalence 0.02/1000

*Defects of lipid metabolism (all show severe intellectual impairment and die young)*
Tay–Sach's disease: birth prevalence 0.04/1000 in Ashkenazi Jewish communities; rare elsewhere
Batten's disease: frequency uncertain

*Defects of mucopolysaccharide metabolism (all show severe intellectual impairment)*
Hurler's syndrome: birth prevalence 0.03/1000

*Defects of hormone system*
Sporadic congenital hypothyroidism: birth prevalence 0.1–2.0/1000 (IQ variably but seriously affected unless treated from very early infancy)

*Mechanism not clear (effect on IQ very variable)*
Epiloia (tuberous schlerosis): birth prevalence 0.01/1000
Neurofibromatosis (Von Recklinghausen's disease): birth prevalence 0.33/1000
Some cases of microcephaly

---

size, immaturity and pre-existing abnormality. Other factors lie in the mother and in the quality of midwifery and neonatal care. Postnatal causes include encephalitis and encephalopathy from communicable disease, trauma and metabolic disasters in infants.

## Major aetiological entities and groups

### Down's syndrome

Down's syndrome is responsible for a significant proportion of severe intellectual impairment in all communities. About 94% of cases are due to non-disjunction of trisomy 21 and about 3–5% are familial, due to translocation, and should be identified after birth for genetic counselling. Of the non-disjunctions, 1–3% show mosaicism, which probably explains the rare Down's person of normal intelligence and achievements.

---

**Box 2.6** Aetiology of secondary organic syndromes (i.e. damaged after conception) related to intellectual impairment (frequencies are approximate and sometimes insecure) (adapted from Fryers, 1984, with permission)

*Antenatal factors*
Iodine deficiency disorders: cretinism – frequency of severe intellectual impairment very variable; can be more than 10% of whole populations (see text)
Neural tube defects: birth prevalence 1–8/1000, possibly 10% are intellectually impaired
Rhesus incompatibility: intellectual impairment varies
Communicable diseases: very varied frequency of infection and of brain damage after infection (see text)
Alcohol: foetal alcohol syndrome – many cases show severe intellectual impairment
Drugs, irradiation, heavy metals: no satisfactory data

*Perinatal factors*
Gross trauma, hypoxia, hypoglycaemia and cerebral thrombosis
Often associated with cerebral palsy and epilepsy (definitions are problematic and the frequency of damage is virtually unmeasurable)

*Postnatal factors*
Physical trauma; accidents
Communicable diseases – meningitis and encephalitis or encephalopathies (see text)
Chemical agents: lead may reduce intelligence a little
Nutritional/metabolic: high-solute baby feeds combined with fever (all very variable in frequency)

---

Among non-disjunctions 75–85% are of maternal origin, mostly from the first meiotic division, and therefore occurring in the mother's foetal life. Prevalence at birth increases with maternal age (0.7/1000 at 20–24 years to 4.5/1000 at 35–39, 16/1000 at 40–44 and over 55/1000 at 45–49). Between 5% and 20% of non-disjunctions are of paternal origin, also mostly at the first division. These may arise just prior to fertilisation, and it is possible that occupational exposures are relevant.

Overall prevalence at birth is lower where maternal age has diminished (McGrother & Marshall (1990) estimated a 45% reduction in the UK since 1941) and where amniocentesis and abortion programmes have had an impact. However, these are reversible, and the data suggest little change in prevalence at birth recently. There is very high mortality of Down's foetuses early in gestation; it is likely, but not certain, that prevalence at conception is also related to maternal age. In developed countries, postnatal survival has increased from about 50% at 1 year 40 years ago to 80–90% at 10 years now, most deaths being among the 25–40% with serious heart defects (Hayes *et al*, 1997).

Generally, the Down's population has an IQ range of 20–55. There is increased survival into middle and old age, where Alzheimer's dementia is common and of early onset. Demographic changes in the UK have affected family structures: 'typical' mothers used to be elderly with several children; they are now often having their first child in their 30s (Gath, 1990).

## Fragile-X syndrome

Fragile-X syndrome is an important contributor to severe intellectual impairment, although not all those with the condition exhibit low intelligence. Fragile-X may be as common as Down's syndrome but prevalence figures vary substantially between studies. It has generally been thought that birth prevalence is 0.5–1/1000 male live births, but recent evidence suggests that it may be substantially lower (Morton *et al*, 1997).

Fragile-X syndrome is usually associated with an expansion in a gene called FMRI, which is located on the X chromosome at the Xq27.3 'fragile' locus, and consists of multiple CGG trinucleotide triplet repeats. In normal individuals there are fewer than 54 repeats, but phenotypically and cytogenetically normal carriers have between 50 and 150 (so-called 'pre-mutations'). Through trans-generational progression, these CGG repeats may expand and proceed to a full mutation, in excess of 200 repeats (Turk, 1995).

Intelligence may be impaired, and about 80% of affected boys will have an IQ <70, including some with IQ <50. About 30% of girls with the mutation have an IQ of 50–69, rarely lower, while 70% of girls are unaffected carriers, half of whose male children and one-sixth of whose female children will be affected (Simon *et al*, 1990). Twenty per cent of males with fragile X syndrome have epileptic seizures, usually presenting in childhood. Nuclear magnetic resonance imaging studies have revealed anatomical abnormalities in the cerebellar vermis.

Because the behaviour of many children with fragile X syndrome fulfils diagnostic criteria for autism, a link between them has been proposed. However, evidence suggests that only 2–3% of autism can be shown to be associated with fragile X syndrome. According to some studies, children with fragile X syndrome appear to be hyperactive, restless and to have poor concentration. The most subtle effect of the fragile X gene may involve personality characteristics, causing shyness and a predisposition to depression (Einfeld & Hall, 1994).

## Sporadic congenital hypothyroidism

Congenital hypothyroidism occurs sporadically in all communities (0.1–2.0/1000 live births), unrelated to iodine deficiency. Unless identified very early (preferably before the age of 3 weeks) by screening, and treated with L-thyroxine, cretinism will result. Since the late 1970s, neonatal screening programmes have been established in countries with advanced health care systems. Before this, affected children could not be diagnosed and treated until after the neonatal period, by which time lack of thyroid hormone would have seriously affected neurological development. Late treatment resulted in impaired intelligence and a range of abnormalities of neurological function, especially poor motor coordination.

It is now clear that even the earliest treatment cannot preclude all such problems, possibly because of low prenatal levels of thyroid hormone, but research so far has been inconsistent. A British study of early-treated congenital hypothyroidism at age 10 found evidence of lowered IQs and a variety of significant deficits in learning, motor skills and behaviour in more severe cases, less so in milder cases (Simons et al, 1994, 1997). Coordination problems appeared diminished, if not eliminated, children sometimes having minor problems with balance or fine manipulation (Grant, 1995). However, a major study in the USA (New England Congenital Hypothyroidism Collaborative, 1981) found no apparent loss of intellectual function at any age in those treated early, and no relationship between severity and outcome.

From a public health perspective, the congenital hypothyroidism screening programme provides the model for a population approach to a sporadically occurring disorder. Screening is usually shared with that for phenylketonuria and other, rarer metabolic disorders.

## Phenylketonuria

Phenylketonuria (PKU) is the most frequent and the most studied of the inborn errors of metabolism, in which the absence of an enzyme prejudices metabolism of certain proteins, carbohydrates or lipids in the normal diet. Toxic brain damage and severe intellectual impairment arise if the hazardous dietary component is not excluded from infancy. Phenylketonuria is an autosomal recessive condition with a prevalence of 0.05–0.2/1000 live births. It is genetically complex, with over 40 different mutations of the phenylalanine hydroxylase gene recognised. Untreated, various degrees of neurological disorder, such as epilepsy, become apparent from early infancy. The Guthrie test, applied to the blood of all newborn infants, identifies those at risk so that a phenylalanine-free diet can be offered. Treatment needs to start within 20 days of birth.

The intellectual status of early-treated subjects is not necessarily normal; subtle, global intellectual impairments that have been documented are largely determined in pre-school years, long before questions of relaxing the diet may arise (Medical Research Council Working Party on Phenylketonuria, 1993). For women with treated phenylketonuria there is a high risk of foetal damage in their offspring, but dietary intervention before conception appears to have a favourable outcome.

## Other inherited disorders of metabolism

Because of the remarkable story of phenylketonuria, other similar inherited disorders of metabolism have been sought. A number have been found, but little effective intervention has proved possible. Tay–Sachs disease is epidemiologically important because its high prevalence is restricted to a very specific population – Ashkenazi Jews. About 1/30 are heterozygous for the gene, compared with 1/300 in other populations. Lipid metabolism is disordered and results in early death. Fortunately, genetic screening now permits pre-marital counselling.

The mucopolysaccharidoses form a group of rare disorders characterised by deficiency of specific lysosomal enzymes, commonly known by eponymous titles (e.g. Hurler's, Hunter's, San Filippo). The total prevalence of all types has been estimated at 0.05–0.1/1000 live births. The most common is MPS III (San Filippo syndrome), in which apparently normally developing children subsequently present with a severe neurological disorder accompanied by deterioration of intellectual function and major behavioural disturbance. The prevalence of the most common sub-type (MPS III A) is approximately 0.05/1000 live births. In the UK, the Society for Mucopolysaccharide Diseases provides mutual support for parents and encourages research.

## Other autosomal recessive genetic disorders

These disorders are especially frequent (up to 5% of total births) where there are high rates of consanguinity; usually communities isolated by geography or social status, or with cultural traditions of consanguinity. To date, 138 autosomal recessive conditions have been reported in association with intellectual impairment, but they are mostly extremely rare and the total number of affected individuals is therefore small. Prevention requires both education and wider opportunities for marriage.

Rett syndrome is a neurologically progressive syndrome that only affects females. It may present as early as 5 months. The child shows regression of intellectual function, curious stereotypical hand-wringing movements, and then progressive motor disabilities. There appears to be geographical variation; prevalence rates of about 0.1/1000 girls have been reported in Scotland, Sweden and Australia, where very high rates of consanguinity among both parents' ancestors were recorded (Hagberg, 1993). Clusters of cases in Norwegian islands and northern Tuscany also suggest a genetic origin, but this is not yet proven.

## Autosomal dominant genetic disorders

Forty-one autosomal dominant disorders have been reported to be associated with intellectual impairment. The most common is tuberous sclerosis, which can cause epilepsy and a degree of intellectual impairment. The true prevalence is unclear because clinical expression is so varied, but it has been estimated at 0.17/1000 live births (Webb & Osborne, 1995). Most children present with seizures and among children with infantile spasms some will be found to have tuberous sclerosis. Many affected children are only identified after a more severely affected sibling has been diagnosed. Population DNA screening might be possible in the future.

## Neural tube defects

Neural tube defects vary geographically in frequency, and dietary deficiency of folic acid is a major cause (Department of Health Expert Advisory Group, 1992). Education to change the diet, or the provision of folate supplements, can prevent defects, but folate sufficiency must be established before conception because the defects arise extremely early in foetal development, usually before a women discovers that she is pregnant. Supplementation should always be provided for women after one baby with a neural tube defect, as risks of recurrence are high. Making folates available together with health education for all fertile women have proved disappointing, and general supplementation, like other vitamins, in common foods such as cereals and flour, is probably also necessary (Murphy *et al*, 2000).

## Foetal alcohol syndrome

Foetal alcohol syndrome is extremely variable in frequency and exhibits a variety of physical and intellectual impairments. There is no known 'safe' dose during pregnancy, and there is evidence of lesser degrees of foetal damage, including intellectual impairment, even when the full syndrome does not arise (Forrest & Florey, 1991). The best advice remains to avoid alcohol completely during pregnancy (Bradley *et al*, 1998).

## Iodine deficiency disease

Iodine deficiency disease in the UK (endemic cretinism and goitre) has now been largely forgotten, and few remember why table salt is 'iodised'. Throughout the world this is by far the most frequent cause of severe intellectual impairment, especially important because it is preventable (Micronutrient Deficiency Information System, 1993). It affects large parts of Asia, Africa and South America, but especially Himalayan communities and various mountain areas of China, where over 10% of some villages showed frank cretinism and goitre was even more rife before the iodine supplementation programmes of the past 20 years

(Hetzel, 1989). The most common medium for iodine supplementation is salt, where supplies are well controlled. Iodised oil injections given to fertile or pregnant women can be successful, with effects lasting about 3 years (Delange, 1996). Oral iodised oil may eventually prove to be a more effective intervention.

### Perinatal factors

Causal processes around birth are a complex of factors affecting vulnerability, the hazards of birth and survival. Epidemiologically, there are very serious difficulties in relating specific factors to specific outcomes (Fryers, 1990; Escobar et al, 1991). Precise definition and accurate measurement of exposure and outcome variables are extremely difficult, even impossible. Comparing outcomes with relevant norms is prejudiced by inadequate population data. It is difficult to know the status of babies before they enter the perinatal period; many syndromes, for example those associated with cerebral palsy, long considered perinatal in origin, are now thought in some cases to arise earlier. Evaluation of the perinatal period is affected by increases in amniocentesis and abortion, and changes in fertility and mean maternal age.

The dynamic relationships between healthy survival, damaged survival and death make even basic numbers hard to estimate. Communities in which major perinatal problems abound are likely also to have high mortality. Other communities have fewer hazards and lower mortality. This has virtually precluded evaluation of changes in perinatal care; decreased mortality is certain, but morbidity rates among survivors are disputed. There is no doubt, however, that the overall birth frequencies of serious and minor impairments and disabilities have increased (e.g. Colver et al, 2000). No statistics can be recommended with confidence (Aylward et al, 1989); though see Pharoah et al (1998) and Cans (2000). Few doubt that perinatal causes contribute importantly to intellectual impairment in most communities.

## Programmes to prevent impairments

### Universal screening of neonates

This is now common for phenylketonuria, several similar disorders treatable by diet, and sporadic hypothyroidism. It has been extremely effective in the UK in preventing intellectual impairment, and is cost-effective, but organisational improvements could increase its effectiveness still further (Pollitt et al, 1997; Streetly & Corbett, 1997).

### Screening healthy adult populations

This was successful for Tay–Sach's disease in Ashkenazi communities in the USA, where the implications of pre-marital genetic counselling were accepted, but not elsewhere. Tay–Sach's is now almost eliminated from American Jewish populations. Genetic registers may eventually play a role in other conditions.

## Antenatal screening: Down's syndrome

Screening for foetal abnormalities, especially Down's syndrome, has become an increasingly important part of antenatal care. When amniocentesis was first introduced, it was confined to women in high-risk groups, specifically those aged 35 or over (Green, 1994). Those found to be carrying a foetus with Down's syndrome or another serious abnormality were offered an abortion. In population terms, the programme was judged a failure; the reduction of Down's births in England and Wales was estimated to be only 10% between 1980 and 1985 (Vyas, 1994). Data from the Office of National Statistics also suggest little change in prevalence at birth. However, more recently some reports have indicated much greater changes (e.g. in South Australia; Cheffins *et al*, 2000).

New serum testing techniques in 1992 permitted all women to be offered antenatal tests for Down's syndrome at 16–18 weeks of pregnancy. Three assays are made, maternal alpha foeto-protein, unconugated oestriol and human chorionic gonadotrophin, from each of which a risk can be calculated. Those whose test results indicate high risk are offered amniocentesis or chorionic villi sampling, to be followed by the option of abortion if positive. Women can therefore know their individual risk. Women must make a decision at three points, before the serum tests, before amniocentesis and before termination, but it is difficult to turn back once the process has started. Adequate counselling is essential before any of these, to allow an informed choice on whether to undertake the whole process. Serum testing is now offered to 70% of pregnant women in the UK (Wald *et al*, 1999*a*); triple-test screening is recommended as the most effective (Wald *et al*, 1999*b*), but doubts have been expressed about the adequacy of the counselling available (Marteau & Croyle, 1998).

Antenatal testing raises a variety of ethical issues (Advisory Committee on Genetic Testing, 2000; Ward, 2001). A decade ago, the Nuffield Council on Bioethics (1993) took the view that in order to justify the implementation of a screening programme, the condition had to be 'serious'. The classification of Down's syndrome as 'serious' is contentious (Chadwick, 2001). The situation facing parents who have been told that they are at high risk of having a Down's syndrome child is no longer clear-cut. Doctors cannot advise parents that a child with Down's syndrome is destined for a life in institutional care with few achievements and a poor quality of life. It is now appreciated that children with Down's syndrome may grow up to have fulfilled lives, to enjoy companionship with others, perhaps even have a job and a home of their own. If parents are to make informed decisions, they will need information, genetic counselling and an opportunity to decide without being put under duress (Russell, 2001).

## Antenatal screening for other conditions

Amniocentesis and abortion are not truly preventive, but are accepted in many communities, not only in respect of Down's syndrome, but also for the abortion of foetuses affected by rubella or a neural tube defect. Serum screening for alpha foeto-protein enables the detection of neural tube defects, and ultrasound can detect other foetal abnormalities.

## Postnatal testing of mothers

To avoid further affected children with a familial disorder, postnatal testing of mothers of affected babies can detect familial (translocation) Down's syndrome and carrier status in fragile X syndrome, to facilitate counselling and choice concerning subsequent pregnancies. If not identified earlier, postnatal tests after a first child should identify rhesus-negative mothers so that they can be immunised against sensitisation by rhesus-positive cells in subsequent pregnancies.

## DNA screening of selected populations at high risk

Over the past decade, fragile X syndrome has been recognised to be a significant cause of learning disability. Recent technical advances in DNA diagnostic methods have made it possible to consider screening populations at risk. This should enable all potentially affected families to be forewarned (Sabaratnam *et al*, 1994). The inheritance has an unusual X-linked pattern; although the majority of males inheriting the mutation are affected, in about 20% the gene is non-penetrant. Their intellect and appearance are normal, but they are, nevertheless, carriers. Thirty per cent of females who inherit the mutation have some degree of intellectual impairment, but there are no specific dysmorphic features. The 70% of females who are intellectually normal show no indications of their carrier status, and it is often only after a second child with learning disabilities is born that a genetic cause is suspected. Screening for carriers is therefore clearly important. DNA-based screening for fragile X syndrome is now technically feasible and is being carried out in some special schools (Slaney *et al*, 1995). A checklist is used to identify a subset of children at particularly high risk. Female relatives can be counselled and further conceptions avoided, and accurate prenatal diagnosis and selective abortion of affected foetuses can also be offered. Wider population screening, however, is not yet feasible (Murray *et al*, 1997).

## Communicable diseases

Although no one organism is numerically important in learning disability, they are collectively important, not least because of the potential for prevention (Dudgeon *et al*, 1985). Rubella syndrome arises during early foetal life and can be prevented by immunisation. Cytomegalovirus is common, but so is natural immunity and vaccine development is incomplete. For toxoplasmosis, there is insufficient information on the frequency of infection, the disease rate after intra-uterine infection and the frequency of specific impairments. Only rough estimates of risk are possible, though they vary from place to place and are probably mostly small. Antenatal screening is carried out in some countries, but this is generally considered unjustified (Hall, 1992). Antenatal treatment is partially successful. There is no consensus on intervention, other than advocating avoidance of cat litter and poorly cooked meat products.

Tuberculosis and syphilis have been important in all countries. Early diagnosis and effective treatment almost eliminated them from developed countries, but continued vigilance remains important, and multiple-drug-resistant tuberculosis has appeared to be associated with AIDS in some communities. Other countries continue to experience both, and the neurological and intellectual impairments resulting from them.

Malaria should not be ignored in countries where it is prevalent. The various causes of meningitis and encephalitis or encephalopathy include measles, mumps, pertussis and haemophylus influenzae, all of which are preventable by immunisation, which reduces individual risk. However, it is more important to minimise communicability by achieving heard immunity, generally requiring about 95% coverage of the population. Rubella, measles, mumps and pertussis are important causes of intellectual impairment. Effective immunisation for measles will also prevent late-onset subacute sclerosing pan-encephalitis.

## Nutrition, dietary supplementation, advice and education

Dietary advice and education are important to improve nutrition in general, especially during pregnancy. In poor communities everywhere, the general health of women and children are still major issues and affect vulnerability to disease and damage. Specific dietary advice on folates depends upon supplementation programmes to be widely effective in preventing neural tube defects. Where there is endemic iodine deficiency disease, community programmes of salt iodisation or alternatives require high levels of political will, and effective community organisation and education. Health promotion to avoid alcohol consumption during pregnancy is variable in effect, but very important where alcohol consumption is generally high or where it is common for women to drink alcohol during pregnancy.

## Environmental issues: accidents and pollution

Accidents, and therefore accident prevention, represent very complex behavioural, environmental, economic and political factors. There have been some successes and some failures. Prevention of non-accidental injury to children is even less certain, although very properly the subject of much professional concern. Avoidance of specific environmental toxins, particularly heavy metals, may be important in some communities. Only lead has been much investigated; it does not create recognised intellectual impairment, and evidence of a general reduction in intelligence of a few IQ points is still disputed.

# Disabilities and social disadvantages related to intellectual impairment

## Related syndromes: mostly disabilities

Certain disorders are prominent in all groups of people with intellectual impairment. Epilepsy and cerebral palsy, syndromes of neurological impairments and specific disabilities may arise as part of the same aetiological process as intellectual impairment, before, during or after birth. Proportions necessarily vary, but a range gives rough guidelines. Epilepsy, often fully-controllable by drugs, is reported in 20–50% of people with severe intellectual impairment, cerebral palsy in 5–40%, serious visual problems in 10–30%, hearing problems in up to 5% and serious problems with speaking in 60–85%. These illustrate the multiple disabilities and multi-disciplinary needs that characterise the group. Groups with lesser degrees of intellectual impairment have much lower frequencies of these disorders, but they are still important contributors to overall dependency.

The pervasive developmental (autistic) disorders are disability syndromes which overlap severe and mild intellectual impairment. Prevalence of autistic spectrum disorder as defined by Wing's triad of impairments (Wing, 1980) is currently estimated at 1–2/1000 (Fombonne, 1999). Recognition as a clinical entity, however, does not imply a single aetiology. Many psychiatric disorders may also be conceived as syndromes of disability in the absence of known organic impairments. Studies usually show more psychiatric problems in people with intellectual impairment than in the general population, but if behavioural disorders are excluded, a true excess of clearly defined psychiatric illness is less certain, given the difficulties of assessment and comparison in people with learning disabilities (Turner, 1989).

## Measuring disabilities

The taxonomy and measurement of disabilities in populations has received little attention, and it is difficult to discriminate between discrete syndromes and to standardise instruments. Clinical and behavioural observation scales can provide useful individual profiles for professional practice, but are difficult to handle for research; they include the AAMD Adaptive Behaviour Scales (Nihira *et al*, 1993), the Vineland Social Maturity Scale and the Development Record (Sparrow *et al*, 1984), among others. Wing's Handicaps, Behaviour and Skills Schedule, developed for research, has been used successfully in community studies in several countries (Wing, 1980). Derived from this, a short Disability Assessment Schedule (Holmes *et al*, 1982) has been used for both service and research applications. There are computer analysis programs for both. There is a need for more epidemiological studies of disability related to normal populations, and evaluation research on procedures and programmes intended specifically to minimise disability. There is a very useful summary of the assessment instruments available in Mittler (1992).

## Individual social disadvantages: elements of dependency

This is a little-explored field for epidemiology. Most social disadvantages are not specific to people with learning disabilities, although they may experience a unique combination of them. There is no accepted taxonomy, few measures and little interest in research. A long-term project following up all those identified as 'mentally retarded' in Aberdeen in the 1950s is one of the few sources of information on adult problems of those identified in childhood. Papers by Richardson and his colleagues have examined marriage, peer relationships and work experience (Richardson & Koller, 1996). We need more studies to reinforce this one and validate its representativeness. There have also been a few studies of economic and other burdens on families with severely handicapped children with learning disabilities. We need data on disadvantage and dependency, because to diminish these is the ultimate aim of all services, and we need the tools with which to evaluate those services.

# References

Advisory Committee on Genetic Testing (2000) *Prenatal Genetic Testing – Report for Consultation*. London: Human Genetics Commission.

American Psychiatric Association (1995) *Diagnostic and Statistical Manual of Mental Disorders* (4th edn) (DSM–IV, International Version). Washington, DC: APA.

Aylward, G. P., Pfeiffer, S. I., Wright, A., *et al* (1989) Outcome studies of low birth weight infants published in the last decade: a meta-analysis. *Journal of Paediatrics*, **115**, 515–520.

Berger, M. & Yule, W. (1985) IQ tests and assessments. In *Mental Deficiency: The Changing Outlook* (4th edn) (eds A. M. Clarke, A. D. B. Clarke & J. M. Berg), pp. 53–96. London: Methuen.

Bradley, K. A., Badrinath, S., Bush, K., *et al* (1998) Medical risks for women who drink alcohol. *Journal of General Internal Medicine*, **13**, 627–639.

Cans, C. (2000) Surveillance of cerebral palsy in Europe: A collaboration of cerebral palsy surveys and registers. *Developmental Medicine & Child Neurology*, **42**, 816–824.

Chadwick, R. (2001) Whose choice? Whose responsibility? Ethical issues in prenatal diagnosis and learning disability. In *Considered Choices: The New Genetics, Pre-Natal Testing and People with Learning Disabilities* (ed. L. Ward), pp. 89–90. Kidderminster: British Institute of Learning Disabilities.

Cheffins, T., Chan, A., Haan, E. A., *et al* (2000) The impact of maternal serum screening on the birth prevalence of Down's syndrome and the use of amniocentesis and chorionic villus sampling in South Australia. *British Journal of Obstetrics & Gynaecology*, **107**, 1453–1459.

Colver, A. F., Gibson, M., Hey, E. N., *et al* (2000) Increasing rates of cerebral palsy across the severity spectrum in north-east England 1964–1993. *Archives of Disease in Childhood: Fetal & Neonatal Edition*, **83**, F7–F12.

Delange, F. (1996) Administration of iodized oil during pregnancy: A summary of the published evidence. *Bulletin of the World Health Organization*, **74**, 101–108.

Department of Education (1993) *Code of Practice on the Identification of Special Educational Needs*. London: HMSO.

Department of Health (2001) *Valuing People – A New Strategy for Learning Disability for the 21st Century*. London: Department of Health.

Department of Health Expert Advisory Group (1992) *Folic Acid and the Prevention of Neural Tube Defects*. London: Department of Health.

Dudgeon, J. A., Peckham, C. S. & Robinson, R. O. (1985) Infectious agents in the aetiology of mental retardation. In *Scientific Studies in Mental Retardation* (ed. J. Dobbing), pp. 203–232. London: Royal Society of Medicine/Macmillan.

Durkin, M. S., Hasan, Z. M., & Hasan, K. Z. (1998) Prevalence and correlates of mental retardation among children in Karachi, Pakistan. *American Journal of Epidemiology*, **147**, 281–288.

—, Khan, N. Z., Davidson, L. L., *et al* (2000) Prenatal and postnatal risk factors for mental retardation among children in Bangladesh. *American Journal of Epidemiology*, **152**, 1024–1033.

Einfeld, S. L. & Hall, W. (1994) Recent developments in the study of behaviour phenotypes. *Australia and New Zealand Journal of Developmental Disabilities*, **19**, 275–279.

Emerson, E. & Hatton, C. (1999) Future trends in the ethnic composition of British society and among British citizens with learning disabilities. *Tizard Learning Disability Review*, **14**, 28–31.

—, Azmi, S., Hatton, C., *et al* (1997) Is there an increased prevalence of severe learning disabilities among British Asians? *Ethnicity and Health*, **2**, 317–321.

Escobar, G. J., Littenberg, B. & Petitti, D. B. (1991) Outcome among surviving very low birth-weight infants: a meta-analysis. *Archives of Disease in Childhood*, **66**, 204–211.

Fernell, E. (1998) Aetiological factors and prevalence of severe mental retardation in children in a Swedish municipality: the possibility of consanguinity. *Developmental Medicine and Child Neurology*, **40**, 608–611.

Fombonne, E. (1999) The epidemiology of autism: A review. *Psychological Medicine*, **29**, 769–786.

Forrest, F. & Florey, C. du V. (1991) The relation between maternal alcohol consumption and child development; the epidemiological evidence. *Journal of Public Health Medicine*, **13**, 247–255.

Fryers, T. (1984) *The Epidemiology of Severe Intellectual Impairment: The Dynamics of Prevalence*. London: Academic Press.

— (1990) Pre- and perinatal factors in the aetiology of mental retardation. In *Reproductive and Perinatal Epidemiology* (ed. M. Kiely), pp. 171–204. Boca Raton, FL: CRC Press.

— (1993) Epidemiological thinking in mental retardation: issues in taxonomy and population frequency. *International Review of Research in Mental Retardation*, **19**, 97–133.

**45**

—— (1996) Mental retardation. In *Psychiatry for the Developing World* (eds D. Tantam, L. Appleby & A. Duncan), pp. 258–290. London: Gaskell.

—— (2001) Mental retardation: public health approaches to intellectual impairment and its consequences. In *Oxford Textbook of Public Health* (4th edn) (eds R. Detels, J. McEwen, R. Beaglehole, *et al*). Oxford: Oxford University Press.

Gath, A. (1990) Down's syndrome children and their families. *American Journal of Medical Genetics* (suppl.), **7**, 314–316.

Gilbert, P. (1992) *The A–Z Reference Book of Syndromes and Inherited Disorders*. London: Chapman & Hall.

Grant, D. B. (1995) Congenital hypothyroidism: optimal management in the light of 15 years' experience of screening. *Archives of Disease in Childhood*, **72**, 85–89.

Green, J. M. (1994) Serum screening for Down's syndrome: experiences of obstetricians in England and Wales. *BMJ*, **309**, 769–772.

Hagberg, B. (ed.) (1993) *Rett Syndrome: Clinical and Biological Aspects* (Clinics in Developmental Medicine, No. 127). Cambridge: Cambridge University Press.

Hall, S. M. (1992) Congenital toxoplasmosis. *BMJ*, **305**, 291–297.

Hayes, C., Johnson, Z., Thornton, L., *et al* (1997). Ten-year survival of Down syndrome births. *International Journal of Epidemiology*, **26**, 822–829.

Hetzel, B. S. (1989) *The Story of Iodine Deficiency; An International Challenge in Nutrition*. Oxford: Oxford University Press.

Hogg, J. & Moss, S. (1993) Characteristics of older people with intellectual disabilities in England. *International Review of Research in Mental Retardation*, **19**, 71–96.

Holmes, N., Shah, A. & Wing, L. (1982) The disability assessment schedule: a brief screening device for use with the mentally retarded. *Psychological Medicine*, **12**, 878–890.

Luckasson, R., Coulter, D. L., Polloway, E. A., *et al* (1992) *Mental Retardation: Definition, Classification and Systems of Supports*. Washington, DC: American Association on Mental Retardation.

Marteau, T. & Croyle, R. T. (1998) The new genetics: psychological responses to genetic testing. *BMJ*, **316**, 693–696.

McDonald, G. & McKay, D. N. (1996) The prevalence of learning disability in a health and social services board in Northern Ireland. *Journal of Intellectual Disability Research*, **40**, 550–556.

McGrother, C. W. & Marshall, B. (1990) Recent trends in incidence, morbidity and survival in Down's syndrome. *Journal of Mental Deficiency Research*, **34**, 49–57.

——, Thorp, C., Taub, N., *et al* (2001) Prevalence, disability and need in adults with severe learning disability. *Tizard Learning Disability Review*, **6**, 4–13.

Medical Research Council Working Party on Phenylketonuria (1993) Phenylketonuria due to phenyl-alanine hydroxylase deficiency; an unfolding story: review of report. *BMJ*, **306**, 115–119.

Micronutrient Deficiency Information System (1993) *Global Prevalence of Iodine Deficiency Disorders. Working Paper 1*. Geneva: WHO.

Mittler, P. (1992) Assessing people with mental retardation. In *Assessment of People with Mental Retardation*, pp. 1–11. Geneva: WHO.

Morton, J. E., Bundey, S., Webb, T. P., *et al* (1997) Fragile-X syndrome is less common than previously estimated. *Journal of Medical Genetics*, **34**, 1–5.

Murphy, M., Whiteman, D., Stone, D., *et al* (2000) Dietary folate and the prevalence of neural tube defects in the British Isles: The past two decades. *British Journal of Obstetrics & Gynaecology*, **107**, 885–889.

Murray, J., Cuckle, H., Taylor, G., *et al* (1997) Screening for fragile X syndrome. *Health Technology Assessment*, **1**, 4.

National Assembly for Wales (2001) *Fulfilling the Promise – Proposals for a Framework for Services for People with Learning Disabilities*. Cardiff: National Assembly for Wales.

New England Congenital Hypothyroidism Collaborative (1981) Effects of neonatal screening for hypothyroidism: prevention of mental retardation by treatment before clinical manifestations. *Lancet, ii,* 1095–1098.

Nihira, K., Lelland, H. & Lambert, N. (1993) AAMR *Adaptive Behaviour Scales – Residential and Community* (2nd edn). Austin, TX: American Association on Mental Retardation.

Nuffield Council on Bioethics (1993) *Genetic Screening: Ethical Issues.* London: Nuffield Council on Bioethics.

Pharoah, P. O. D., Cooke, T., Johnson, M. A., *et al* (1998) Epidemiology of cerebral palsy in England and Scotland, 1984–9. *Archives of Disease in Childhood: Fetal & Neonatal Edition,* **79,** F21–F25.

Pollitt, R. J., Green, A., McCabe, C. J., *et al* (1997) Neonatal screening for inborn errors of metabolism: cost, yield and outcome. *Health Technology Assessment,* **1,** 7.

Richardson, S. A. & Koller, H. (1996) *Twenty-Two Years: Causes and Consequences of Mental Retardation.* Cambridge, MA: Harvard University Press.

Rumeau-Roquette, C., Granjean, H., Cans, C., *et al* (1997). Prevalence and time trends of disabilities in school-age children. *International Journal of Epidemiology,* **26,** 137–145.

Russell, O. (2001) Supporting families to make informed decisions; how can we safeguard genetic diversity while respecting parents' right to choose? In *Considered Choices: The New Genetics, Prenatal Testing and People with Learning Disabilities* (ed. L. Ward). Kidderminster: British Institute of Learning Disabilities.

Sabaratnam, M., Laver, S., Butler, L., *et al* (1994) Fragile-X syndrome in north east Essex: toward systematic screening: clinical selection. *Journal of Intellectual Disability Research,* **38,** 27–35.

Scottish Executive (2000) *The Same as You? A Review of Services for People with Learning Disabilities.* Edinburgh: Scottish Executive.

Simon, V. A., Abrams, M. T., Freund, L. S., *et al* (1990) The fragile X phenotype: cognitive, behavioural and neurobiological profiles. *Current Opinion in Psychiatry,* **3,** 581–586.

Simons, W. F., Fuggle, P. W., Grant, D. B., *et al* (1994) Intellectual development at 10 years in early treated congenital hypothyroidism. *Archives of Disease in Childhood,* **71,** 232–234.

—, —, —, *et al* (1997) Educational progress, behaviour and motor skills at 10 years in early treated congenital hypothyroidism. *Archives of Disease in Childhood,* **77,** 219–222.

Slaney, S. F., Wilkie, A. O. M., Hirst, M. C., *et al* (1995) DNA testing for fragile X syndrome in schools for learning difficulties. *Archives of Disease in Childhood,* **72,** 33–37.

Sparrow, S. S., Balla, D. A. & Cicchetti, C. (1984) *Vineland Adaptive Behaviour Scales.* Circles Pines, MN: American Guidance Service.

Smith, I., Cook, B. & Beasley, M. G. (1991) Review of neonatal screening programme for phenylketonuria. *BMJ,* **303,** 333–335.

Streetly, A. & Corbett, V. (1997) *The National Newborn Screening Programme: Summary of an Audit of Phenylketonuria and Congenital Hypothyroidism Screening in England and Wales.* London: Department of Public Health Medicine, UMDS Guy's and St Thomas's Medical Schools.

Tao, K.-T. (1988) Mentally retarded persons in the People's Republic of China: a review of epidemiological studies and services. *American Journal on Mental Retardation,* **93,** 193–199.

Turk, J. (1995) Fragile-X syndrome. *Archives of Disease in Childhood,* **72,** 4–5.

Turner, T. H. (1989) Schizophrenia and mental handicap; an historical review with implications for further research. *Psychological Medicine,* **19,** 301–314.

Vyas, S. (1994) Screening for Down's syndrome. *BMJ,* **309,** 753–754.

Wald, N., Watt, H. C. & Hennessy, C. F. (1999*a*) Down's syndrome screening in the UK in 1998. *Lancet,* **354,** 1264.

—, — & Hackshaw, A. K. (1999b) Integrated screening for Down's syndrome based on tests performed during the first and third trimesters. *New England Journal of Medicine*, **341**, 461–467.

Ward, L. (ed.) (2001) *Considered Choices: The New Genetics, Prenatal Testing and People with Learning Disabilities*. Kidderminster: British Institute of Learning Disabilities.

Webb, D. W. & Osborne, J. P. (1995) Tuberous sclerosis. *Archives of Disease in Childhood*, **72**, 471–475.

Wing, L. (1980) MRC Handicaps, Behaviour and Skills (HBS) Schedule. *Acta Psychiatria Scandinavica* (suppl.), **62**, 275–284.

World Health Organization (1980) *International Classification of Impairments, Disabilities and Handicaps*. Geneva: WHO.

— (1992) *The ICD–10 Classification of Mental and Behavioural Disorders: Clinical Descriptions and Diagnostic Guidelines*. Geneva: WHO.

— (2001) *International Classification of Functioning, Disability and Health (ICIDH–2)*. Geneva: WHO.

## Further Reading

British Psychological Society (2001) *Learning Disability – Operational Definitions in Clinical, Legal and Other Contexts*. Leicester: British Psychological Society.

Emerson, E., Hatton, C., Felce, D., *et al* (2001) *Learning Disabilities – Fundamental Facts*. London: Foundation for People with Learning Disabilities.

# CHAPTER 3

# Genetics and learning disability*

Walter Muir

## Relevance of genetics to learning disability

Molecular medicine is increasingly becoming the dominant mode of understanding pathology. The impact of molecular genetics on our understanding of disease processes has been enormous, and is likely to increase with the historic publication of the draft DNA sequence for the complete set of human chromosomes, the genome. This is a remarkable race between private (Venter *et al*, 2001) and public (Lander *et al*, 2001) consortia. It is a starting point rather than an end in itself. The genome map and sequence may be near complete and the total number of genes in man perhaps surprisingly small. Genes can be seen as regions of DNA that code for proteins, along with the initiation and regulatory DNA elements that control the process. However, genes in themselves are not the key functional structures. Their direct coding sequences, exons, are transcribed into messenger RNA (mRNA or message), which may itself have a regulatory role without further processing. The complete set of mRNAs at a given time in any cell is termed the transcriptosome – which, unlike the set of genes, has a short-acting dynamic rather than changing across generations. Messenger RNA is, of course, more commonly translated into proteins and these make up the functional powerhouse of the cell.

Differential splicing and post-transcriptional processing of messages are two of many ways that variations in protein structure can be produced from a limited set of genes. The resultant subtle changes in amino-acid sequence can lead to major changes in a protein's activity, raising the available complexity by several magnitudes beyond that apparently dictated by the genome alone. Thus, there is really no need to have huge numbers of genes to produce the complexity of the human organism. The total set of proteins expressed by a cell at any one time is termed its proteome. Efforts to characterise and understand the forces that shape this shifting dynamic will, if anything, produce even more important and exciting results than the genome project has done.

---

* See pp. 319–327 for a glossary of the molecular genetics terms used in this chapter.

The result of interactions between genes, their products and the environment is usually termed the phenotype. This need not be restricted to physical features; cognitive performance and behaviours are also highly important outcomes (behavioural phenotypes).

There are two related areas to be covered within this chapter, which will therefore be selective. I will discuss rare conditions if they illuminate mechanisms, and avoid some common ones if they are not well understood at present. Overall, I will try to convey some of the excitement and the pace of discovery that is happening in the field at present.

# Basic genetics

It is obvious that inheritance is a major factor in many conditions that are associated with learning disability. From the viewpoint of intellectual functioning alone, the main determinant of mild learning disability seems to be the largely random allocation of genes from both parents with the additive summation or interaction of effects from many genes (polygenic inheritance), taken together with the influences of internal (biochemical) and external environments. Where each gene of influence contributes only a small part towards any particular phenotype, they are often called quantitative trait loci (Flint & Mott, 2001). There is increasing interest in how such loci can be identified and their relative contributions estimated, but the focus here shall be on those conditions that result from large structural rearrangements of chromosomes, or where one (monogenic) or a few (oligogenic) major genes operate. These individually, of course, tend to be much rarer than complex multifactorial disorders but the total number known is very large and increasing, and it is through our understanding of them that much of our knowledge about the genetics of conditions associated with learning disability has arisen.

With the current pace of gene discovery for conditions associated with learning disability, any attempts at numerical estimates must be treated with some caution. There is a definite ascertainment bias towards monogenic conditions, which are more easily mapped, but out of over 3000 currently known genetic disorders (some 70% monogenic), nearly 40% are associated with a learning disability. The X chromosome alone harbours loci associated with over 200 disorders related to learning disability, of which approximately 40% have learning disability as the only (currently) detectable phenotypic outcome (the so-called non-syndromal X-linked mental retardations or MRX). Thus, learning disability can result from a legion of individual and multiple gene disruptions; the term has little specificity in itself and does not signify a particular disorder. With the vast number of genetic conditions involved, it is neither useful nor possible to present a comprehensive survey. Instead, I will focus on conditions that illuminate our understanding of the genetic processes involved and show us how genetics is rapidly transforming the biology of our field of interest.

Monogenic conditions may not show classical Mendelian-pattern inheritance. In fact, it is becoming evident that clear dominant or recessive patterns are the exception rather than the rule in conditions associated with learning disability. Genes are usually expressed on both chromosomes of a pair (biallelic expression). In rare cases, a mutant product from one aberrant gene may suppress the transcription of the normal gene on the other chromosome, leading to a dominant-negative effect. Usually, however, gene disruptions on one chromosome of a pair will only reduce the amount of product made (haploinsufficiency). The severity of this reduction to the organism will determine whether a disorder is inherited in a dominant or recessive fashion. The penetrance of an inherited disorder can be thought of as a measure of how often a given mutant genotype will result in a detectable phenotype. In a fully (100%) penetrant disorder, a person carrying one copy (heterozygote) of the mutant gene for a dominant condition, or two copies (homozygote) for a recessive condition, was thought always to express the full clinical disorder (such as in Huntington's disease). However, clinical variability in the expression of even fully penetrant genes is often striking. In some inherited eye conditions (aniridia), the expression within a single family can range from full iris abnormality through to subtle changes in the lens. The eye is easy to see, but more commonly a clinical outcome cannot be detected in people who must be carriers of the mutant genotype by virtue of their position in a family, and the disorder is said to have partial penetrance. This results either from our current inability to detect specific clinical features that are actually present, or from the interacting influences of environment and other genes to fully suppress all aspects of the clinical disorder. The body's homoeostatic mechanisms apply from the gene level up, through biochemistry to adaptive behavioural interactions with the environment, and only when this homoeostatic buffering capacity is exceeded is pathology clinically expressed – so partial penetrance is the rule rather than the exception.

Humans are diploid organisms in that we each usually inherit 23 pairs of chromosomes, one of each pair deriving individually from our father or mother. One pair of chromosomes, the sex chromosomes that determine genetic sex and in most cases also biological sex, have particular differences in form and structure that lead them to be classified separately from the 22 other pairs that are termed autosomes. When we talk of chromosomes, we usually think of the metaphase structures that play only a small part in the normal cycle of the cell's activity. Mostly, chromosomes are held in the nucleus at interphase – in the form of extended filaments containing active genes producing the mRNA that is moved to cytoplasmic ribosomes for translation into the proteins that both dynamically and structurally form the basis of the cell's function. However, at cell division a set of phasic changes takes place and the chromosomes form compacted, dense, coiled structures, with well-defined central regions (the centromeres).

In mitotic division, the diploid number of chromosomes in each cell is preserved. The nuclear envelope disappears and the condensed chromosome pairs replicate to form into discrete pairs of sister chromatids. The centromeric kinetochores of these pairs link to filaments (astral microtubules) that grow out from the spindle poles, and the chromatids separate and move towards the opposite poles by an energy-dependent interaction with the microtubules.

In meiotic division that forms germ cells (gametes), two stages of division occur. In meiosis 1, sister chromatids pair with their homologues at the equator of the spindle structure, where recombination (crossing-over of DNA from one chromosome of the pair to the other) occurs, as visualised by chiasmata or synaptic bridges. The chromatids do not separate at this division; instead, each chromosome of the pair moves into a separate cell that then divides again (meiosis 2) and the chromatids segregate into gametes without further duplication (forming four sperm, or an egg and three redundant polar bodies). Thus, each gamete has half the chromosome count (haploid) of the parent cell – the full diploid number is restored at fertilisation. There is a delay (checkpoint 1) after meiosis 1 to allow the catch-up of other chromatid pairs that are moving at an uneven rate towards the pole, which delays anaphase until the correct number of chromosomes are present at the pole.

The textbook picture of a chromosome is of one condensed in the pre-division state of metaphase, but a normal somatic cell spends little time in this state. Metaphase architecture has immense practical importance, however, and classical cytogenetics uses it to distinguish chromosomal abnormalities. Certain DNA binding dyes such as Giemsa will produce a pattern of light and dark bands down the metaphase chromosomes that have been numbered to identify specific positions. From the centromere, the bands on the shorter ($p$) chromosome arms and the long ($q$) arms are numbered consecutively towards the telomeres. If we stretch the chromosome out before applying a dye, then single bands resolve into finer sub-bands and these are further numbered (high-resolution banding). These bands represent differences in the regional composition of the underlying chromosome. Light bands in general have higher gene numbers and the genes tend to be associated with long, repeated stretches of cytosine–guanosine nucleotide pairs (CpG islands). Those light bands that are immediately subtelomeric (R bands) can have very high gene densities, and their involvement in subtelomeric rearrangements are an important cause of learning disability, occurring in over 7% of children with moderate-to-severe learning disability and 0.5% of those with mild learning disability (Knight *et al*, 1999). Currently, the methods of detection of these are rather complex, but clinical pointers that increase the likelihood of such a rearrangement being present include familiality of the learning disability and prenatal-onset growth retardation (de Vries *et al*, 2001).

It is conceptually useful to consider how things can go wrong with DNA at different levels of scale. The scale of the anomaly does not necessarily mirror the severity of the associated clinical condition or degree of learning disability, however, and it is important to remember that it is the whole system that reacts to mutation with its buffering capacity from our other inheritance, and from internal (biochemical) and external (environmental) factors.

# Disorders involving dosage effects of large number of genes – trisomies, monosomies and other large structural rearrangements

Human reproduction seems to be extremely inefficient, with around 40% of conceptions terminating spontaneously during pregnancy. Much of this early foetal loss is due to major chromosomal abnormalities. The survival to term where a foetus is aneuploid (the overall number of chromosomes differs from the normal) for an autosome may depend on the gene content of the chromosome concerned. Chromosome 21 was the second human chromosome to have its complete sequence documented (Hattori *et al*, 2000) and is remarkably gene-poor compared with the first to be sequenced, chromosome 22, although they differ little in overall size. This may be a major factor in survival of trisomy (three copies) of chromosome 21 that results in Down's syndrome. Gene poverty may also explain the relatively frequent survival of trisomies of chromosomes 13 and 18, although the clinical constellations (Patau's and Edwards' syndromes) are much more severe than trisomy 21. The cellular origins of aneuploidy, the key to which is usually abnormal recombination patterns between paired chromosomes, may differ between individual forms and also depend on the parental derivation of the chromosome (Hassold *et al*, 2000). Trisomy 21 is usually associated with maternal meiosis 1 errors with a decrease in the numbers of chiasmatic exchanges, especially around the centromere. This also holds for the rarer paternal meiosis 1 errors. If the error is in maternal meiosis 2, however, the number of exchanges seems to be increased, and in paternal meiosis 2 errors there may be little change in the number of chiasmata. For trisomy 16, there is an overall alteration in the placement of chiasmatic exchanges along the chromosome, and individual differences exist for other trisomies. Thus, although the net effect may be similar – non-disjunction of one complete chromosome – the underlying factors involved in its production may be specific to the chromosome, parent-of-origin and meiotic division. For meiosis 1 errors, a factor may be dysfunction of the MAD2 protein, which is an essential part of the spindle meiosis checkpoint 1 in lower organisms (Shonn *et al*, 2000), though its homologous functioning in humans has still to be explored.

Trisomies (and monosomy XO or Turner's syndrome) of the sex chromosomes are surprisingly common (each trisomy has frequency of between 1:1000 and 1:1500 newborns; Turner's occurs in around 1:3000 live births and may account for around 10% of foetal loss). In normal cells, one of the X chromosomes is randomly inactivated by a process involving hypermethylation of chromatin. (The process is termed Lyonisation after Mary Lyon who investigated it. Such condensed X chromosomes form densely-staining Barr bodies, originally described in buccal cells.) Inactivation of the X chromosome is under control of a regulatory structure, the XIC (X inactivating centre at Xq13) of at least four genes. One of these genes, XIST (X inactive-specific transcript) codes for an RNA that is not translated into any protein, but instead is retained in the nucleus and may be the primary signal that initiates the X inactivation, starting at the XIC and spreading down the chromosome, perhaps requiring certain repeat sequences (LINES) to act as signals for further hypermethylation. The effect is not X chromosome-specific, and will spread to an autosomal chromosome if the X chromosome is involved in a reciprocal translocation. Since all X chromosomes in a cell are inactivated save one, there must be a counting mechanism. Again, genes for this are hypothesised to occur in the XIC (Avner & Heard, 2001). Not all genes are inactivated, however, and around 15% remain active in regions mainly on the short arm that are called pseudo-autosomal, as in inheritance they behave in a similar manner to genes on autosomes. The clinical effects of the trisomy may involve gene dosage disruption of the limited number of unmethylated, transcriptionally active genes on any additional X or Y chromosomes.

Trisomy X and Klinefelter's syndrome (XXY) lower the average IQ score by around 10 points and the affected population will have an excess of learning disability compared with the normal population. In fact, the sex chromosome aneuploidies show well the deleterious effects of increasing gene dosage. Tetrasomy X (XXXX) and pentasomy X (XXXXX) are associated with increasingly severe degrees of learning disability. Since all but one X chromosome is Lyonised in these conditions, the phenotype is presumably due to an increased dosage of active pseudoautosomal regions. Many people with sex chromosome aneuploidies are in fact mosaic – that is, they have more than one clonal cell line, often with one being normal in karyotype, and in such cases the phenotype may be less severe. The effects of multiple Y chromosomes are less well understood. The Y chromosome is much less autosome-like than the X, and save its pseudoautosomal regions has extensive regions that do not recombine. Recombination is essential to genomic health, and this has led to evolutionary shrinkage and accumulations of retroviral and heterochromatin sequences. Non-recombining Y genes often show multiple copies, perhaps as a compensation mechanism against mutation, with selective persistence of genes with male-specific functions such as the SRY (sex-determining region Y) gene (Lahn *et al*, 2001).

Autosomes do not show extensive condensation in interphase. Most genes are expressed biallelically and will show dosage effects in trisomy, of which Down's syndrome (1:700 to 1:1000 live births) is the classical case and the most common. The intellectual impairment associated with Down's syndrome is on average moderate in degree (IQ mean around 50) and many will have severe or profound learning disability. Much less common than full trisomy 21 are partial duplications of small areas of the chromosome that may arise *de novo*, but are more commonly associated with a balanced reciprocal translocation between two different chromosomes in one or other parent. Their children can have a normal karyotype, inherit both rearranged chromosomes and thus remain balanced carriers; or they may inherit only one of the abnormal (derivative) chromosomes, in which case they will have a partial trisomy or monosomy. In many cases the unbalanced karyotype is highly deleterious and the foetus does not survive to term (often they present as high miscarriage rate without a clinical phenotype in the balanced carrier parent). However, a partial trisomy of chromosome 21 can be associated with survival, and in such cases researchers have tried to estimate the genetic contribution to the clinical picture that the child inherits; not all of the chromosome is needed in trisomy to produce all the clinical features of Down's syndrome. This has led to the concept of a Down's syndrome critical region, and sensitive techniques are now available to accurately measure the copy number (number of active genes) in various tissues by determining levels of the mRNA transcripts. With the complete sequence of chromosome 21 now known, and its genomic content established, the genotype-to-phenotype relationships should become clearer. Certainly the molecular dissection of the wide range of phenotypes in Down's syndrome is now much closer, and it may not be 'too complex' to gain at least a partial understanding.

A crucial event has been the development of tools to insert very large pieces of human DNA into target genomes. Stretches of human chromosome 21 DNA have been inserted into the mouse genome to create a transgenic model using a vector that can handle stretches of DNA in the order of a megabase – the YAC (yeast artificial chromosome) vector. In this way, the behavioural phenotype of such experimental partial trisomies can be explored (Smith *et al*, 1997). In one case where the gene *Dyrk1a* (which is the mammalian homologue of the *Drosophila* neural gene 'minibrain') was expressed in trisomy, subtle and reproducible effects on learning were seen in the mouse. Although learning deficits in mice cannot be directly mapped to the learning disability in Down's syndrome, the model opens the way for experimental manipulations of trisomies of various genes in parallel, and the influence of environmental modulation under controlled conditions (Reeves *et al*, 2001). This will complement the examination of the very rare cases of human partial trisomy. The techniques continue to advance, and more stable and defined bacterial artificial chromosome (BAC) vectors (which can handle stretches of DNA around 100–200 kbp long) have now been used successfully to create similar mouse models (Chrast *et al*, 2000).

In contrast to the trisomies, the only common full monosomy is that of Turner's syndrome, and although associated with a specific pattern of cognitive changes, these do not amount to learning disability. Other full chromosome monosomies are rare. It is interesting that monosomy 21 shows many features in common with trisomy 21 – it could be that the gene dosage is critical within a certain window to allow correct development.

Partial monosomies are more common. Cri-du-Chat involves loss of the whole or part of the long arm of chromosome 5. Although this can be in association with a balanced rearrangement in the parents, it often occurs *de novo*. The learning disability is usually severe. Chromosome 4 short-arm loss leads to Wolf–Hirschhorn syndrome – again with severe learning disability. Surprisingly, and for reasons that are not clear, the large deletions of chromosomes, producing Cri-du-Chat Syndrome (5p-), Wolf–Hirschhorn syndrome (4p-) and the 18p- syndrome, also show a disproportionate derivation from paternal chromosomes. The consequences of such large loss of chromosomal material may be better understood through the creation of mouse models. A promising technique is to use gene targeting to insert tailored DNA sequences into the genome of mouse stem cells that then permit chromosome engineering by specific recombination when exposed to a DNA recombinase enzyme (the Cre-LoxP system; where Cre is a site-specific recombinase that operates between pairs of inserted LoxP sequences, a 34 bp nucleotide). This can be used to create deletions and other chromosomal rearrangements between precisely defined boundaries, and the detailed phenotype can then be explored for rearrangements involving many genes at once (Mills & Bradley, 2001).

Smaller deletions or duplications of parts of chromosomes are also known. Of special interest are microdeletions (or microinsertions) that have become increasingly well defined and understood in the past few years. In general, these involve abnormalities of several genes that lie in series in the area affected by the abnormality – thus the term 'contiguous gene syndrome' has been coined for these conditions.

## Contiguous gene syndromes

An increasing number of syndromes are being shown to be associated with intrachromosomal deletions, or more rarely duplications, that are often sub-microscopic in size and rely on detection using the more sensitive method of fluorescent *in-situ* hybridisation (FISH), where a complementary DNA (cDNA) probe is tagged with a fluorophore. Minute deletions are revealed when only one signal is present rather than signals from both chromosomes. The WAGR syndrome (Wilms' tumour, aniridia, genitourinary anomalies and mental retardation), due to a constitutional deletion at 11p13, is one of the best understood. The renal tumour and anomalies of the genitourinary tract are due to deletion of the WT1 (Wilms' tumour suppressor 1) gene and the aniridia is due to loss of the PAX6 gene. The cause of the learning disability is less certain, and although in patients with specific PAX6 mutations magnetic resonance imaging has shown anterior commissure, frontal cortex and callosal changes, the effects could be due to another gene or depend on interactive effects of several missing genes.

The velocardiofacial syndrome is the most common contiguous gene syndrome and comprises a huge spectrum of anomalies, including neural crest cell derivatives – commonly conotruncal heart anomalies and specific facial appearance. Importantly, they can generate a behavioural phenotype including learning disability and a psychosis that resembles schizophrenia (Shprintzen, 2000). Its clinical spectrum overlaps the more severe DiGeorge syndrome, where hypocalcaemia presents early, and taken together they are the most common cause of congenital heart abnormalities after Down's syndrome. Velocardiofacial and DiGeorge syndromes are nearly always associated with microdeletions at chromosome 22q11.2. Although the entire region has been cloned and sequenced, a single human gene whose haploinsufficiency is enough to cause the syndrome has not yet been isolated. However, the Cre/loxP system has been used to remove both copies of the TBX1 transcription factor gene (T-box 1 gene) in the mouse, resulting in most of the systemic, if not behavioural features of the two syndromes (Jerome & Papaioannou, 2001). In humans, however, there are cases through translocations, with breakpoints relatively far away in molecular terms from this gene. Either other genes are at work or a position effect is occurring, whereby architectural disruption of the chromosome can influence the transcription of genes a considerable distance away (Kleinjan & Van Heyningen, 1998).

Lissencephaly (literally 'smooth brain') is the name given for a group of conditions where there is formation failure of a correctly layered cerebral cortex, leading to varying degrees of agyria/pachygyria. The contiguous gene syndrome due to microdeletions at 17p13.3, the Miller–Dieker syndrome, is a classical lissencephaly where the thickened cortex has four layers rather than the normal six. It seems that a specific gene is responsible for the lissencephaly in this case (LIS1, which also has a role in platelets as PAFAH1; Vallee et al, 2001), but its role in neuronal migration is unclear. Several other genes for lissencephaly have been described including doublecortin (DCX) on the X chromosome, which causes an inversion of the cortex layering (normally the youngest cells are most external, migrating past older cells – an 'inside-out' arrangement). The gene codes for a neural migration signalling protein, and seems to interact with LIS1 (Caspi et al, 2000).

Williams' syndrome is another microdeletion-associated disorder (at 7q11.23) that has been the focus of much recent interest. In addition to dysmorphic features, infantile hypercalcaemia, cardiac and connective tissue changes, there is a well-defined behavioural phenotype and 75% will have a learning disability. The cognitive deficits are fascinating and specific, with poor visuo-motor integration and the relative sparing of language function (Mervis & Klein-Tasman, 2000). Although haplo-insufficiency of the elastin gene is probably responsible for the systemic features of the condition (Morris & Mervis, 2000), at least 16 genes are deleted and LIM-kinase 1 has been suggested as a candidate for producing the visuo-spatial deficits.

In contrast to those contiguous gene syndromes associated with deletions, the Beckwith–Wiedemann syndrome (neonatal gigantism, macroglossia, exomphthalmos, increased tumour risk and sometimes learning disability) usually involves partial duplication of 11p. It is associated with complex imprinting mechanisms including uniparental disomies, aberrant methylation patterns and in some cases imprinting switch disturbances (Bliek et al, 2001). Such mechanisms will be discussed later under the Prader–Willi/Angelman syndromes.

It is likely that these varied syndromes are the tip of the iceberg and that many more deletion and duplication contiguous gene syndromes will be discovered in the next few years.

## Disorders involving single genes

Mutations directly involving particular genes can take several forms. Point mutations change single base pairs of DNA, and are a major player in gene mutations. By changing the triplet sequence of the genetic code, they may cause several types of misreading, such as substitution of different bases in mRNA (and thus amino acids in proteins), premature stop codons, and changes in regulatory and initiation elements within the gene structure. Insertions of small stretches of DNA by transposable elements (transposons) also seem to be fairly common sources of direct mutation and, again, disruption to the reading of the underlying code may result.

Spontaneous mutations within germ lines are influenced strongly by gamete type. In general, germline mutations occur much more frequently in males than in females, and since this is related to the number of germ cell divisions that occur (spermatogenesis continues throughout life), the effect is also more pronounced with increasing paternal age (Crow, 2000). There are exceptions (the maternal age effect on the risk of having a child with Down's syndrome is the most striking), but in general for single base pair mutations, the paternal origin effect dominates. It is important to place direct mutation in context; not all mutations are deleterious, many are neutral or may even be advantageous. In fact, they provide vital substrates for evolutionary selection; in the Darwinian model, we adapt through our organism's homoeostatic buffering capacity to changes in given internal and external environments. Exceeding that capacity will be deleterious, but mutation may also allow the capacity itself to be increased or altered. We can also alter the buffering by external therapeutic intervention.

Many of the severe 'inborn errors of metabolism' are due to direct gene mutations. If dietary phenylalanine restrictions are started early, then mutations in the phenylalanine hydroxylase gene that lead to phenylketonuria (1:10000 newborns) seldom today produce the severe learning disability formerly seen, and such knowledge was the stimulus to introducing blood screening of newborns for a variety of genetic diseases. Guthrie's inhibition test was originally a bacterial assay, but sophisticated DNA or mass spectroscopy assays hold the potential to screen for many more inborn errors. Over 400 mutations are known in the phenylalanine hydroxylase gene, and some produce much more mild phenotypes than full phenylketonuria. This variability in phenotype due to the type of mutation is vividly seen in those of the human L1 gene (Xq28), which codes for one of the important neural cell adhesion molecules. The effects of mutations within the same gene can vary between severe hydrocephalus, complicated spastic periparesis, callosal agenesis and MASA syndrome (the CRASH spectrum of disorders). Mutations in the gene that codes for the extracellular part of the protein lead to its truncation or absence, and a severe phenotype. Mutations in the region coding for the cytoplasmic domain lead to a much milder disorder with minimal ventricular dilatation (Fransen *et al*, 1998). Differential effects of direct mutation are thus one cause of intrasyndromic variation in phenotype. As our understanding of the genome increases, the other factors involved, such as multiple background genes and environmental influences, should be more readily investigated, these being crucial to the design of targeted therapeutic interventions to prevent phenotypic outcomes in mutation carriers.

## Strategies for finding genes for inherited conditions associated with learning disability

When we have no clues as to the position of genes from chromosomal rearrangements, or where we know nothing about the underlying biology of a condition that would give us proteins to target (and thus candidate genes), the methods of linkage analysis have long been applied. Recombination at meiosis is much more likely if two pieces of DNA are far apart on a chromosome than if they are close together, so two pieces that are close together will tend to be inherited together. If we know the position of a piece of DNA on a given chromosome and have a mechanism through which we can track its inheritance within a family, then a strong co-segregation with an inherited disease in the family would suggest a piece of DNA involved in the expression of that disease lies close by. Crudely, this is the basis of linkage analysis.

The identification of mechanisms by which we can track the descent of pieces of DNA was one of the most crucial steps in modern genetics. Its usefulness lies in the variability of the underlying composition of stretches of DNA in the population, which are inherited in a stable fashion within any given family (where a piece of DNA differs between chromosomes it is said to show different alleles). The first such useful markers were termed restriction fragment length polymorphisms (RFLPs). These are single nucleotide base-pair differences between individuals that change the pattern of specific DNA signatures that a DNA-digesting enzyme (a restriction endonuclease) recognises, thus altering the site at which the enzyme 'cuts' the DNA (the restriction site). The lengths of the fragments generated (which represent differences in the position of the restriction sites) thus differ between individuals, and since size is related to mobility under an electrical potential gradient, the fragments can be separated after enzymic digestion by gel electrophoresis. Denaturing this DNA on the gel renders it single-stranded and the separated pattern of single-stranded DNA (ssDNA) can be transferred by capillary action to a nylon membrane (Southern blotting). Membrane-bound ssDNA can then be hybridised with a radioactivity- or fluorescence-labelled single-stranded piece of cDNA (a molecular probe) and variations in separated length investigated from the pattern of hybridisation. The key to the method's success is having a probe that is highly variable in the population, reducing the chances of two parents carrying the same variants and thus increasing the accuracy by which a polymorphism's descent within a family can be traced. Although RFLPs were important in identifying chromosomal regions for many important diseases, more informative markers have since been developed.

Repeated blocks of nucleotides exist where the copy number is highly variable (variable-number tandem repeats or minisatellites have long-sequence repeats, whereas microsatellites usually have a repeated two-nucleotide motif; all of these are now generally grouped as simple tandem repeats). These are usually detected after amplification using the polymerase chain reaction (PCR), the development of which was one of the most significant technical advances in molecular genetics. The key here is the use of a heat-stable DNA-copying enzyme, *Taq* polymerase, that can specifically catalyse the formation of complementary DNA across genomic regions whose boundaries have been marked by the binding of externally synthesised short unique sequences of DNA (oligonucleotide primers, the sequence of the DNA flanking that to be amplified, which must be already characterised). By heating, DNA can be made single-stranded (denatured), freeing the system for another round of primer ligation and DNA formation, with the capability of amplifying specific DNA sequences from tiny amounts of starting material. The amplified DNA can be analysed directly for length variation using standard (and now automated) electrophoresis or sequencing methods. Once a locus has been defined by linkage analysis, the cloning and characterisation of underlying genes can now be rapidly advanced by knowledge of the human genome sequence (Evans *et al*, 2001). However, additional information through chromosomal analysis may still be vital, as has been shown in detecting schizophrenia genes (Blackwood *et al*, 2001). The well-known over-representation of schizophrenia in adults with mild learning disability may be due mainly to genetic factors, and there is an increased incidence of chromosomal abnormalities in this group that may point to disrupted genes (Muir, 2000).

Such methods have also been successful in delineating areas of linkage in autism. Twin and family studies have indicated that the predisposition to autism has a strong genetic component and several genome scans of large sets of families have been undertaken. Although a locus has been implicated on chromosome 13q (Collaborative Linkage Study on Autism, 1999), the best current linkage evidence points to a locus on the long arm of chromosome 7q from both family data and sib-pairs (International Molecular Genetic Study of Autism Consortium, 2001). This chromosomal locus also contains a putative region for some of the problems in autism in the shape of SPCH1 at 7q31 that is implicated by translocations associated with speech and language disorder (Lai *et al*, 2000). More recently, another locus has been implicated for autism on the long arm of chromosome 2 (Buxbaum *et al*, 2001). To try to create a more homogenous subgroup, they found that restricting the analysis to families where individuals with autism with a delayed onset (after age 3 years) who were also late in using phrased speech further increased the significance. Although there are problems with this approach, it does seem likely that there will be more than one susceptibility gene for autism. As with so many other neuropsychiatric conditions, it is likely that we will have to redefine the term 'autism' as a useful clinical rubric for a group of conditions with heterogeneous aetiologies. Another region of interest is that at the Prader–Willi/ Angelman region of chromosome 15q11-13. Duplications of this area seem to have no obvious consequences if they arise on the chromosome 15 inherited from the father; however, maternal 15q duplications lead to a variety of language disorders and autistic-spectrum phenotypes (Cook *et al*, 1997), and a candidate brain-expressed gene has been described (see below).

Most recently, PCR technology in combination with automated genotyping methods have meant that single-nucleotide polymorphisms (SNPs; an RFLP is one type of SNP that happens to alter the position of a restriction site) that occur very frequently throughout the genome can be directly and easily assayed. Their information content individually is fairly low, but their density means that they can be used to finely screen large stretches of the genome. SNPs usually lie in non-coding regions, so are useful in linking to a nearby locus. They can, however, also have functional consequences on the expression of genes if they lie directly in coding or regulatory elements (hence the term 'functional polymorphisms'). There are many ways of genotyping SNPs, and the most efficient method depends on the analysis attempted; however, there is a noticeable bias towards direct sequencing after PCR amplification (Gray *et al*, 2000). A massive SNP detection effort, combining commercial and charitable scientific endeavours (the 'SNP Consortium', which has already met its target and produced over 500 000 SNPs), has produced an extremely detailed SNP map across the human genome. This will be coupled to genotyping on array technology (see below) to maximise throughput, and one eventual ambitious aim is the advent of individual genetic profiling where therapeutic interventions will be tailored to the patient. Such dense SNP maps are useful in performing association studies. These are usually case–control studies of populations with and without a given phenotype, looking for different frequencies of alleles of a given polymorphism that would imply either that there was a candidate gene nearby (linkage disequilibrium) or that a cohort effect was taking place with all cases derived from a common ancestral population. Other approaches include looking at sib-pairs and parent-affected offspring trios. Association and linkage studies often look in the region of candidate genes, which may also be directly screened for mutations. The number of brain-expressed genes is huge, and the choice of candidates for learning disability difficult. However, important proteins involved in hippocampal development play key roles in learning, memory and cognition, and their pathways are being actively explored (the 'hebbesome'; Husi & Grant, 2001).

Although complex, the effects of variable penetrance, expressivity, dominance modification and pleiotropy are starting to be susceptible to analysis. Modifier genes can alter the expression of a genetic trait in addition to individual variation at the gene locus itself (allelic hetero-geneity), or environmental effects can act in a monogenic, oligogenic or multigenic fashion (Naldeau, 2001). A whole range of different phenotypes within a given family segregating for a single gene has been repeatedly described, and indeed such variability may be the rule rather than the exception for most human inherited disease. Although much more amenable to exploration in inbred mice strains, where the genome is near homozygous, there are an increasing number of human conditions where specific genetic modifiers have been identified and help us understand the homoeostatic mechanisms that work to buffer the deleterious effects of mutation. For example, in a family where non-syndromic deafness was segregating several individuals who were homozygous for the DFNB26 deafness gene, some were found to have normal hearing due to a dominant modifier locus that protects against deafness separately inherited on chromosome 7 (Riazuddin *et al*, 2000). Our biochemical understanding of such interactions is at an early stage but is vitally important in helping to understand how we could possibly alter the outcomes of genetic mutation.

# Developmental gene cascades

The past few years have seen great advances in our understanding of the essential role that genes play in embryonic brain development. Complex and interacting cascades of proteins that are involved in signalling or that regulate gene transcription have been defined, and mutations in specific genes within these pathways can lead to a variety of developmental conditions, many associated with learning disability. Holoprosencephaly is a term for a variety of conditions where midline structures of the brain and head fail to separate. In its most severe form, it involves a complete lack of hemispheric separation, resulting in a single midline eye. Such severe forms may be a frequent cause of prenatal foetal loss, but are not common at birth (1:16 000). However, much milder variant phenotypes exist right down to simple hypertelorism. Like other developmental conditions, holoprosencephaly can have several genetic aetiologies. One major form is due to sporadic or inherited mutations in the human form of sonic hedgehog gene (hSHH). This gene was originally defined in *Drosophila*, where mutations produce a larval form with a spiky underbelly – hence the name (fruit fly gene nomenclature unfortunately does not always translate well when human counterparts are found, and there are many such oddly named genes). The gene is active in producing a signalling protein in the notochord and floorplate of the early developing neural tube (and also later in the brain, limb buds and gastrointestinal tract), and seems crucial in coordinating successful early brain development. The protein produced by hSHH is processed into an active form and modified by the addition of a cholesterol group – linking this path to the disorders of cholesterol synthesis that characterise the Smith–Lemi–Opitz syndrome, which has a phenotypic overlap with the holoprosencephalies and other hedgehog pathway disorders.

Hedgehog protein binds the membrane-bound receptor PATCHED-1, which interacts with another transmembrane protein, SMOOTHENED, and sets off a cascade of signalling within the cell. This involves the proteins of the GLI pathways, which have been described as mutated in several human cancers and developmental disorders with multiple dysmorphic features sometimes associated with learning disability (Villavicencio *et al*, 2000). Mutations in GLI-3, for instance, are involved in producing the Grieg and Pallister–Hall syndromes. GLI-3 interacts with CREB-binding protein that has been mutated in Rubenstein–Taybi syndrome, and GLI-1 seems to interact with the protein of the TWIST gene that may link the sonic hedgehog cascade to the Saethre–Chotzen syndrome. All of these syndromes have overlapping clinical features. Other such gene regulation and signalling cascades are known, and it is probable that commonalities in the phenotypic outcome of many genetic disorders that produce learning disability, currently thought to be entirely separate, will be linked by our increased understanding of developmental biology. The genes in such pathways tend to be highly conserved across species and, even if the eventual outcomes are very different, the hedgehog system has shown that it is useful to study their interactions in species such as *Drosophila* and *Caenorhabditis elegans*. These species are genetically manipulated much more easily than humans are.

## From genetics to epigenetics: dynamic mutations, imprinting and other mechanisms

Epigenetic effects on gene expression are those that, although inherited, are not directly controlled by the sequence information in the DNA of chromosomes. In the normal cell, they largely operate by inhibiting or silencing the expression of genes. Such repression can involve recognition of certain DNA sequences, with subsequent direct chemical modification (often methylation of cytosine residues; Robertson & Wolffe, 2000). This then alters DNA polymerase activity or acts by other mechanisms, such as alterations in chromosome-associated protein structure (e.g. histones). To be effective, imprinting needs to be heritable from one generation of cells to another and re-methylation of replicating DNA strands is achieved very rapidly by the presence of a methyltransferase enzyme directly at the replication fork during the cell division. Why epigenetic effects should have evolved at all is becoming clearer through our understanding of the cell's defence mechanisms against the integration of foreign DNA, from endogenous retroviruses and other parasitic transposable elements, into the genome (Prak & Kazazian, 2000). Over a third of the human genome is in the form of such mobile repeats and methylation tends to occur in such regions to suppress unwanted activity. Some of this methylation may be RNA-mediated, by double-stranded RNA intermediates that then direct the methylation of multiple copies of unwanted homologous sequences. In addition, direct epigenetic regulation of transcribed RNA without change in underlying DNA has been documented in several organisms and is a potential additional epigenetic control mechanism in humans (Wolffe & Matzke, 1999).

Several important human disorders that produce learning disability have been instrumental in our understanding of epigenetic effects.

## Fragile sites and learning disability: fragile-X syndrome and FRAXE mental retardation

### The genetics of fragile-X

Fragile-X syndrome is a relatively common disorder (occurring in around 1:4000 men and 1:6000 women), with a highly variable and often quite subtle clinical phenotype, especially when the condition is partially penetrant in female carriers. The term itself is derived from the appearance of a culture artefact when growing cells are deprived of folate (Lubs, 1969). Folate deprivation delays DNA replication in a specific region on X chromosome (Xq27.3) and thus normal DNA condensation at metaphase here is absent, leaving a thin interphase-like stalk joining two condensed regions near the end of the long arm. Such regions are called rare fragile sites and there are 29 known in the human genome, of which 22 are folate-sensitive. They are to be distinguished from common fragile sites (87 known) that have been implicated as cancer cell chromosome break-point sites, but in general are thought not to be associated with pathology (Sutherland & Baker, 2000). Of the rare fragile sites, only three have been definitely implicated in human disorders – FRAXA and FRAXE on the X chromosome, and FRA11B on chromosome 11q that has been implicated in a subset of patients with Jacobsen syndrome.

FRAXA is the site of the genetic alteration that produces fragile-X syndrome. It is the paradigm of a class of human inherited disorders that involve dynamic mutations, where the length of runs of repeated triplets of nucleotides alters between generations. These disorders can show an increasingly severe degree of learning disability down generations (termed anticipation – an effect originally used to describe earlier age at onset of conditions, but now more widely applied to increasing severity). The outcome is determined by the biological sex of the parent through which the mutation is inherited. Prior to the discovery of the gene involved, these effects were very difficult to explain by standard Mendelian laws, although imprinting had been suggested by Laird as early as 1987, and a methylated CpG island was shown to lie near the fragile site. The gene, termed FMR1 (fragile site mental retardation 1) was isolated in 1991, and shown in patients with fragile-X syndrome to contain a lengthy series of CGG triplets within the untranslated end of exon 1 near the promoter element. (A note on nomenclature – strictly speaking, CCG would be a more consistent term with respect to other triplets, but of course CGG is its anti-parallel complement, and identical and more frequently used). A greatly expanded triplet repeat (to between 200 and 600 triplets or more) is the most common cause of fragile-X syndrome, but rare deletions involving part or all of the gene, and a point mutation in a key coding region, can also produce the full clinical syndrome. This implies that it is the FMR1 gene that is causal, rather than the expanded repeat itself. Along with the expanded number of triplets, the CpG island becomes methylated, surrounding histones de-acetylated, and the binding of DNA polymerase to the nearby promoter is inhibited, silencing the gene. Why this happens is not clear, but again it may be a cellular defence against the intrusion of mobile repeat elements. Chemical de-methylation leads to transcription of the gene, whether an expanded repeat is present or not It is also transcribed in individuals with mutations in methylation. The fragile site itself is related directly to the presence of the repeat, however, and de-methylation does not affect its expression in culture.

The number of copies of the CGG triplet that exist in the general population, who are non-carriers of fragile-X, is around 30 (range 6–54); in carriers the number of repeat copies is higher at 52–200, in most cases without clear phenotypic effect. The remarkable feature of this repeat, however, is that any copy number over 52 is meiotically unstable if passed through a female meiosis – in other words during oogenesis. Thus, daughters of a man who carries a pre-mutation will only have a pre-mutation on one of their X chromosomes. Daughters and sons of women with a pre-mutation will have a massive further expansion in the repeat copy number (from 100 to 1000 added triplets), resulting in a full mutation. For female offspring this is usually less deleterious than for males, since random inactivation of one X chromosome of the pair leaves 50% remaining to express the FMR1 gene. In males there is no such compensation and the outcome, in terms of learning disability, is much more severe. There are complications to this story and non-random shutdown of the X chromosome has been postulated to explain differences in the phenotype of monozygotic female twins carrying the full mutation (Willemsen *et al*, 2000). In addition, a small proportion of affected males (12%) and females (6%) are actually mosaic for the mutation, with some of their cells carrying only the pre-mutation, but the size of the expansion is larger in mosaic men than in mosaic women. It has been argued that the absolute size of the repeat expansion relates to the degree of learning disability and other phenotypic features, and that smaller mutations may not always silence the gene. As well as gene silencing, the presence of an expanded repeat alters (delays) the timing of replication of a large chromosomal region around FRAXA on the X chromosome during cell division. The causes of the expansion itself are unclear. Slippage or looping of DNA when chromosomes replicate may play a part in increasing the copy number of repeats from the normal range into the pre-mutation size. Interruptions of the CGG sequence by AGG triplets reduce the risk of expansion. The level of variation of the repeat sequence relates to a population's genetic history, with a high degree of within-population conservation suggesting founder effects.

There are still many unexplained phenomena, such as the extremely low incidence of fragile-X syndrome in Nova Scotia (Beresford *et al*, 2000). Previously, pre-mutation carriers were thought not to have any clinical phenotype, but this is incorrect. Women with a pre-mutation but not a full mutation are more at risk of premature ovarian failure (defined as menopause before the age of 40 years; Sherman, 2000). There have been several studies on cognitive and psychological functioning in male and female premutation carriers and suggestions that deficits correlate with the size of the pre-mutation (Mazzocco, 2000). However, socio-economic factors in explaining this genotype–phenotype relationship have still not been fully excluded. The process of change from a pre-mutation to a full mutation probably cannot be explained by simple slippage of DNA polymerase at replication, but may involve the looping-out of a single strand of DNA in a hairpin fashion and depend on DNA repair mechanisms (Sinden, 2001). Exactly when this process occurs and why it is specific to female transmission is poorly understood.

Explanations for the parent-of-origin effect assume different mechanisms if the expansion is believed to be post- or pre-zygotic (Salat *et al*, 2000). Post-zygotic expansion would need an imprinting mechanism to distinguish paternal from maternal pre-mutations. In contrast, pre-zygotic expansion in both male and female gametocytes could occur with expansion removal only in developing sperm (either selective removal of sperm containing full expansion or a direct contraction of the expansion back to a smaller size). Sperm cells undergo multiple divisions through life, oocytes do not, and one suggestion is of an initial mosaicism for the full mutation. Normal sperm would then be at an advantage because of FMR1 protein's support of cell proliferation. Interestingly, men with fragile-X syndrome who have the full expansion in their somatic cells have only a premutation in their germ cell line (as studied by foetal testicular biopsy or directly on sperm). In the oocytes of female full-mutation carriers, the expansion process continues forming enormous repeats.

The FMR1 gene has 17 exons and the mRNA transcribed from these can be spliced together in different ways to produce at least four different protein isoforms. The FMR1 protein contains sequences that are characteristic of RNA-binding proteins. It is part of a family of similar proteins (that includes two interacting homologues, FXR1 from chromosome 3q28 and FXR2 from 17p13, the latter with an action in nucleosomes) that are involved in RNA regulation, association with polyribosomes and in shuttling between cytoplasm and nucleoplasm. Of these, FMR1 protein has an additional specific effect to inhibit translation (Laggerbauer et al, 2001) and also co-localises strongly with another protein, NUFIP (nuclear FMRP-interacting protein) in the cortex, hippocampus and cerebellum. This indicates that, yet again, FMR1 protein may be a component of a complex system of intracellular signalling and gene activity control. Men with large pre-mutations (>100 triplets) have high levels of FMR1 mRNA but reduced levels of FMR1 protein, indicating complex regulation of translation and transcription (Tassone et al, 2000). The temporal expression of the FMR1 gene also changes strikingly at different times of mammalian development. In the foetus, it is expressed from an early age in the dividing and migrating neuroblasts of the brain as well as in other non-neural tissues.

## FRAXE

Another folate-sensitive fragile site, FRAXE, exists at Xq28, very close to FRAXA. Again the underlying feature is an unstable repeat involving CGG triplet expansion (Gecz, 2000). The associated gene is FMR2 and the transcription of this is silenced when the triplet copy number exceeds 250. Normal copy number is from 4 to 39 and the pre-mutation size is considered to range from 31 to 60. The effects of the full mutation are very variable, from mild learning disability (perhaps better classified as a behavioural phenotype including speech delay and over-activity), through to no learning disability and this is really an example of a non-specific X-linked mental retardation (MRX2 see below). The best estimates (Youings et al, 2000) indicate that around 1 in 23 500 males may be clinically affected, but the carriage rate of the full mutation may be higher due to those with no clinical phenotype. The repeat lies in the untranscribed region of the FMR2 gene and expansion results in methylation of an associated CpG island and gene silencing. The function of FMR2 is less well characterised than FMR1, but it is a large 22-exon gene whose protein is one of a family that localises in the cell nucleus and also includes genes mutated in cancer. It seems to be a potent activator of gene transcription linking this to other signalling genes of the MRX series of disorders (Hillman & Cecz, 2001). In mammals, it is highly expressed in the hippocampus and amygdala (Chakrabarti *et al*, 1998).

## MRX disorders

In normal female cells, genes (save the pseudoautosomal ones) are only actively expressed on one of the X chromosomes, the other X chromosome being randomly inactivated. Thus, there is a 50% chance that a deleterious mutation in a gene will not be expressed if it is on the X chromosome that is compacted. In contrast, in normal male cells the Y chromosome does not offer such compensation. Males will therefore be more likely to express the results of an X-linked mutation and this is one source of the increased incidence of learning disability in males. This excess has been known for a considerable time; it was described by Johnson (1897) in the USA, by Luxenburger (1932) in Germany and again by Penrose (1938) in the UK. However, the causal assumptions (ascertainment bias, higher aggression leading to institutionalisation) were later shown to be incorrect and the male bias largely due to sex-linked genetic disorders.

Over 200 heritable X-linked disorders associated with learning disability are known, and may affect up to 1 in 600 of the total male population (Chiurazzi *et al*, 2001). Fragile-X syndrome (15–20%), and other conditions with dysmorphic or systemic features (syndromal mental retardation or MRXS), account for a large percentage. However, up to half may be non-syndromic conditions with learning disability as the only phenotypic feature (Tariverdian & Vogel, 2000). These have been grouped together as the MRX disorders (non-specific mental retardation) and the effects of such gene mutations are thought to be largely restricted to the central nervous system. The X-chromosome location has been identified for 59 families segregating MRX and the genes for seven have been isolated. Many appear to be genes involved in cellular signalling or in the control of transcription. Some are due to variant mutations in genes that are normally associated with dysmorphic conditions. For instance, one syndrome of X-linked mild learning disability, MRX19, is produced by a specific mutation that reduces expression from the gene (RPSKA3 at Xp22) that, when completely silenced, leads to the Coffin–Lowry syndrome. This indicates a threshold effect for the action of this gene in a protein kinase signalling cascade. The gene for another signalling kinase in the Rho-GAP cascade, PAK3 (Xq21-24), is mutated in four separate MRX families as well as other neurological conditions. PAK3 is highly expressed in hippocampus and cerebral cortex, but MRI findings indicate that the actions may be subtle, perhaps on axonal outgrowth (Allen *et al*, 1998). Mutations in another Rho-GAP signalling gene, RABGDIA (Xq28; formerly oligo-phrenin 2), are the cause of the learning disability in MRX41 and 48, and again we are beginning to see the linking together of such conditions by study of functional signalling cascades. Finally, to emphasise the point, MRX1 is caused by mutations in the IL1RAPL1 gene that produces a novel protein involved in the interleukin signalling pathways very important to cognitive functioning (Carrie *et al*, 1999).

## Polyalanine tract expansion

A recently identified type of repeat expansion is that of polyalanine tracts within HOX genes. Originally described in *Drosophila*, where they play fundamental roles as transcription factors in the formation of the segmental body plan, there are four separate chromosomal clusters of human HOX genes (HOXA to HOXD) that contain a total of 39 genes. These code for proteins all containing a highly conserved DNA binding motif – the homoeodomain – that interacts with specific target DNA sequences and forms protein complexes regulating transcription of the bound gene. Human malformation syndromes have been described that involve alterations in HOXD13 (synpolydactyly) and HOXA13 (hand–genital–foot syndrome). In addition to classical direct mutations of the DNA homoeobox (codes for homoeodomain), a new class of mutation – an expansion of triplet nucleotide sequences that code for alanine – was discovered. It was first seen in synpolydactyly, but has now also been described in other transcription factors such as in the ZIC2 gene which leads to one form of holoprosencephaly (Goodman & Scambler, 2001). These expansions are in regions of the previously little-understood areas of the protein and are meiotically stable, fairly short and probably generated by unequal crossing-over at recombination between two misaligned regions of homologous DNA. Their actions may be through a dominant negative effect, dimerising with the normal wild-type protein from the other chromosome when the mutation is hemizygous. Another syndrome, similar to the hand–genital–foot, but also including other system malformations and mild learning disability, has been described in a patient with a deletion on chromosome 7p that removes the entire HOXA cluster. Although there only a few human HOX-associated and polyalanine expansion disorders, these are sure to increase in number as we continue to explore the contents of the human genome. HOX genes also link into other gene cascades through interaction of HOXA5 with p53 (see below).

## Rett syndrome

Rett syndrome, a severe degenerative multisystem disorder of childhood associated with increasingly severe learning disability and stereotyped hand movements, illustrates the opposite bias to most sex-linked disorders – it is almost exclusive to females. The brain (disorder of neurones in cortical layers 5 and 6), the heart (increased QT interval) and bones (osteopaenia is common and in the rare affected males severe growth retardation) are all affected. Classical Rett syndrome is usually sporadic and rare males are much more severely affected than females. A set of small families with dominant inheritance had alleles of probes from Xq28 that were conserved between them, and this positional information led eventually to the identification of MECP2 (Amir *et al*, 1999) as the gene responsible. MECP2 produces a methyl-CpG-binding protein, linking it to epigenetic imprinting phenomena, since MECP2 is involved in the recruiting of histone deacetylases to regions of methylated DNA and altering chromatin structure. MECP2 mutations are largely inherited through the male germline, explaining the female predominance (Girard *et al*, 2001). Already, MECP2 is known to harbour over 70 different mutations (Dragich *et al*, 2000). There are also mutations in some MRX families and individual MRX patients (Couvert *et al*, 2001). This is an exciting result, as numerically the number affected by MECP2 mutations in the MRX population was comparable to that of expansions in FMR1.

## Prader–Willi/Angelman and imprinting

Save for the sex chromosomes, the expression of most of our genes is biallelic. There is a small but increasing number of known genes that are expressed from only one chromosome (monoallelic). For some of these genes, expression is not a random choice but preferential for a chromosome of a pair inherited from one or other parent. Some form of chromosomal marking mechanism must exist to distinguish the parent-of-origin and this marking has attracted the term genomic imprinting (Reik & Walter, 2001). These imprints are established in the germ line cells and thus, assuming no subsequent DNA changes take place, are transferred to all derived cells after fertilisation. Here we have a mechanism that changes the inherited pattern of gene expression, but is not inherent in the genome DNA sequence itself – an example of an epigenetic effect. Imprinted genes often lie close – CpG islands are flanked by other unique repeat sequences that may be involved in flagging up the region to be imprinted. In contrast to our near-complete lack of knowledge about nature of the primary imprint that distinguishes male and female parent-derived regions, we know a considerable amount about the major human imprinting maintenance mechanism – the methylation of the cytosine nucleotide at a CpG pair. The gene promoter region that is necessary for DNA polymerase binding and thus replication of DNA often has a high density of such pairs and their methylation often silences the gene. Since the chromosomes inherited from parents will initially contain the imprints that they themselves have established (i.e. distinguishing between their own parents (the patient's grandparents)) it will be clear that the imprints have to be 'reset' in the germ cell lines (ova and sperm). The old imprints are 'erased' at an early stage of germ cell development, probably by a genome-wide demethylation that is complete by around embryonic day 12. *De novo* differential re-methylation then takes place, directed by some form of primary imprint over a much longer time span (still continuing in the germ cells after birth).

Around 20 human conditions are known to be associated with alteration of imprinted gene function and this number will probably rise considerably as our understanding of the control of gene expression improves. Silencing of a gene or, more usually, a group of genes on one parent-specific chromosome leaves the genes on the other chromosome as the only active copies (monallelic expression). A germ line insult to these active genes (whether through deletion, direct mutation or other effect) will thus cause complete gene silencing. Post-zygotic changes will give outcomes dependent on their timing and on which somatic cell clone they alter, with potentially more restricted outcomes (Hanel & Wevrick, 2001).

The best-studied imprinting disorders are those on the long arm of chromosome 15 which result in Prader–Willi syndrome or Angelman syndrome, depending on which particular chromosome of the pair is affected. Although these disorders are rare (Prader–Willi syndrome birth frequency is around 1:15 000; Angelman syndrome 1:30 000), they are paradigms of our understanding of epigenetic effects and are worth considering in some detail. Prader–Willi syndrome was very clearly described in 1864 and photographed by Langdon Down who called the condition polysarcia (Ward, 1998). There is a clear behavioural phenotype – compulsive overeating – combined with a variable degree of learning disability, emotional lability, short stature, microcephaly and hypogonadism. It has been known for around 20 years that deletions of a small region of chromosome 15 (15q11-13) occur in Prader–Willi syndrome, and it was discovered soon after that they always seemed to occur on the chromosome 15 inherited from the patient's father.

However, only in the past decade have the mechanisms that underlie this been more clearly understood.

Most (70%) of cases of Prader–Willi syndrome are sporadic and associated with deletion on the chromosome 15 of paternal origin, perhaps through unequal crossover in paternal meiosis or through the formation of an intra-chromosomal loop that is then excised. Genes in the deleted region are normally only expressed from the paternally derived chromosome and those on the maternally derived chromosome are normally silenced by an imprinting mechanism. Thus, from the functional point of view, there is a complete lack of expression of the genes within the deleted region, resulting in Prader–Willi syndrome. Since multiple genes are involved, Prader–Willi syndrome is properly considered a contiguous gene, though the effects of one or two genes may predominate. Key candidates are the nectin and nectin-like genes (NDN and MAGEL2) that encode brain-expressed transcription-factor-binding proteins. Most (around 30%) of the non-deletion cases of Prader–Willi syndrome are due to the inheritance of two chromosome 15s that are derived from only one parent. This situation is described as uniparental disomy, and most usually results from the formation of an initial chromosome trisomy that is then reduced in number to two. In the case of Prader–Willi syndrome, both chromosome 15s are maternal in origin, and with a maternal pattern of imprinted silencing of genes at 15q11-13, the result is similar to a deletion on the paternally derived chromosome. Maternal meiosis I non-disjunction seems to be involved (and this relates to maternal age), followed by a 'trisomy rescue' to form a disomy. Chorionic villus sampling has shown a mosaic pattern of trisomy 15 cells (confined placental mosaicism) in mothers of children with uniparental disomy Prader–Willi syndrome. In addition to chromosome 15, uniparental disomy is now known to occur in 17 other human chromosomes.

The reciprocal mechanisms, a deletion in the maternally derived chromosome 15 or uniparental disomy of paternal chromosomes results in the clinically completely different disorder Angelman syndrome. Learning disability is severe, associated with epilepsy in most cases and with other features including paroxysmal outbursts of laughter, ataxia, prognathism, macrostomia and protruding tongue. Over 70% have a maternal deletion. The only known genes in the region that are solely expressed from the maternal chromosome 15 are UBE3A, an ubiquitin ligase (see below), and ATP10C, a phospholipid transport gene (Herzing *et al*, 2001). Both these genes are expressed biallelically in most tissues but only monoallelically in the brain. Point mutations that silence UBE3A on the maternally derived chromosome produce classical Angelman syndrome and it is likely that most of the clinical syndrome is accounted for by this. However, deletion cases are said to be more severe and other genes may modify the situation through haploinsufficiency.

## The Prader–Willi syndrome/Angelman syndrome imprinting centre

Rare cases of Prader–Willi syndrome and Angelman syndrome are familial. Some of these result from unbalanced inheritance of a chromosomal translocation leading to a monosomy of the region or in some cases to a balanced form with a partial uniparental disomy. Others arise from imprinting centre mutations.

As in the X chromosome, an imprinting centre is now known to control the methylation pattern in the Prader–Willi syndrome/ Angelman syndrome region, and microdeletions of this centre lead to failure to reset the imprint of chromosome 15 during gamete formation (in essence, it retains the grandparental imprint which will determine whether the imprint pattern is 'female' or 'male' in type). There seem to be two overlapping parts to the imprinting centre, one controlling the paternal methylation pattern and the other the maternal, with the common part of the imprinting centre being centred around a complex transcription unit (SNRP–SNURF; Wirth *et al*, 2001) which codes for peptides that are associated with ribonucleoproteins. Studies of human deletions and transgenic experiments in mice (Shemer *et al*, 2000; Buiting *et al*, 2001) have shown that that the promoter/ exon 1 of SNRPN and a small 1 kbp segment nearby are enough to confer proper methylation patterns and parent-of-origin effects. The best current model is that the two parts of the centre must establish the correct methylation and that the UBE3A on the paternal chromosome may be silenced by an antisense RNA produced by a UBE3A antisense gene on the paternal chromosome (Chamberlain & Brannan, 2001).

Mutations in the imprinting centre will alter or prevent the correct methylation pattern, leading to either Prader–Willi syndrome (very rare) or Angelman syndrome (around 6% of cases). Angelman syndrome is only one of the many human conditions that are linked to the metabolic activities of ubiquitin. Ubiquitin is a small protein that, as its name suggests, is involved in a huge number of cell activities via its conjugation with other proteins (ubiquitylation). Classically, it binds proteins that will be broken down by the intracellular proteasome complex. However, it also has signalling and other complex functions. Angelman syndrome itself is due to disorder of an enzyme that modifies ubiquitin and is part of a group of proteins that range from the well-known tumour-suppressor gene p53, through to proteins that interact with epithelial channels (mutations in the binding domains which can give rise to one type of inherited hypertension). Other variants or ligands of the ubiquitin families include those responsible for juvenile-onset Parkinson's disease and BRCA-1 involved in breast and ovarian cancer. In fact, ubiquitin regulation is essential to virtually every eukaryotic cell process, and undoubtedly there will be many more conditions that result in learning disability, representing disorders of some part of its multi-faceted biology (Weissman, 2001).

# The human genome mapping project and learning disability: now and into the future

## Advances in genetic technology

Many of the recent discoveries in learning disability genetics would not have been possible without great important technical advances. The polymerase chain reaction has already been mentioned, as have the large insert size cloning vectors (YACs, BACs). These methods of amplifying and handling DNA were combined with high throughput (and highly automated) DNA sequencing methodologies to provide large numbers of partial sequence, upon which the human genome sequence was constructed. The assembly of these into overlapping, linearly arranged stretches of DNA ('contig building') required the development of new computer algorithms and is one part of the explosion in the new science of bioinformatics (Searls, 2000). Much of the way forward, as we move from genomics to proteomics, will be through the development of technologies to process large sample sets in parallel (Mir & Southern, 2000). Leading the field at the moment are microarrays. Attachment of cDNAs or oligonucleotides to a substrate to produce a Cartesian grid of single-stranded molecules for hybridisation experiments has become a fine art. Substrates are various (glass, gold, plastic) and are often labelled 'genechips' – borrowing both terminology and photo-deposition methodology from the semiconductor industry. Dense arrays with over 10 000 different cDNAs per $cm^2$ are now both realisable and repeatable, representing huge numbers of genes that can then be probed, for example with labelled mRNA from a given tissue or organ to report on its current expression pattern, the transcriptosome (Lockhart & Winzeler, 2000). Mutations can be detected by looking for mis-matched binding to complementary sequence or, inversely, DNAs representing the mutations when known can be used to quickly characterise a sample. All the multiple mutations causing cystic fibrosis, for example, have now been hung onto a single chip. Peptides and proteins will be the next molecules to be arrayed, allowing us to study the proteome of an organ or cell, fingerprinting its characteristics and how it changes over time. This opens up the potential to directly study the complex multiple actions of therapies at the gene, message and protein levels, and some indicate that this is a harbinger of individualised pharmacogenetics with drug therapy being tailored to the individual's constitutional characteristics (Roses, 2000).

**75**

## Genotype to phenotype

Other developments important to learning disability will emerge from our understanding of genotype–phenotype axes and the multiple genes involved, especially in signalling. New reporter molecules such as the jellyfish-derived green fluorescent protein (Chamberlain & Hahn, 2001) can be attached to normal protein to form a fully functional chimaera that 'lights up' under fluorescence. This can be used to directly visualise the activities and distributions of a protein – vital factors in exploring the effects of gene modification in animals. The experimental gene manipulations most relevant to learning disability are those done in mice (Nolan, 2000). Transgenic constructs inserting mutated human genes into the system, as well as direct knockouts or knockins of altered mouse homologous genes, are powerful ways to study aberrant and normal biology, and key to the development of targeted therapies for components of learning disability-associated syndromes. The reversal of a dictated phenotype by insertion of an altered construct into a mouse containing a mutated gene (gene rescue) shows how we can change outcomes by genetic methods (or gene products – the use of proteins). Another powerful way of studying gene control is through RNA interference. Double-stranded RNA complementary to the gene sequence is synthesised and injected into a cell, where it is broken down into short strands that specifically induce the degradation of the targeted gene's message, allowing the outcome of phenotype to be readily and rapidly evaluated. Although widely used in lower organisms, differences in mammalian RNA processing have, until recently, limited its application. However, Elbashir *et al* (2001) have circumvented some of the problems, and its use to create mammalian models would be a major advance in terms of cost and utility over direct transgenic models. The goal of gene therapy for our patients, however, is still a long way off (and in some cases may never be reached; Ye *et al*, 2001). Ethical issues in learning disability are discussed elsewhere in this volume. However, as in the fields of prenatal diagnosis and genetic testing in general for inherited disease, we must be very careful that developments such as gene therapy do not outpace our ethical thinking about conditions associated with learning disability. It is a salutary reminder that among the strongest supporters of the discredited eugenics movement were scientists and psychiatrists. The few human conditions (e.g. severe combined immune deficiency) where gene therapy has been used have generated mixed results, and a much greater understanding of the complex developmental biological processes involved is needed before progress can be made using either this or more standard therapeutic tools. However, with the major current genetic advances, the door to achieving this with respect to gene and protein function is wide open.

## *Where will all this lead?*

From the viewpoint of the psychiatrist in learning disability, many of these ideas may feel unfamiliar and strange. However, although often embedded in offputting language and terminology, the beauty of the most important molecular genetic findings lies in their simplicity. Our understanding of the key genetic elements that shape the multitude of conditions that we still tend to gather together using the term 'learning disability' advances at a furious pace and the learning disability itself is usually only one epiphenomenon of the causative process. For many psychiatrists, all this will mean a serious rethink about the basic definition and use of the term learning disability.

We also should not (and those of us who have ever visited Hadamar Psychiatric Hospital overlooking the Rhine cannot) forget the past, the eras of eugenics and the horrific misuse of genetics in social control. Partly the ideas of the scientists themselves, many from the UK, were to blame – genetics was assumed to have a total determinism that even then was completely unsupported and we should still be on our guard against a re-emergence of such views. Instead, however, our increased valid genetic knowledge will allow us to start to study how the interplay between genetic substrates, our life-span experiences, and the world in which we live dictates our behavioural and cognitive processes, and our own uniqueness, and thus opens the way to the valid design of therapies (psychological as well as pharmacological) for the problems that arise through having a condition that generates a learning disability. Knowing the genetics goes a great way towards isolating and understanding the environmental (and modifiable) contributions to such disorders.

The publication of the first draft of the human genome sequence is as much a watershed for us in the field of learning disability as for the scientific community as a whole, as we enter a new and exciting era of molecular psychiatry.

# References

Allen, K. M., Gleeson, J. G., Bagrodia, S., *et al* (1998) PAK3 mutation in nonsyndromic X-linked mental retardation. *Nature Genetics,* **20**, 25–30.

Amir, R. E., Van Den Veyver, I. B., Wan, M., *et al* (1999) Rett syndrome is caused by mutations in X-linked MECP2 encoding methyl-CpG-binding protein 2. *Nature Genetics,* **23**, 31–35.

Avner, P. & Heard, E. (2001) X-chromosome inactivation: counting, choice and initiation. *Nature Reviews Genetics,* **2**, 59–67.

Beresford, R. G., Tatlidil, C., Riddell, D. C., *et al* (2000) Absence of fragile-X syndrome in Nova Scotia. *Journal of Medical Genetics,* **37**, 77–79.

Blackwood, D. H. R., Fordyce, A., Walker, M., *et al* (2001) Cosegregation of schizophrenia and affective disorders with a translocation that directly disrupts brain expressed genes at chromosome 1q42: clinical and P300 findings in a family. *American Journal of Human Genetics*, **69**, 428–433.

Bliek, J., Maas, S. M., Ruijter, J. M., *et al* (2001) Increased tumour risk for BWS patients correlates with aberrant H19 and not KCNQ1OT1 methylation: occurrence of KCNQ1OT1 hypomethylation in familial cases of BWS. *Human Molecular Genetics*, **10**, 467–476.

Buiting, K., Barnicoat, A., Lich, C., *et al* (2001) Disruption of the bipartite imprinting center in a family with Angelman syndrome. *American Journal of Human Genetics*, **68**, 1290–1294.

Buxbaum, J. D., Silverman, J. M., Smith, C. J., *et al* (2001) Evidence for a susceptibility gene for autism on chromosome 2 and for genetic heterogeneity. *American Journal of Human Genetics*, **68**, 1513–1520.

Carrie, A., Jun, L., Bienvenue, T., *et al* (1999) A new member of the IL-1 receptor family highly expressed in hippocampus and involved in X-linked mental retardation. *Nature Genetics*, **23**, 25–31.

Caspi, M., Atlas, R., Kantor, A., *et al* (2000) Interaction between LIS1 and doublecortin, two lissencephaly gene products. *Human Molecular Genetics*, **9**, 2205–2213.

Chakrabarti, L., Bristulf, J., Foss, G. S., *et al* (1998) Expression of the murine homologue of FMR2 in mouse brain and during development. *Human Molecular Genetics*, **7**, 441–448.

Chamberlain, C. & Hahn, K. M. (2001) Watching proteins in the wild: fluorescence methods to study protein dynamics in living cells. *Traffic*, **1**, 755–762.

Chamberlain, S. J. & Brannan, C. I. (2001) The Prader–Willi syndrome imprinting center activates the paternally expressed murine Ube3a antisense transcript but represses paternal Ube3a. *Genomics*, **73**, 316–322.

Chiurazzi, P., Hamel, B. C. J. & Neri, G. (2001) XLMR genes: update 2000. *European Journal of Human Genetics*, **9**, 71–81.

Chrast, R., Scott, H. S., Madani, R., *et al* (2000) Mice trisomic for a bacterial artificial chromosome with the single-minded 2 gene (Sim2) show phenotypes similar to those present in the partial trisomy 16 mouse models of Down syndrome. *Human Molecular Genetics*, **9**, 1853–1864.

Collaborative Linkage Study on Autism (1999) An autosomal genome scan for autism. *American Journal of Medical Genetics (Neuropsychiatric Genetics)*, **88**, 609–615.

Cook, E. H. Jr., Lindgren, V., Leventhal, B. L., *et al* (1997) Autism or atypical autism in maternally but not paternally derived proximal 15q duplication. *American Journal of Human Genetics*, **60**, 928–934.

Couvert, P., Bienvenu, T., Aquaviva, C., *et al* (2001) MECP2 is highly mutated in X-linked mental retardation. *Human Molecular Genetics*, **10**, 941–946.

Crow, J. F. (2000) The origins, patterns and implications of human spontaneous mutation. *Nature Reviews Genetics*, **1**, 40–47.

de Vries, B. B. A., White, S. M., Knight, S. J. L., *et al* (2001) Clinical studies on submicroscopic subtelomeric re-arrangements: a checklist. *Journal of Medical Genetics*, **38**, 145–150.

Dragich, J., Houwink-Manville, I. & Schanen, C. (2000) Rett syndrome: a surprising result of mutation in MECP2. *Human Molecular Genetics*, **9**, 2365–2375.

Elbashir, S. M., Harborth, J., Lendeckel, W. *et al* (2001) Duplexes of 21-nucleotide RNAs mediate RNA interference in cultured mammalian cells. *Nature*, **411**, 494–498.

Evans, K. L., Muir, W. J., Blackwood, D. H. R., *et al* (2001) Nuts and bolts of psychiatric genetics – building on the human genome project. *Trends in Genetics*, **17**, 35–40.

Flint, J. & Mott, R. (2001) Finding the molecular basis of quantitative traits: successes and pitfalls. *Nature Reviews Genetics*, **2**, 437–445.

Fransen, E., Van Camp, G., D'Hooge, R., *et al* (1998) Genotype–phenotype correlation in L1 associated diseases. *Journal of Medical Genetics*, **35**, 399–404.

Gecz, J. (2000) The FMR2 gene, FRAXE and non-specific mental retardation: clinical and molecular aspects. *Annals of Human Genetics*, **64**, 95–106.

Girard, M., Couvert, P., Carrie, A., *et al* (2001) Parental origin of de novo MECP2 mutations in Rett syndrome. *European Journal of Human Genetics*, **9**, 231–236.

Goodman, F. R. & Scambler, P. J. (2001) Human *HOX* gene mutations. *Clinical Genetics*, **59**, 1–11.

Gray, I. C., Campbell, D. A. & Spurr, N. K. (2000) Single nucleotide polymorphisms as tools in human genetics. *Human Molecular Genetics*, **9**, 2403–2408.

Hanel, M. L. & Wevrick, R. (2001) The role of genomic imprinting in human developmental disorders: lessons from Prader–Willi syndrome. *Clinical Genetics*, **59**, 156–164.

Hassold, R., Sherman, S. & Hunt, P. (2000) Counting cross-overs: characterising meitotic recombination in mammals. *Human Molecular Genetics*, **9**, 2409–2419.

Hattori, M., Fujiyama, A., Taylor, T. D., *et al* (2000) The DNA sequence of human chromosome 21. *Nature*, **405**, 311–319.

Herzing, L. B. K., Kim, S.-J., Cook, E. H. Jr, *et al* (2001) The human aminophospholipid-transporting ATPase gene ATP10C maps adjacent to UBE3A and exhibits similar imprinted expression. *American Journal of Human Genetics*, **68**, 1501–1505.

Hillman, M. A. & Cecz, J. (2001) Fragile-XE-associated mental retardation protein (FMR2) acts as a potent transcription activator. *Journal of Human Genetics*, **46**, 251–259.

Husi, H., & Grant, S. G. (2001) Proteomics of the nervous system. *Trends in Neuroscience*, **24**, 259–66.

International Molecular Genetic Study of Autism Consortium (2001) Further characterization of the autism susceptibility locus AUTS1 on chromosome 7q. *Human Molecular Genetics*, **10**, 973–982.

Jerome, L. A. & Papaioannou, V. E. (2001) DiGeorge syndrome phenotype in mice mutant for the T-box gene, Tbx1. *Nature Genetics*, **27**, 286–291.

Johnson, G. E. (1897) Contribution to the psychology and pedagogy of feeble-minded children. *Journal of Psychoasthenic*, **2**, 26–32.

Kleinjan, D. J. & Van Heyningen, V. (1998) Position effect in human genetic disease. *Human Molecular Genetics*, **7**, 1611–1618.

Knight, S. J. L., Regan, R., Nicod, A., *et al* (1999) Subtle chromosomal rearrangements in children with unexplained mental retardation. *Lancet*, **354**, 1676–1681.

Laggerbauer, B., Ostareck, D., Keidel, E.-M., *et al* (2001) Evidence that fragile-X mental retardation protein is a negative regulator of translation. *Human Molecular Genetics*, **10**, 329–338.

Lahn, B. T., Pearson, M. M. & Jegalian, K. (2001) The human Y chromosome, in the light of evolution. *Nature Reviews Genetics*, **2**, 207–216.

Lai, C. S., Fisher, S. E., Hurst, J. A., *et al* (2000) The SPCH1 region on human 7q31: genomic characterisation of the critical interval and localization of translocations associated with speech and language disorder. *American Journal of Human Genetics*, **67**, 357–368.

Lander, E. S., Linton, L. M., Birren, B., *et al* (2001) Initial sequencing and analysis of the human genome. *Nature*, **40**, 860–921.

Lockhart, D. J. & Winzeler, E. A. (2000) Genomics, gene expression and DNA arrays. *Nature*, **405**, 827–836.

Lubs, H. A. (1969) A marker X chromosome. *American Journal of Human Genetics*, **21**, 231–244.

Luxenburger, H. (1932) Endogener schwachsinn und geschlechtsgebundener erbang. *Zeitschrift für Neurologie und Psychologie*, **140**, 320–332.

Mazzocco, M. M. M. (2000) Advances in research on the fragile-X syndrome. *Mental Retardation and Developmental Disabilities Research Reviews*, **6**, 96–106.

Mervis, C. B. & Klein-Tasman, B. (2000) Williams syndrome: cognition, personality, and adaptive behavior. *Mental Retardation and Developmental Disabilities Research Reviews*, **6**, 148–158.

**79**

Mills, A. A. & Bradley, A. (2001) From mouse to man: generating megabase chromosomal rearrangements. *Trends in Genetics*, **17**, 331–339.

Mir, K. U. & Southern, E. M. (2000) Sequence variation in genes and genomic DNA: Methods for large-scale analysis. *Annual Review of Genomics and Human Genetics*, **1**, 329–360.

Morris, C. A. & Mervis, C. B. (2000) Williams syndrome and related disorders. *Annual Review of Genomics and Human Genetics*, **1**, 461–484.

Muir, W. J. (2000) Genetic advances and learning disability. *British Journal of Psychiatry*, **176**, 12–19.

Naldeau, J. H. (2001) Modifier genes in mice and humans. *Nature Reviews Genetics*, **2**, 165–174.

Nolan, P. M. (2000) Generation of mouse mutants as a tool for functional genomics. *Pharmacogenomics*, **1**, 243–255.

Penrose, L. S. (1938) *A clinical and genetic study of 1280 cases of mental defect (the Colchester Survey)*. Medical Research Council London Special Report Series No. 229. London: Medical Research Council.

Prak, E. L. & Kazazian, H. H. (2000) Mobile elements and the human genome. *Nature Reviews Genetics*, **1**, 134–144.

Reeves, R. H., Baxter, L. L. & Richtsmeier, J. T. (2001) Too much of a good thing: mechanisms of gene action in Down syndrome. *Trends in Genetics*, **17**, 83–88.

Reik, W. & Walter, J. (2001) Genomic imprinting: parental influence on the genome. *Nature Reviews Genetics*, **2**, 21–32.

Riazuddin, S., Castelein, C. M., Ahmed, Z. M., *et al* (2000) Dominant modifier DFNM1 suppresses recessive deafness in DFNB26. *Nature Genetics*, **26**, 431–434.

Robertson, K. D. & Wolffe, A. P. (2000) DNA methylation in health and disease. *Nature Reviews Genetics*, **1**, 11–19.

Roses, A. (2000) Pharmacogenetics and the practice of medicine. *Nature*, **405**, 857–865.

Salat, U., Bardoni, B., Wöhrle, D., *et al* (2000) Increase of FMRP expression, raised levels of *FMR1* mRNA, and clonal selection in proliferating cells with unmethylated fragile-X repeat expansions: a clue to the sex bias in the transmission of full mutations? *Journal of Medical Genetics*, **37**, 842–850.

Searls, D. B. (2000) Bioinformatic tools for whole genomes. *Annual Review of Genomics and Human Genetics*, **1**, 251–279.

Shemer, R., Hershko, A. Y., Perk, J., *et al* (2000) The imprinting box of the Prader–Willi/Angelman syndrome domain. *Nature Genetics*, **26**, 440–443.

Sherman, S. L. (2000) Premature ovarian failure in the fragile-X syndrome. *American Journal of Medical Genetics*, **97**, 189–194.

Shonn, M. A., McCarroll, R., Murray, A. W. (2000) Requirement of the spindle checkpoint for proper chromosome segregation in budding yeast meiosis. *Science*, **289**, 300–303.

Shprintzen, R. J. (2000) Velo-cardio-facial syndrome: a distinctive behavioral phenotype. *Mental Retardation and Developmental Disabilities Research Reviews*, **6**, 142–147.

Sinden, R. R. (2001) Origins of instability. *Nature*, **411**, 757–758.

Smith, D. J., Stevens, M. E., Sudanagunta, S. P., *et al* (1997) Functional screening of 2 Mb of human chromosome 21q22.2 in transgenic mice implicates minibrain in learning defects associated with Down's syndrome. *Nature Genetics*, **16**, 28–36.

Sutherland, G. R. & Baker, E. (2000) The clinical significance of fragile sites on human chromosomes. *Clinical Genetics*, **58**, 157–161.

Tariverdian, G. & Vogel, F. (2000) Some problems in the genetics of X-linked mental retardation. *Cytogenetics and Cell Genetics*, **91**, 278–284.

Tassone, F., Hagerman, R. J., Taylor, A. K., *et al* (2000) Elevated levels of FMR1 mRNA in carrier males: a new mechanism of involvement in the fragile-X syndrome. *American Journal of Human Genetics*, **66**, 6–15.

Vallee, R. B., Tai, C.-Y. & Faulkner, N. E. (2001) LIS1: cellular function of a disease-causing gene. *Trends in Cell Biology,* **11**, 155–160.

Venter, J. C., Adams, M. D., Myers, E. W., *et al* (2001) The sequence of the human genome. *Science,* **291**, 1304–1351.

Villavicencio, E. H., Walterhouse, D. O. & Iannaccone, P. M. (2000) The sonic hedgehog-patched-gli pathway in human development and disease. *American Journal of Human Genetics,* **67**, 1047–1054.

Ward, O. C. (1998) *John Langdon Down, A Caring Pioneer.* London: Royal Society of Medicine Press.

Weissman, A. M. (2001) Themes and variations on ubiquitylation. *Nature Reviews Molecular Cell Biology,* **2**, 169–178.

Willemsen, R., Olmer, R., Otero, Y. D. D., *et al* (2000) Twin sisters, monozygotic with the fragile-X mutation, but with a different phenotype. *Journal of Medical Genetics,* **37**, 603–604.

Wirth, J., Back, E., Huttenhofer, A., *et al* (2001) A translocation breakpoint cluster disrupts the newly defined 3' end of the SNURF-SNRPN transcription unit on chromosome 15. *Human Molecular Genetics,* **10**, 201–210.

Wolffe, A. P. & Matzke, M. A. (1999) Epigenetics: regulation through repression. *Science,* **286**, 481–486.

Ye, X., Mitchell, M., Newman, K., *et al* (2001) Prospects for prenatal gene therapy in disorders causing mental retardation. *Mental Retardation and Developmental Disabilities Research Reviews,* **7**, 65–72.

Youings, S. A., Murray, A., Dennis, N., *et al* (2000) FRAXA and FRAXE: the results of a five year survey. *Journal of Medical Genetics,* **37**, 415–421.

# Internet resource

Online Mendelian Inheritance in Man – http://www.ncbi.nlm.nih.gov/Omim/

# CHAPTER 4

# Behavioural phenotypes

Tom Berney

Advances in genetic techniques mean that more and more people with learning disabilities can expect an aetiological diagnosis. The progress in laboratory precision has pressed for a matching clarity in our clinical definition of phenotype, both somatic and psychological. Although this chapter focuses on the latter, the two are so closely intertwined that the somatic component cannot be ignored. However, most syndromes are very pervasive, leaving few systems untouched, so that any catalogue of stigmata is lengthy and requires depiction by photograph (Jones, 1996).

## Assessment

Assessment of the psychological phenotype has tended to concentrate on ability and skills – the *cognitive phenotype* – in terms of both specific disabilities and overall intellectual impairment; of level of function as well as potential abilities. A central component is language function and personality assessment, contentious enough in the rest of the population and hampered here by limited communication. With access to subjective perceptions and attitudes blocked, the emphasis shifts to one of the more observable aspects of personality – behavioural style or temperament. This, the characteristic manner in which different individuals approach and respond to the world around them, can be dissected into a number of variables. Ideally independent of each other, variables such as the quality of mood, the intensity of reaction, the level of activity and attention span can be grouped to give recognisable categories such as 'easy', 'difficult' or 'slow to warm up'. Alternatively, the variables may be summed to give dimensions such as 'emotionality', 'activity' and 'sociability' (Goldsmith *et al*, 1987; Ganiban *et al*, 1990).

The *behavioural phenotype* includes temperament as well as all other facets of behaviour such as attention span, unusual interests, stereotypies, and sleeping and eating habits. Some distinction may be made from the *psychiatric phenotype*, which includes symptoms such as depression, obsessive–compulsive phenomena or frank psychosis. These outward signs of an inward congenital predisposition unfold with development, shaped by other, innate factors (such as the mix and degree of mental, physical and sensory disabilities) and by interaction with the environment. Consequently, breakdown into phenotypical components is arbitrary but conceptually convenient.

The main environmental influence is usually the family. It can be difficult to determine the extent to which the family is responding to the proband's behaviour (the genotype creating its own environment) or whether the members carry a variant of the disorder in themselves. There is therefore the potential to treat family interaction as a phenotypical character. In addition, if specific sites influence different elements of a phenotypical character, there is the potential for the genotype to exert a dosage effect on the outcome (Osborne & Pobert, 2001).

In the end, after some elements have been amplified and others muted, a single aetiology can produce such a wide range and variety of behaviours (the phenomenon of pleiotropy) as to make it hard to discern any common thread without taking into account a large number of people. After that, further assessment will be hindered by the common expectation that every person with that syndrome will have that phenotype. In practice, relatively few people will have the 'full hand' of features in their full intensity; most will have a paler reflection or fragments of the phenotype, if indeed it surfaces at all. The essential distinction between diagnostic criteria and associated characteristics must be kept in mind when determining the diagnosis of ambiguous cases. A number of methodological problems complicate the study of behavioural phenotypes (Hodapp & Dykens, 2001).

(1) There are a large number of assessment schedules designed for use by observation, interview or questionnaire. Many are poorly validated and no single schedule will encompass the full range of abilities, skills and behaviour. Therefore, thought must be given to the appropriate instrument (O'Brien, 2001).

(2) Behavioural assessment requires a balance to be struck between the use of direct observation, necessarily for brief periods, and the reports of carers, which will draw on a longer period of time and a wider variety of circumstances. Unfortunately, carers' reports are usually coloured by their own view of the behaviour: one person's restless overactivity might be another's healthy inquisitiveness. Allowance must be made for this, for example, by obtaining a consensus account from several carers.

(3) There are relatively few forms for symptoms to manifest, therefore it is unusual for one to be specific to a disorder – for example, hyperphagia is not pathognomonic of Prader–Willi syndrome, nor

is hand-wringing diagnostic of Rett syndrome. Studies are becoming more precise about the exact features of a symptom to see whether it differs with disorder. For example, a study of self-injury that previously would have recorded simply its frequency and intensity might now include its topography and function (Rojahn, 1986). Furthermore, it is the combination of symptoms rather than any symptom itself that is associated with a syndrome. How to combine the intensity and prevalence of the symptom can be a problem. An ersatz lumping, by summing arbitrarily weighted scores, can leave the resultant phenotype coloured by a few outliers.

(4) Behavioural phenotypes are age-specific and must be seen in the context of both chronological and developmental ages as well as taking account of environment – for example, where a group has grown up in an institution, any innate predisposition might be hidden by a spurious uniformity.

(5) Although a phenotype has to be defined against some standard, there is no single comparison group that is entirely satisfactory, a frequent choice being whether to match for age or for ability. Should not the control group have a comparable degree of disability then, although an attribute might be specific to the syndrome studied? Equally, it might be simply characteristic of learning disability. Selecting a suitable group can be complicated further by disparities between verbal and non-verbal ability or between receptive and expressive language. Where a group is being compared against itself, as in a longitudinal study, the instruments used must be sufficiently standardised for age for the results to be comparable.

(6) Comparison with another syndrome of specific aetiology, frequently Down's syndrome, allows both age and ability to be matched. However, any differences are relative, being attributable either to their presence in the syndrome under study or to their absence in Down's syndrome.

(7) The rarity of many syndromes has encouraged the use of small samples of widely varied age and ability.

(8) Selection pressures have led to unrepresentative samples, biased by the severity of disturbance or learning disability, such as is seen in hospital or clinic populations. Adding to this is the distorting effect of a publication bias that favours positive findings.

All of these have led to the growth of a phenotypical mythology, founded on tentative conclusions awaiting confirmation, and the hunt is on, with phenotypes being identified for any discernible syndrome.

There follow some examples that have been selected for the lessons that can be drawn from them. Further detail may be obtained from specialist texts (O'Brien & Yule, 1995; O'Brien, 2001).

## Down's syndrome

This syndrome is unusual in that the obvious somatotype allows diagnosis at birth, laboratory confirmation is readily available and there is a widespread awareness of the disorder and its characteristics. Although long recognised and with a high prevalence, much of the large body of research is spoiled by methodological shortcomings.

Although no system is unaffected, there is no single abnormality, other than the trisomic genotype, that is invariable or characteristic of Down's: indeed, there is a substantial overlap between all the autosomal trisomies.

The pattern of development comprises a complex mixture of elements such as IQ, self-help and social and language skills. Overall, there is a downward shift of IQ by about 50 points, and subsequent slowing in the developmental trajectory results in a widening gap between children with Down's syndrome and their unimpaired peers. Although there is no loss of skills, their acquisition progressively diminishes until a static state is reached in late childhood. This is a simplification, as, for example, visual short-term memory strengthens in comparison with auditory. Although dementia may be feared as the child's performance progressively falls behind, some of this reflects an inability to exploit the environment unaided. There is an impassioned debate as to how far this can be offset by intensive tuition or enrichment, as in the Headstart and Doman–Delacato programmes. Unfortunately, later on comes the early onset of true dementia, apparent in about 45% of those aged over 45 years.

Behaviour and IQ cannot be divorced from the somatic phenotype; for example, cognitive and language development are limited by deafness and are predicted by the degree of hypotonia. Childhood behavioural disorder, sleep disturbance and eventual maternal stress are linked with disability and poor health, notably recurrent respiratory problems. Hypothyroidism occurs frequently, is usually borderline in degree and is probably autoimmune in type (with raised levels of anti-thyroid and antimicrosomal antibodies).

In a society that places a high value on physical attractiveness, individuals with Down's syndrome may suffer as a result of their characteristic appearance. Anything that enhances this is likely to have a widespread effect on the whole of their self-esteem, social development and integration. In theory, it should be worthwhile to use cosmetic surgery to modify the facial appearance, which brands a person with Down's syndrome. In addition, it is argued, reduction of the over-large tongue will help the articulation and tone of speech, reduce drooling, improve breathing and the ability to eat, as well as reducing the proneness to infections. Although parents and doctors have found cosmetic surgery to be extremely successful in general, their accounts indicate that specific improvements were less obvious. More-rigorous studies, using controls, photographs, videotapes and external raters, not only failed to find any significant improvement but even hinted at adverse effects. Speech difficulties have proved to be cognitive rather than anatomical in origin. Educational methods, including behavioural training in speech, social and assertive skills, might be a more cost-effective approach to tongue protrusion, eating difficulties, and social behaviour and integration; surgery would then be an adjuvant to these techniques rather than a replacement for them (Katz & Kravetz, 1989). Although less emotive than sterilisation, it is an elective, irreversible procedure and requires equal scrutiny where there is any doubt about the ability to obtain valid consent.

Is there a characteristic behavioural phenotype? Langdon Down, demarcating this group from that of congenital hypothyroidism, gave a vivid description of children who were humorous and good-natured mimics, albeit stubborn. The stereotype has been confirmed by subsequent case reports, encapsulated as the 'happy puppy' description, and established by Tredgold as 'a group of cheerful and happy disposition who are affectionate and easily amused'. Only lately has this been tested by more systematic studies. One such study found school children with Down's syndrome to be clownish, sociable, affectionate and self-confident. The non-Down's comparison group, of similar age and ability, were more often confused, nervous, tense, unstable and uncooperative, although the contrast might merely indicate a high level of unease in other forms of learning disability. Other studies, although identifying temperamental characteristics such as 'impassivity' and a 'readiness to approach novel circumstances', emphasise the wide scatter of characteristics and the overall similarity to children without disabilities. This applies particularly where comparison with siblings allows compensation for the family climate (Ganiban et al, 1990).

Pervasive developmental disorder occurs in about 5% of people with Down's syndrome, about half of the prevalence to be expected, given the degree of learning disability, suggesting its neuropathology to be more selective than that of other disorders.

## Fragile-X syndrome

The identification of this syndrome brought together laboratory scientist and clinician with geneticist, dysmorphologist, psychologist, psychiatrist and language therapist – it is the exemplar of a multi-disciplinary approach.

The well-known somatic characteristics, which include testicular enlargement, a large head circumference, long and prominent ears and a high arched palate, emerged as part of a wider connective-tissue disorder with lax joints, flat feet, cave chest and mitral valve prolapse.

Although the degree of intellectual disability varies greatly, it usually lies in the mild to moderate range. As in Down's syndrome, there is a flattening trajectory of cognitive development in late childhood, reflecting difficulty with the development of abstract reasoning. The profile is misleadingly uneven, visuomotor and spatial deficits being combined with relative strengths in verbal and adaptive behaviour: the heterozygote (female) carrier has a similar selective impairment of a range of abilities, as well as a predisposition to depression and other psychiatric disturbances. All of these features vary in extent and degree, with no apparent penetrance in about one-fifth of males and half of females. Although the genetic basis is now clear, it has not been possible to show a quantitative link with the clinical features (Turk *et al*, 1994).

That fragile-X syndrome might be linked with autism has sparked a vigorous debate about research methodology. Although various studies found 5–46% of people with fragile-X to show autism and 0–16% of people with autism to have fragile-X, these were mostly of small groups, selected for their disturbed (autistic) behaviour and lacking control comparison. Any association might simply be the chance overlap to be expected from the study of two conditions that are overrepresented in populations with learning disabilities – in short, from ascertainment bias. However, as fragile-X might be only one of a number of causes of autism and as most people with Fragile-X will not have autism, this would swamp any association, making it imperceptible.

Alternatively, imprecise observation may have contributed to an illusory similarity. Fragile-X syndrome is characterised by social avoidance and gaze aversion (particularly marked in greeting) – but these are rooted in shyness rather than autistic indifference or a preference for peripheral vision. The speech is abnormal, with a fast, garbled quality and articulation difficulties. However, it is characterised by perseveration rather than echolalia, litanic pitch rather than monotony, as well as by an anxious interest in communication which hurries the person into a repetitive unintelligibility. Together with other characteristics (not specific to fragile-X syndrome) such as hyperactivity, impulsiveness, distractibility and wrist-biting, they make for a behavioural phenotype that has a superficial similarity to autism. In the end, much will depend on the clarity and tightness of the criteria used to identify autism. This comparison of the way in which symptoms present across a number of different disorders has made for better diagnostic definition.

## Prader–Willi syndrome (PWS)

The somatic phenotype was described in 1956 and includes obesity, hypogonadism, short stature, small extremities and poor muscle tone.

Subsequent studies fleshed out a picture of a pervasive and puzzling dystrophy with a characteristic facies, sleep apnoea (with daytime drowsiness) and frequent spinal deformity, with friable connective tissue, increased bleeding and softer bone increasing the risks of corrective thoracotomy. The intellectual impairment varies in degree, but usually lies in the mild to moderate range, coupled with an expressive language disorder and poor articulation. By contrast, visual perceptual skills are potentially good and may extend to hyperlexia.

An initial hypotonia leads to feeding difficulties and poor weight gain, but from about 3 years old it turns to the insatiable hunger drive that, together with a defective sense of satiety, soon leads to the obesity (and its complications) that comes to dominate the picture. In comparison with other forms of obesity, the proportion of fat (30–40%) is unusually high but is not reflected in skin-fold measurements. The fat-free mass is small relative to height, weight, surface area and age and may explain the lower metabolic rate that suggests a contributory reduction in calorific requirement.

Outbursts of violent temper result from thwarting the appetite, but non-food-related belligerence also occurs. In fact, from early childhood, against a mixed background of stubbornness and impulsiveness, explosiveness and inactivity, there is a high incidence of psychiatric disturbance, with incessant skin-picking, compulsive and anxious neuroses and occasional reports of later, self-limiting psychotic episodes.

The aetiology is clearly genetic in its lack of a paternal 15q11–13, usually the result of deletion but occasionally of maternal disomy. The latter is associated with higher verbal ability and fewer behavioural problems, indicating a syndromal subtype. There is also a remarkably high frequency of problems in pregnancy that leads us to question how often there is a genetic basis for the perinatal problems often blamed for the impairment in other forms of learning disability.

Therapies abound, with behavioural control a central component. Drug treatments have had mixed results, the ubiquitous selective serotonin reuptake inhibitors (SSRIs) producing as much adversity as improvement. There are isolated reports of success with risperidone and stimulants that improve both obesity and mood. Trials of potential satiety factors, whether pancreatic polypeptide, cholecystokinin or sucrose, have proved ineffectual, as has treating the opioid system with naltrexone.

## Sex aneuploidy

Klinefelter's syndrome (XXY) and its variants occur in 1/2000 male neonates. Additional X chromosomes result in a degree of impairment that is variable, debatable and perhaps limited to a specific language deficit. Also reported are increased passivity, apprehensiveness, shyness, impulsiveness and, unsurprisingly, poor relationships with others. There is hypogonadism and infertility, with reduced levels of testosterone and increased gonadotrophins. Many symptoms are said to respond to supplementary testosterone.

Additional Y chromosomes occur in 1/1000 male neonates. People with XYY syndrome, although more assertive and restlessly impulsive, probably have more in common with, than differing from, those with XXY. Both syndromes make for a tall individual, possibly with a degree of cognitive deficit and some immaturity of personality. Consequently, it might be expected that there should be a raised prevalence if screening is limited to tall men and/or to the inhabitants of institutions, including prisons.

The female equivalent, Turner's syndrome (XO), occurs in about 1/2500 female neonates after a high rate of spontaneous abortion. There are widespread somatic stigmata and growth retardation. Although overall intelligence is unimpaired, there is a specific cognitive phenotype, comprising a strong verbal ability with visuomotor and spatial difficulties. Social impairment, on occasion amounting to frank autism, is specific to those whose X chromosome is maternally derived (Skuse *et al*, 1997).

## Tuberous sclerosis (epiloia)

This well-recognised syndrome, which peppers the body with hamartomata, is associated with hyperkinetic and autistic features. Infantile spasms tend to identify those children who will be left with the more severe learning disabilities and the most intractable epilepsy. Difficult behaviour is frequent, with sleep problems, hyperactivity, aggression and self-injury, and a non-compliant obsessiveness. All of this, as well as a strong association with autism, may be specific to tuberous sclerosis. However, it might represent a common link with the combination of severe learning disability and severe epilepsy. The site of the intracranial hamartomata is probably relevant, the temporal lobes and cerebellum being cited, but family studies hint at the possibility of a more direct genetic predisposition. Disentangling these issues and, in particular, the nature of secondary autism, requires further studies that control for these interlaced variables and include the characteristics of immediate relatives.

## Cornelia de Lange syndrome

This sporadic syndrome probably has a genetic basis, with a variable and age-dependent expression. It comprises a moderate to severe learning disability, growth retardation, limb abnormalities and a distinctive facies with a small, turned-up nose, a down-turned mouth and eyebrows that meet in the middle (synophrys). The personality is likely to be coloured by the many physical problems, but particularly by the discomfort and danger of gastro-oesophageal reflux (gastrointestinal malformation and malfunction being frequent).

De Lange syndrome was one of the earliest disorders to be ascribed a behavioural phenotype. This included self-injurious and autistic behaviour, as well as other characteristics associated with severe learning disability. It has been impossible to sort out the significance of their co-occurrence, but earlier and more effective treatment, together with studies of the more able members, are needed to reveal the true phenotype.

## Williams syndrome

The main features, including mild to moderate learning disabilities and a characteristic 'elfin' facies, are only the beginning of a progressive, multisystem syndrome. Cardiovascular complications are frequent and include hypertension, arterial stenoses and mitral valve prolapse. There is physical deformity with kyphoscoliosis and contractures. A variety of urinary and gastrointestinal problems, particularly constipation, contribute to chronic ill-health and discomfort. Calcium levels may be raised, especially in infancy, and this syndrome overlaps with the idiopathic infantile hypercalcaemia caused by hypervitaminosis D.

The cognitive and personality profile is peculiar. In contrast to other forms of learning disability, there is an extraordinary verbal facility that has been compared with the 'cocktail-party speech' of hydrocephalic children. The latter, while fluent, well-articulated and over-familiar, is made superficial and meaningless by its litter of stereotyped phrases and clichés, repetitive responses and irrelevant personal experiences. Although Williams syndrome does indeed have a hyperverbal subgroup, its speech is meaningful rather than empty chatter, with a tendency to remember and use adult phrases and vocabulary. The overall impression of ability is misleading, masking severe visuospatial and motor deficits. There is also a hypersensitivity to sound, expressed in an exaggerated startle reflex, with a resultant anticipatory anxiety, distractibility and hyperactivity. Earlier reports stressed a polite and gentle charm, but more recent work suggests a more difficult temperament that had passed unnoticed in the brief, formal interview where an over-friendly, disinhibited sociability stood in contrast to the avoidance so frequently associated with learning disability. Nevertheless, there is a unique quality of enthusiastic happiness associated with this syndrome that make for a distinctive phenotype. Alongside many of the more adverse traits, this might be the natural consequence of coping with the combination of unrecognised cognitive handicaps, physical discomfort and hyperacusis.

## Rett syndrome

Rett's original description was published in German in 1966. It is only in the past 20 years that the syndrome has gained general recognition and been distinguished from other pervasive developmental disorders. Occuring only in females, it is thought to arise as a mutation in the *MeCP2* gene at Xq28 – an abnormality that is likely to be lethal in males, as they lack the compensatory allele. Rett syndrome is still defined by its clinical presentation of slowed head growth and dementia after 6–18 months of relatively normal development. Typically there is an autistic withdrawal accompanied by seizures, hand stereotypies (notably hand-wringing), agitation and breathing irregularities (a pattern of alternate hyperventilation and breath-holding that is absent in sleep). Then follow ataxia, spasticity and dystonia, to leave a person with severe mental and physical disabilities, although, as in other conditions, this classical picture is only the focus of an ever-widening clinical phenotype. Therapeutically, some improvement has been reported with both L-carnitine and magnesium.

The difficulty with identifying a behavioural phenotype specific to Rett syndrome is that many of its features, particularly those associated with autism, might simply be a function of the severity of the learning disability; few studies include an effective control group (Mount *et al*, 2001).

## Lesch–Nyhan syndrome

This holds a particular interest as compulsive self-mutilation, the scourge of individuals with more severe disabilities, here has a specific biochemical basis. It is an X-linked syndrome that is almost exclusive to males. The classic picture is one of normal development in early infancy except perhaps for orange, uricosuric sand in the nappy. Hypotonia then heralds a progressive motor deterioration to spasticity, choreo-athetosis, dysarthria and dysphagia, with seizures occurring in about 50% of cases. The compulsive self-mutilation that follows seems to be as distressing to the child as to the observer and there is a preference for imposed restraint, making it qualitatively different from other forms of self-injury. Over time this waxes and wanes, perhaps improving in early adolescence. There is also a more generalised aggression, with tantrums directed against objects and people. In time there emerges moderate learning disability, marked growth retardation and a failure of secondary sexual development, with respiratory or renal failure bringing death in early adulthood.

The disorder is spectral, with its severity closely related to the degree of deficiency in hypoxanthine–guanine phosphoribosyl transferase (HPRT), an enzyme essential to the process of salvage in purine synthesis. Unable to recycle the enzyme, there is a greater reliance on *de novo* synthesis and the basal ganglia, which appear particularly vulnerable to this distortion, develop deviant dopaminergic terminals. Uric acid is released in excess, but the use of allopurinol to reduce its levels yields no psychological benefit. Animal models suggest the self-injury to be mediated by supersensitive $D_1$ receptors, so there is the potential for their selective blockade. Clinically, the issue is less clear-cut, with reports of a deficit in dopaminergic transmitters contrasting with an increase in serotonin metabolite. There are few studies and, although fluphenazine has been reported as dramatically successful, other accounts indicate a more mixed and idiosyncratic response to this as well as to a variety of compounds, including anti-epileptics, tetrabenazine, carbidopa–levodopa, bromocryptine, hypoxanthine and xanthine oxidase. Other measures include splinting, extraction of the primary teeth and behavioural measures, the last being even less successful than in other forms of self-injury.

## Smith–Magenis syndrome

A chromosomal deletion at 17p11.2 underlies a subtle characteristic facies, short stature and a variety of abnormalities that can affect most systems, coupled with an overlay of secondary symptomatology – for example, chronic otitis media can add a conductive element to the sensorineural hearing loss. The degree of learning disability is very varied but mostly moderate. The disorder presents at an early age with severe management problems that include attention-deficit hyperactivity disorder (ADHD), sleep disturbance, bruxism and behaviour that is stereotypical (hand- and object-mouthing, and page-flicking) and self-injurious (biting, slapping, and picking at the skin or nails). The result is a child whose inexplicable behaviour, particularly the self-injury, is particularly distressing for sleep-deprived parents. Diagnosis brings understanding and a more rational management programme, and, to that extent, is the start of a remedy.

## Phenylketonuria (PKU)

An autosomal recessive disorder underlies a variable deficit in hepatic phenylalanine hydroxylase. The resultant rise in phenylalanine levels gives a spectrum of disorder that ranges from benign hyperphenylalanin-aemia (with levels sufficiently low for it to be doubtful whether treatment is merited), through mild PKU, to classic PKU. Quite distinct is atypical PKU, which arises from a deficit in the synthesis of biopterin (a coenzyme of the hydroxylase) and is unresponsive to diet. PKU can be detected by routine screening in the second week of life, allowing the early restriction of dietary phenylalanine.

Untreated, the consequences can be severe, with microcephalic mental impairment, autism and epilepsy. Phenylalanine affects myelination, and the immature central nervous system (CNS) is most vulnerable, although susceptibility continues into adulthood. This might be the effect of a combination of direct neurotoxicity, competitive blockade of the uptake of other amino acids (notably valine, leucine and isoleucine) and, lacking tyrosine and tryptophan, a reduction in the synthesis of serotonin and dopamine.

The focus of management, a restricted and expensive diet, inevitably affects family functioning, particularly in adolescence when it is compounded by changing dietary requirements and the issue of independence. In family studies there is little that distinguishes them from the general population except for a suggestion that they are less cohesive and more inflexible and routine. There is a considerable variation within this population but one potentially useful categorisation might be into 'child-centred' and 'PKU/diet-centred' families. Although it has yet to be substantiated, there is hope that a dietary supplement of deficient and competing amino acids (blocking phenylalanine uptake) might provide a more acceptable and palatable regimen.

Even with the effective control of phenylalanine levels, there can be a degree of irritability, anxiety and social isolation, with a reduction in concentration and cognitive ability, particularly in visuomotor and spatial abilities. This may represent either pre-diet damage or the failure to hold to a very narrow therapeutic window – too low a level of phenylalanine also carries a cognitive penalty. Frequently the diet is discontinued, usually in adolescence, occasionally to be followed by a delayed global deterioration. This ranges from the subtle to the gross and includes upper motor neuron abnormality, which is reflected centrally by delayed visual evoked potentials, slowing of the electroencephalogram (EEG) spectrum and abnormality on magnetic resonance imaging (MRI) scan. In addition, there are sufficient reports of a general improvement in previously untreated adults to warrant a trial of treatment even where severe learning disabilities and abnormal behaviours appear entrenched. These go to suggest that only life-long control is safe.

Maternal hyperphenylalaninaemia causes cardiac defects and microcephaly, often with learning disabilities in the non-PKU foetus. This means that dietary control must be in place before conception; a painful confrontation for many who thought that they had outgrown, or were even unaware of, their disorder and its restrictions.

## Foetal alcohol syndrome

In addition to the characteristic facies, growth deficiency and multiple systemic impairments that characterise this syndrome, there is a mild learning disability with speech and language problems, particularly in expressive language, although this is often camouflaged by a prolific verbal output. Starting with an infantile withdrawal syndrome that ranges from hypertonic jitteriness to frank seizures, the later picture is one of irritability and hyperactivity.

This syndrome has been proposed as one of the more common identifiable causes of learning disability in the Western world and, as such, to pose a huge challenge in public health. However, it is questionable as to whether it is as prevalent as suggested: many of the effects ascribed to it might have as much to do with the associated disease, social deprivation and cigarette smoking. The diagnosis is often missed, as the expression is neither consistent nor specific to prenatal alcohol. Damage probably depends on a combination of the amount, duration and timing of alcohol intake relative to the pregnancy, binge drinking being especially suspect.

## Congenital hypothyroidism (cretinism)

In the developed world this is usually the consequence of an innate deficit in the foetus which, if discovered by neonatal screening, is effectively remedied by early and energetic treatment with thyroxin. Elsewhere, foetal iodine deficiency disorder reigns as a common but often unrecognised cause of intellectual impairment. The clinical picture ranges from visuomotor deficits, through a more pronounced (albeit euthyroid) neurological disorder, to the widespread intellectual impairment of myxoedematous hypothyroidism. The outcome depends on the timing and degree of maternal iodine deficit, genetic predisposition and, in the myxoedematous form, an underlying autoimmunity. Furthermore, geographical differences indicate rather more than a simple elemental deficiency as the iodine uptake is affected by other goitrogens specific to the geological site.

# Psychiatric issues

Many clinical problems do not coincide with the aetiological diagnosis, but run as themes through these phenotypes. Notable are sleep and feeding problems, attentional, depressive and obsessional disorders, and self-injury, as well as recurrent idiosyncrasies.

## Autism

This protean diagnosis often leads to confusion. The term 'autism' is often used indiscriminately for the primary (genetic) disorder as well as for the behavioural syndrome (of which 10–20% of cases are secondary to other disorders). Although autism can arise in any condition that causes cerebral dysfunction, some disorders (e.g. untreated PKU, tuberous sclerosis and fragile-X syndrome) are more closely associated with it than are others (e.g. Down's and Williams syndromes). There is no laboratory test to determine the presence of autism and so it remains uncertain whether there is more than a superficial similarity between the primary and secondary syndromes.

Sotos syndrome of cerebral gigantism exemplifies this confusion. Although there is a wide range and variety of cognitive impairment, common threads can be found in the frequent aggressive outbursts and deficits in socialisation, which may extend to autism. However, the entity of Sotos syndrome itself is under attack as further studies reveal that it too might have a varied aetiology, including fragile-X.

## Self-injurious behaviour

This can be more frequent, or simply more pronounced, in syndromes such as Prader–Willi and de Lange. It remains to be determined how frequent and how specific is self-mutilation, as well as the extent to which it is linked to an altered awareness of pain or to autism. Also unclear is the relationship between self-injury, self-stimulation, stereotypies and compulsion.

## Other psychiatric disorder

We are beginning to discern links with psychiatric disorder, both within the individual and in the family. Examples are the associations between fragile-X syndrome and depression, between autism and bipolar disorder and between Down's syndrome and dementia. Affective disorder and obsessive behaviour are recurrent familial themes, which might indicate common faults in neurotransmitter systems.

## Physical illness

Most syndromes are associated with chronic and distressing physical disorders such as gastrointestinal disturbance. Although often un-noticed by the literature, these may well contribute to disturbance and even be the major factor in syndromes such as de Lange and Williams. Active epilepsy most likely contributes to many phenotypes.

# Conclusions

Diagnosis of a syndrome carries the risk that those affected will be expected to conform to their stereotype, living up to their label. Against this must be balanced the help that it can bring.

A genetically defined disorder is merely the starting point of a pattern of development in which the person defines his or her environment and, in turn, is altered by it. The result is an evolving, interactive system that encourages great variability within the groups, allows effective intervention and takes the study of behavioural phenotypes far from the genetic determinism that its critics claim.

With diagnosis comes genetic counselling and a more focused approach, with better definition of the individual's disabilities and targeted treatment, whether medical, surgical or educational. Prognosis and acceptance of the disability are subsequently put on a firmer footing.

A diagnosis also gives eligibility for support or contact groups (for the individual, the parent and the siblings), which can bring a number of advantages and, in particular, alleviate the sense of isolation. They put the features of the disorder onto a more concrete footing: you can see how others have turned out and the range of possible variation. Furthermore, there is the opportunity to discover which remedies have worked or failed for others.

The recognition of behavioural traits specific to a syndrome is particularly valuable where the parent or the individual has felt responsible for what is, in reality, a bruising mismatch of temperaments. It encourages aspects of disturbed behaviour to be seen as innate rather than wilful.

The national networks and their documentation can be of great help to the psychiatrist, both when faced with an unusual syndrome (of which he or she might see only a few cases) and as a source of fresh ideas for the more prevalent disorders such as Down's syndrome or autism.

Finally, a syndromal diagnosis encourages a collaborative approach to problems in both parents and professionals, driving forward the development of better services and further research. The conferences of groups such as the de Lange Foundation are highly sophisticated events that are parent-led and enlist international scientific expertise and enthusiasm.

This is a burgeoning field, reflected in the rapid growth of the Society for the Study of Behavioural Phenotypes, established in 1990. There is the risk of following Sheldon's path and, with the eye of enthusiasm, imposing a behavioural phenotype where only a somato-typical link exists. This is particularly problematic where a recurrent disability or discomfort gives a spurious uniformity to behaviour, for example where social isolation follows deafness or irritability follows gastrointestinal pain. Would these secondary phenomena constitute a behavioural phenotype or should we accept only traits that have a direct genetic link? Should the term be restricted to those disorders associated with a substantial learning disability (as distinct from the omnipresent specific learning disabilities), thereby excluding disorders such as Turner and Kleinfelter syndromes?

# References

Ganiban, J., Wagner, S. & Cicchetti, D. (1990) Temperament and Down's syndrome. In *Children with Down's Syndrome: A Developmental Perspective* (eds D. Cicchetti & M. Beeghly), pp. 63–100. Cambridge: Cambridge University Press.

Goldsmith, H. H., Buss, A. H., Plomin, R., *et al* (1987) What is temperament? Four approaches. *Child Development*, **58**, 505–529.

Hodapp, R. M. & Dykens, E. M. (2001) Strengthening behavioral research on genetic mental retardation syndromes. *American Journal on Mental Retardation*, **106**, 4–15.

Jones, K. L. (1996) *Smith's Recognizable Patterns of Human Malformation* (5th edn). Philadelphia, PA: W. B. Saunders.

Katz, S. & Kravetz, K. (1989) Facial plastic surgery for persons with Down's syndrome: research findings and their professional and social implications. *American Journal of Mental Retardation*, **94**, 101–110.

Mount, R. H., Hastings, R. P., Reilly, S., *et al* (2001) Behavioural and emotional features in Rett syndrome. *Disability and Rehabilitation*, **23**, 129–138.

O'Brien, G. (ed) (2001) *Behavioural Phenotypes in Clinical Practice*. London: MacKeith Press.

—— & Yule, W. (eds) (1995) *Behavioural Phenotypes*. Cambridge: McKeith/Cambridge University Press.

Osborne, L. & Pobert, B. (2001) Genetics of childhood disorders: XXVII. Genes and cognition in Williams syndrome. *Journal of the American Academy of Child and Adolescent Psychiatry*, **40**, 732–735.

Rojahn, J. (1986) Self-injurious and stereotypic behavior of noninstitutionalized mentally retarded people: prevalence and classification. *American Journal of Mental Deficiency*, **91**, 268–276.

Skuse, D. H., James, R. S., Bishop, D. V. M., *et al* (1997) Evidence from Turner's syndrome of an imprinted X-linked locus affecting cognitive function. *Nature*, **387**, 705–708.

Turk, J., Hagerman, R. J., Barnicoat, A., *et al* (1994) The Fragile-X syndrome. In *Mental Health in Mental Retardation: Recent Advances and Practices* (ed N. Bouras), pp. 135–153. Cambridge: Cambridge University Press.

# CHAPTER 5

# Children with learning disabilities and psychiatric problems

Bruce Tonge

The serious handicap of learning disability in children is frequently further complicated by the psychopathology of emotional and behavioural problems. Serious psychopathology affects more than 40% of children and adolescents with learning disabilities, which is a prevalence 2–3 times higher than that in typical children (Rutter, 1989; Einfeld & Tonge, 1996a,b). This psychopathology is identified by parents as the greatest source of stress, even more demanding than the care required by a physically dependent child (Quine & Pahl, 1985). Contributing to this stress are an increased risk of physical injury to the child or other family members; limitations to family activities; household damage; increased likelihood of parental mental health problems, embarrassment and shame; and family and sibling dysfunction and adjustment problems (Shearn & Todd, 1996; Sherrard, 1999). Psychopathology is also a source of significant extra cost to the community, being the single most important cause of residential placement and placement failure (Bruininks *et al*, 1988). Psychopathology also adds considerably to the cost of education and greatly limits or even precludes participation in recreational and educational programmes (Parmenter *et al*, 1998). Unfortunately, these psychiatric disorders in children with learning disabilities are often erroneously regarded as simply a manifestation of the learning disability, rather than an additional and separate problem that might be responsive to treatment (Einfeld & Tonge, 1996a,b). Thus, comorbid psychiatric disorder is a great source of distress to the child and an added burden to the family and community, but one that is amenable to assessment and treatment.

## Approaches to diagnosis

The standard approaches to classification of psychiatric disorders such as the DSM–IV (American Psychiatric Association, 1994) and ICD–10 (World Health Organization, 1992) can be used to define and classify many of the disturbed emotions or behaviours manifest in young people with learning disabilities. These classification systems have not yet been validated for use in this group, and a number of the diagnostic categories, such as obsessive–compulsive disorder, post-traumatic stress disorder and schizophrenia, are difficult to apply when the child lacks adequate verbal communication skills (Einfeld & Aman, 1995; Einfeld & Tonge, 1999). Other conditions such as attention-deficit hyperactivity disorder (ADHD) require that the child's developmental age is taken into account, or the diagnosis is precluded in the presence of a developmental disorder such as autism. Therefore, delays and distortions in cognitive and emotional development and the inability of some children with learning disabilities to inform us of their emotions, thoughts and perceptions means that a greater reliance is placed upon the behavioural criteria of some psychiatric disorders. For example, separation anxiety might be inferred when a child clings to a parent, or suicidal ideas might be implied by some acts of self-harm. It is also recognised that some symptoms that have not yet been formally classified occur more commonly or even exclusively in young people with learning disabilities. An example is the DSM–IV diagnosis of stereotypic movement disorder, with or without self-injurious behaviour. Emotional and behavioural disturbance can also be described in a standardised dimensional manner, using questionnaires usually completed by informants such as parents or teachers. Factor analysis of these questionnaires produces groupings of symptoms that are useful clinically and may be regarded as psychopathological syndromes (Tonge *et al*, 1996). An analysis of six existing rating scales identified that aggression/anti-social behaviour, social withdrawal, stereotypic behaviours, hyperactive disruptive behaviours, repetitive communication disturbance, and anxiety and mood disturbance were relatively consistent groups of symptoms. The Developmental Behaviour Checklist (Einfeld & Tonge, 1992) and the Nisonger Child Behaviour Rating Form (Aman *et al*, 1996) are two carer-completed rating scales, designed specifically for use with young people with learning disabilities, which provide a total score that measures overall psychopathology and factor or syndrome group scores. These questionnaires can be used to screen populations and aid in the application of limited child mental health service resources, and are also of use to the clinician in the diagnosis and assessment of response to treatment of psychopathology in young people with learning disabilities.

## Aetiology of psychopathology

Emotional and behavioural problems in children with learning disabilities are usually the result of a complex interaction of factors. Biological disorders that affect brain function, for example tuberous sclerosis, some genetic disorders with specific behavioural manifestations such as Williams syndrome (Einfeld *et al*, 1997), fragile-X syndrome (Einfeld *et al*, 1994) and Prader–Willi syndrome (Einfeld *et al*, 1999), and heritable temperamental characteristics contribute to psychopathology. Family and social adversity and disadvantage also have an influence. Maternal mental illness, family dysfunction and abusive, inconsistent or neglectful parental treatment have been shown to be associated with behavioural disorder, at least in children with mild learning disabilities, although the independence of these factors from low socio-economic status is still to be determined (Sameroff *et al*, 1987). Young people with learning disabilities are more likely than typical children to have experienced adverse life events such as being placed in care, being bullied, assaulted or abused (Greenbaum & Auerbach, 1998). Furthermore, they are generally more vulnerable to psychosocial adversity than are typical children because of reduced coping skills, learned helplessness and poor self-esteem (Greenbaum & Auerbach, 1998). The normal transitional stages of life, such as the onset of puberty and the move from primary to secondary school, are chronological events for which the young person with learning disability may not be psychologically or cognitively ready.

The level of cognitive ability and profile of skills may contribute to the development and form of psychopathology. For example, children who do not have sufficient language or non-verbal communication skills to indicate their needs or understand their environment may become frustrated and distressed, initiating a cascade of interactional difficulties with their carers. Symptoms of distress are more likely to be similar to those seen more typically in younger children, such as irritable behaviour in a child with depression, or rocking and aggression in an anxious young person (Reiss, 1994). Children with learning disabilities are more likely to have a scatter of cognitive skills. For example, a hyperactive and disruptive child with mild learning disability might have significant impairment in short-term auditory memory. Children with autism usually have relatively better visual, motor and performance skills, but greater difficulty with language and social comprehension tasks (Tonge *et al*, 1994). An understanding of the child's specific cognitive strengths and weaknesses has implications for education and management. For example, the disruptive behaviour of a child with autism may settle when communication is attempted using visual cues such as pictures.

Children with learning disabilities have an increased risk of suffering medical illness due to the association between its specific causes and congenital abnormalities, but also unfortunately due to poor care, neglect and an increased risk of injury (Sherrard, 1999). For example, children with Down's syndrome have an increased risk of cardiac and bowel problems; mitral valve prolapse and aortic stenosis are associated with Williams syndrome (Einfeld *et al*, 1997); and children with autism have a 20% risk of developing epilepsy (Tonge *et al*, 1994). Epilepsy is the most common neurological problem associated with learning disability, but recent studies suggest that children with both learning disabilities and epilepsy are no more likely to experience psychopathology than are children with learning disabilities alone, except perhaps where there is poor seizure control (Coulter, 1993; Lewis *et al*, 2000). Tuberous sclerosis with neuro-cutaneous lesions in the central nervous system is associated with a number of psychiatric problems, including autism, tic disorder and psychosis (Roach, 1988).

Disturbed behaviour in children may also be due to the side-effects of medication. Some drugs used in the treatment of medical conditions may produce dramatic behavioural side-effects. For example, steroids and bronchodilators used in the treatment of asthma may cause mood disturbance and agitation, and anticonvulsants may cause drowsiness and impair learning (Alvarez *et al*, 1998). Overprescribing and a high use of psychoactive drugs occurs in older adolescents and young adults with learning disability (Rinck, 1998). Children with learning disabilities also receive a wide range of psychoactive drugs, for which empirical evidence of effectiveness is often lacking (Rinck, 1998). Psychotropic drugs have the capacity to produce a range of neurological, cognitive, behavioural and emotional side-effects and may also mask a normal emotional response to an adverse life experience such as physical abuse. Children may be unpredictably sensitive to psychotropic medication or may experience paradoxical effects such as stimulation from benzodiazepines. Drug side-effects may masquerade as symptoms of a psychiatric disorder. For example, drowsiness and akathisia are side-effects of neuroleptic medication such as haloperidol. Anxiety, mood disturbance or even psychosis are side-effects of stimulant medications such as dexamphetamine. In the assessment of some children with learning disabilities and complex psychopathology, it may be necessary to systematically observe the child off all but life-saving medication, in order to determine if medication is playing either a positive or an adverse role, or having no effect.

## The treatment of childhood psychiatric disorders

A comprehensive clinical assessment is the necessary foundation of planning a rational management programme. The psychiatric assessment needs to consider the various biological, health, medication, psychological and cognitive, family, environmental and cultural issues referred to earlier that might contribute to the disorder and be responsive to treatment. Information usually needs to be gathered from a variety of sources such as parents and teachers. Observation of the child in different settings, such as at home or at school, may complement the assessment, for example to determine whether the child is aloof from the peer group. The clinical assessment should comprise an interview with the parents or carers, preferably together with the child. If the child can manage the separation, it is essential to see the child individually to undertake a mental state examination using discussion, play, drawing (e.g. draw a person, draw a dream) and structured activities (e.g. formal cognitive assessments, motor skills assessment). A medical and neurological examination and other laboratory and imaging investigations should be conducted when indicated. A comprehensive assessment may require the contribution of a multi-disciplinary team, comprising for example a paediatrician (assessment of health and known causes of learning disability), a psychologist (cognitive assessment), a speech pathologist (language assessment), an occupational therapist (motor and sensory assessment) and a child psychiatrist (for psychiatric assessment, diagnosis and case coordination). The information gathered from the assessment is best summarised in a diagnostic formulation, using the multiaxial approach of either DSM–IV (American Psychiatric Association, 1994) or the modified ICD–10 guide for mental retardation (World Health Organization, 1996). This guide comprises five axes: Axis I, severity of retardation and problem behaviours; Axis II, associated medical conditions; Axis III, associated psychiatric disorders; Axis IV, global assessment of psychosocial disability; and Axis V, associated abnormal psychosocial situations (Einfeld & Tonge, 1999). Structured interview protocols are useful, particularly in the assessment of some specific conditions or for research purposes. Examples include the Anxiety Disorders Interview Schedule (Silverman & Nelles, 1988) and the Autism Diagnostic Instrument (Lord et al, 1994) and companion Autism Diagnostic Observational Schedule (Lord et al, 1989). Following the assessment, a case conference, preferably including the parents, is a helpful step in initiating management and defining roles and responsibilities, particularly in relation to case management, review processes and crisis care.

The management of a disturbed child with learning disability usually begins with involvement of the parents or carers. Caring for a child with learning disability is likely to be difficult and stressful. Parenting and behavioural management skills, and training and education of the parents about learning disability are associated with improved child behaviour, reduced parental stress and an improved sense of parental competence and well-being (Pisterman et al, 1992; Marcus et al, 1997). Parents of children with learning disabilities are themselves at risk of mental health problems, particularly depression. Therefore, the child's behaviour may improve when the parents receive treatment for their own mental health problems (Harris, 1994). Parental and family dysfunction may also be helped with family therapy focusing on communication skills, conflict resolution and parenting skills, although further empirical outcome studies of family therapy are required (Sloman & Konstantereas, 1990; Marcus *et al*, 1997). Parents should also be involved as partners with therapists and teachers in the delivery of speech therapy, physiotherapy and special education programmes.

Interventions based on behaviour modification and operant conditioning techniques are effective in managing a range of difficult and disruptive behaviours. One approach focuses on teaching parents to apply consistent consequences for adaptive and maladaptive behaviours, for example rewarding the child for compliance or using time out and systematically ignoring the child when there is misbehaviour (Sanders & Plant, 1989). Another approach is based on detailed analysis of the antecedents and consequences of disruptive behaviour that may occur to gain attention, obtain a desired object, escape from a demand or stress, or produce a desirable sensory stimulation (Wacker *et al*, 1998). This treatment is based on understanding the function of the behaviour and then providing the child with a better way to achieve his or her purpose. Most studies of the effectiveness of this approach are single case studies (Sigafoos & Meikle, 1996). However, one study of 22 children has produced empirical evidence of effectiveness over a 12-month follow-up period (Wacker *et al*, 1998). The use of augmentive communication techniques such as signing or visual symbols and pictures can also reduce disturbed behaviour resulting from the frustration of communication difficulties (Reiss, 1994; Marcus *et al*, 1997).

Cognitive–behavioural therapy is the empirically supported treatment of first choice for depression and anxiety disorders in childhood (Harrington *et al*, 1998). However, its effectiveness in treating children with learning disabilities, who have internalising disorders such as anxiety and depression, has not yet been established. Modified forms of cognitive–behavioural therapy that take into account the level of language ability and teach relaxation techniques by demonstration and imitation may reduce anxiety and depression, at least in adults with learning disabilities (Lindsay *et al*, 1993). There are also some case reports of the successful use of cognitive–behavioural therapy, including modelling, behavioural relaxation, exposure, desensitisation and the use of positive self statements, in the treatment of anxiety disorders in young people with learning disabilities (Matson, 1981; Luscre & Center, 1996). The use of psychological treatments in children with learning disabilities must be modified to take into account the developmental level and language ability of the child, if they are to have any chance of success.

Empirical evidence for the use of psychotropic drugs to treat emotional and behavioural disorders in children is limited, particularly for children with learning disabilities. The rationale for much pharmacotherapy in childhood is based on studies of drug efficacy in adults, even though pharmacokinetics and drug metabolism may be different in children. A recent international consensus review of psychopharmacotherapy and developmental disabilities indicates that most of the empirical evidence is derived from studies of adults with learning disabilities (Reiss & Aman, 1998). There is, however, empirical evidence for the effectiveness of a number of drugs in the treatment of some specific child psychiatric disorders and therefore it is reasonable to prescribe these medications for children with learning disabilities as a component of a comprehensive management plan (Werry & Aman, 1999). For example, stimulant medication such as dexamphetamine, clonidine, imipramine, buspirone and neuroleptic drugs have empirical support for the treatment of ADHD. Clomipramine and selective serotonin reuptake inhibitors (SSRIs) are effective in the treatment of obsessive–compulsive disorder. Imipramine and perhaps buspirone may be effective in the treatment of childhood anxiety disorders such as separation anxiety. Benzodiazepines are not an effective treatment for childhood anxiety and are likely to produce paradoxical responses, particularly in anxious children who also have disruptive and hyperactive behaviour. The SSRIs are effective in the treatment of depression in young people, but not to the same extent as in adults, and the tricyclic antidepressants are no better than a placebo. Neuroleptics, specifically haloperidol, pimozide or clonidine, are indicated for the treatment of tic disorders.

There is also evidence that drugs are effective in the treatment of disruptive and difficult behaviours that occur more specifically in children with learning disabilities. Neuroleptic drugs such as chlorpromazine, haloperidol and probably the newer neuroleptics such as risperidone act to reduce aggression, impulsiveness, hyperactivity and stereotypic behaviour. Doses should be kept as low as possible and side-effects monitored, given their proclivity to produce drowsiness and extrapyramidal and dystonic side-effects (Werry & Aman, 1999). There is some evidence, mostly from open trials, to support the use of anticonvulsants such as sodium vaproate and carbamazepine, or lithium in the treatment of self-injurious, aggressive, agitated behaviour, particularly of an episodic nature, or when there is a family history of bipolar or cycling mood disorder (Reiss & Aman, 1998). Self-injurious behaviour may be reduced by the opiate antagonists naloxone and naltrexone (Werry & Aman, 1999); beta-blockers and buspirone may also be of some use in managing disruptive and self-injurious behaviour (Reiss & Aman, 1998).

Psychotropic drugs should be used only as part of a more comprehensive management plan involving the school and parents. Regular follow-up is necessary to encourage compliance and to review side-effects and therapeutic response facilitated by the use of parent- and teacher-completed checklists.

# Specific psychiatric disorders in children with learning disabilities

The range of psychopathological symptoms seen in children with learning disabilities cannot be fully encapsulated by the existing ICD–10 and DSM–IV classification systems, particularly when applied to the symptoms of children with more-severe disabilities. However, the emotional and behavioural disturbance of many children with learning disabilities can be adequately classified using ICD–10 or DSM–IV criteria, although some modification or qualification of these criteria might be necessary. Most childhood psychopathological disorders can be subdivided into the two broad groups of internalising and externalising disorders.

## Internalising disorders

### Mood disorders

Depression is more common among children with learning disabilities than among typical children (Schloss *et al*, 1988), but is often under-reported and unrecognised (Jacobson, 1990). Children with learning disabilities who become depressed are more likely to manifest a range of disturbed behaviours, which may be easily misunderstood as being due to other problems such as disobedience. Irritability is a common manifestation of depression in children with learning disabilities (Reiss & Rojahn, 1993), and is recognised in DSM–IV as an equivalent symptom to depressed mood in children with no such disability. The majority of the diagnostic criteria for major depression or dysthymia such as loss of interest and energy, reduced level of activity and disturbed sleep and appetite are manifest as behaviours that can be observed in children without language skills. An increase in self-absorption and regressive behaviours such as pica and rocking may also be behavioural markers of depression (Davis *et al*, 1997). Feelings of worthlessness and recurrent thoughts of death and suicide may be more difficult to assess. However, adolescents with moderate to severe levels of learning disability who possess only limited language skills are capable of making simple negative self-statements such as 'stupid', or 'no good', and may develop self-injurious or dangerous behaviours in depression (Benavidez & Matson, 1993). Some children with learning disabilities have an added biological risk of depression, perhaps through the expression of a behavioural phenotype. Although young people with Down's syndrome have lower rates of psychopathology than other young people with learning disabilities (Collacott *et al*, 1992), they still have higher levels of disruptive behavioural problems than typical children. Depression emerges as an increasing problem in adolescents with Down's syndrome, but may go unrecognised when it is manifest

**105**

as an increase in oppositional and irritable behaviour. Children with autism, particularly those with milder levels of learning disability, are much more likely than typical children and other children with learning disabilities to experience depression, particularly together with other comorbid conditions such as anxiety or ADHD (Bryson & Smith, 1998). The risk of developing a depressive illness increases for young people with autism during adolescence, which is an intriguing finding given the increased association between autism and a family history of affective disorder (Gillberg & Coleman, 1992).

Little is known about the dimensions and nature of the problem of elevated mood and hypomania in children with learning disabilities. Episodic or cycling fluctuations in the disturbed behaviour of children with learning disabilities can occur, and may respond to the use of mood stabilisers such as sodium valproate and lithium (Poindexter *et al*, 1998). Bipolar and unipolar mood disorder is well documented in adolescents with learning disability (McCracken & Diamond, 1988). A daily parent- or carer-completed checklist of mood and activity level helps to confirm the presence of a cycling disorder.

## Anxiety disorders

At least 10% of both boys and girls with learning disability suffer clinically significant symptoms of anxiety (Tonge *et al*, 1996). This is in great contrast to a prevalence of 2–5% in typical children, with twice as many girls as boys affected (Tonge, 1988). Symptoms of anxiety emerge early in life in children with learning disabilities and tend to persist into adolescence (Tonge & Einfeld, 2000). Separation anxiety associated with school refusal and social anxiety are common features of anxiety disorder in children with learning disabilities. Anxiety causes great distress to the child and interferes with concentration, learning and the development of adaptive functioning skills necessary for successful integration into school and the community (Gullone *et al*, 1995). Separation anxiety is more likely to persist in older children with learning disabilities than in typical children and is usually further complicated by school, the provision of speech and occupational therapy and physiotherapy, fears related to the teacher, class performance and other children (Tonge, 1988). The incidence of fears and phobias is at least 2–3 times more common in young people with learning disability than typical children. Fears of things such as the dark, loud noises, insects and animals are more likely to be characteristic of typical younger children (King *et al*, 1994: Gullone *et al*, 1996). There are a number of potential explanations for the high rate of anxiety disorders and phobias and the equal gender distribution in young people with learning disabilities (Ollendick *et al*, 1993). Cognitive and verbal skills, environmental deprivation, traumatic experiences and neglect or parental overprotectiveness may all act to increase the vulnerability of a child with a learning disability to become over-anxious, particularly in stressful situations (Ollendick *et al*, 1993). Separation from parents, school entry, educational demands, and social and peer rejection are all likely to be anxiety-provoking, leading to avoidance, lowered self-esteem and expectations of failure. Anxiety in children with learning disabilities might also be a reaction to the stress of parental mental health problems and family conflict and dysfunction (Larcharite *et al*, 1995). Inherited temperamental characteristics and genetically deter-mined biological vulnerability may also predispose to anxiety as a manifestation of a behavioural phenotype in children with learning disabilities. Children with fragile-X syndrome have social anxiety and shyness (Einfeld *et al*, 1994). Anxiety and fearfulness are a specific feature of Williams syndrome, often associated with hyperactivity, that becomes increasingly more problematic in adolescence (Udwin & Yule, 1991; Einfeld *et al*, 1997). Adolescents with Prader–Willi syndrome experience increasing anxiety and low self-esteem, often associated with their obsessive–compulsive preoccupations with, for example, food and cleanliness (Dykens & Cassidy, 1995). Young people with autistic disorder frequently suffer from anxiety, often in association with attention-deficit hyperactivity symptoms and stereotypic or ritual-istic behaviour and preoccupations (Smalley *et al*, 1995).

The ability to cope with stressful experiences tends to decrease with the level of intellectual ability. Therefore, at least in adults, post-traumatic stress disorder tends to be more prevalent with lower IQ levels (McNally, 1993). This may be due to a reduced cognitive capacity to understand and resolve the traumatic experience. It is likely that young people with learning disabilities are more prone to post-traumatic stress disorder, given their higher risk of experiencing adverse life events such as abuse and institutionalisation (Greenbaum & Auerbach, 1998). Anxious repetitive play, perseverative talk, behavioural regres-sion, and sleep and emotional disturbance might be symptoms of a post-traumatic stress reaction in some children with learning disabil-ities, but this diagnosis has not been systematically studied in such children and is probably underrecognised.

The diagnosis of obsessive–compulsive disorder in young people with learning disability is a clinical challenge. The disorder is defined by the presence of intrusive thoughts and repetitive behaviours, performed to reduce the anxiety associated with obsessional thoughts. Although DSM–IV criteria do not require the presence of insight in children with obsessive–compulsive disorder, it is difficult, if not impossible, in some young people with learning disabilities and limited language ability to determine if they do experience intrusive thoughts and anxiety (Szymanski *et al*, 1998). Some consider that ritualistic and self-injurious behaviour might be a manifestation of obsessive–compul-sive disorder (King, 1993). However, stereotypic and self-injurious behaviours are often performed for self-stimulation or to gain attention rather than to reduce anxiety, and they do not usually respond to standard psychological and pharmacological treatments for anxiety (Reiss, 1994). In cases where a diagnosis of obsessive–compulsive disorder seems likely, a therapeutic response to pharmacotherapy (clomipramine or an SSRI) might be regarded as confirming the diagnosis. However, this approach is not based on any empirical evidence from controlled drug trials in young people with learning disabilities who have obsessions and compulsive or ritualistic and stereotypic behaviour.

## Externalising disorders

### Attention-deficit hyperactivity disorder

The ICD–10 and DSM–IV criteria for ADHD reflect observable behaviours and do not require language ability to make the diagnosis. The diagnosis depends upon the observed behaviour being 'inconsistent' with the developmental level of child (American Psychiatric Association, 1994). Young people with moderate or severe levels of learning disability are likely to have an attention span and activity level consistent with that of a much younger child. Therefore, great care must be taken to ensure that their attention-deficit hyperactivity behaviours are indeed greater than might be expected in a younger child before making the diagnosis of ADHD. Children with learning disabilities may exhibit attention-deficit hyperactivity symptoms as an adjustment reaction to a specific environmental stress, such as parental conflict or bullying at school. These situational reactions usually respond to psychosocial management rather than to psychotropic drugs. Therefore, it is important to ensure that the diagnosis of ADHD is made on the basis of symptoms being present in at least two settings, such as at home and at school. In young people with learning disabilities, symptoms of attention-deficit hyperactivity often occur with other comorbid problems such as anxiety, conduct disorder, and oppositional and defiant behaviour. These comorbid conditions need to be carefully taken into account when planning management, because stimulant medication may precipitate or exacerbate anxiety and emotional distress as a side-effect (Werry & Aman, 1999). Consistent with the developmental trajectory of typical children, attention-deficit hyperactivity symptoms become less prevalent in young people with learning disabilities as they move from childhood through adolescence into early adult life (Tonge & Einfeld, 2000). Problems with attention-deficit and hyperactivity symptoms are also a behavioural phenotype feature in young children with Williams syndrome (Einfeld et al, 1997) and children with Prader–Willi syndrome, who are also generally impulsive (Einfeld et al, 1999). The DSM–IV diagnosis of autistic disorder precludes a comorbid diagnosis of ADHD (American Psychiatric Association, 1994). However, there is evidence that 20–30% of children with autism have attention-deficit hyperactivity symptoms that meet diagnostic criteria for ADHD and are likely to show some therapeutic response to stimulant medication (Reiss & Freund, 1990). Attention-deficit hyperactivity symptoms become less prevalent during adolescence in young people with autistic disorder.

### Antisocial and oppositional defiant behaviour

Persistent antisocial behaviour occurs in approximately 30% of adolescent males with mild or borderline learning disabilities. This association is strongly predicted by inconsistent and aggressive parental care, particularly by fathers, family dysfunction and socio-economic difficulties (Schonfeld *et al*, 1988). The diagnosis of conduct disorder requires that we take into account whether the young person's ability to understand social rules, the concept of ownership of property and the rights of others is sufficient to enable him or her to comprehend the consequences of the behaviour. The diagnosis of conduct disorder or oppositional defiant disorder is not applicable to a non-verbal young person. Some apparently antisocial behaviour may be understood as a response to the environment or context. For example, a young person with a learning disability may copy a parent lighting a fire or mimic the swearing and aggressive behaviour of a child at school, without understanding the inappropriateness or consequences of this behaviour. For some children with learning disabilities, defiance or aggression are their only means of communicating the stress that they experience in a particular situation, such as the demand to produce schoolwork at a level beyond their capacity. For others, non-compliance might be the only means they have available to express an opinion that differs from that of a parent or carer. In this situation, the behaviour might even be viewed as adaptive (Szymanski *et al*, 1998).

### Pica rumination disorder and stereotypic movement disorder

These disorders most commonly occur in association with learning disability and often together with other self-injurious behaviours (American Psychiatric Association, 1994). They become a focus for attention when they are persistent and interfere with daily activities. The behaviours have a driven quality, and self-stimulation and the attention or response of carers might be rewarding and reinforce them. These behaviours may also be exacerbated by anxiety and depression (Szymanski *et al*, 1998).

### Tourette syndrome, tic disorders and stereotypic movement disorder

Children with tic disorders are usually able to describe an urge to make the repetitive movement or vocalisation that can be suppressed, but is ultimately irresistible. It is not always possible for children with learning disabilities to describe these urges. Therefore, it might be difficult to differentiate stereotypic movements and self-stimulating behaviour from tic disorders in these children. Tics are usually rapid, sudden, recurrent and non-rhythmic motor movements or vocalisations, whereas stereotypic movements and self-stimulatory behaviour are usually more complex and apparently intentional (Szymanski *et al*, 1998). There is a comorbid association between autistic disorder and tic disorders. Some intriguing neuropsychological research, which requires replication, suggests that these two conditions might share a common neuropsychological impairment of executive function (Baron-Cohen, 1998). The driven, non-functional motor behaviour or self-injurious behaviour of stereotypic movement disorder occurs in about 2–3% of young persons with more-severe levels of learning disability. These behaviours are more common in institutionalised children and in those with Lesch–Nyhan syndrome, autistic disorder, Cornelia de Lange syndrome and severe degrees of fragile-X syndrome (Szymanski *et al*, 1998). The behaviours may be reinforced because they are self-alerting and stimulating, or act to gain attention or achieve the avoidance of certain tasks and activities (Reiss, 1994). The pain produced by stereotypic movements may also act to maintain levels of endogenously produced opioids, but further empirical evidence to support this theory is required (King, 1993).

## Implications for child mental health service delivery

The likelihood that biological and genetic factors play a major part in determining that at least 40% of young people with learning disabilities suffer from serious psychopathology should not be a counsel of despair. On the contrary, knowledge of the developmental, progressive and accumulative nature of the gene–environment interaction should provide an impetus for the redirection of services towards early intervention with at-risk groups, such as young children with develop-mental delay. Parent skills training and education regarding the disability early in the child's life and at transitional points such as moving to secondary school, combined when necessary with the treatment of parental mental health problems, holds promise for creating a more secure and nurturing family environment. This encourages attachment and child development (Rogers, 1996; Marfo *et al*, 1998). Parents are further supported and have time to focus on their other children when respite care, home help and holiday programmes are available. The provision of speech and occupational therapy and physiotherapy enables the child with a learning disability to improve communication, coordination, sensory motor and play skills, which contribute to adaptation and self-esteem. Individualised education and socialisation programmes with the support of an aide promotes adaptation and confidence. Unfortunately, serious mental health problems in young children with learning disabilities are likely to go unrecognised, with probably only about 10% of these disturbed young people receiving a specialised mental health service (Einfeld & Tonge, 1996b). If undergraduate and post-graduate training of health, education and welfare professionals and general medical practitioners helps them to make a paradigm shift in their understanding and to recognise that young people with learning disability are also likely to have psychiatric disorders, then improvements in mental health services for this at-risk population and their families is likely to follow.

# References

Alvarez, N., Besag, F. & Iivanainen, M. (1998) Use of antiepileptic drugs in the treatment of epilepsy in people with intellectual disability. *Journal of Intellectual Disability Research*, **42**, 1–15.

Aman, M. G., Tasse, M. J., Rojahn, J., *et al* (1996) The Nisonger CBRF: a child behaviour rating form for children with developmental disabilities. *Research in Developmental Disabilities*, **17**, 41–57.

American Psychiatric Association (1994) *Diagnostic and Statistical Manual of Mental Disorder.* Washington, DC: APA.

Baron-Cohen, S. (1998) Modularity in developmental cognitive neuropsychology: evidence from autism and Gilles de la Tourette syndrome. In *Handbook of Mental Retardation and Development* (ed. J. Burack), pp. 334–348. New York: Cambridge University Press.

Benavidez, D. A. & Matson, J. L. (1993) Assessment of depression in mentally retarded adolescents. *Research in Developmental Disabilities*, **14**, 179–188.

Bruininks, R., Hill, B. K. & Morreau, L. E. (1988) Prevalence and implications of maladaptive behaviours and dual diagnosis in residential and other service programs. In *Mental Retardation and Mental Health: Classification, Diagnosis, Treatment, Services* (eds J. A. Stark, F. J. Menolascino, M. H. Albarelli, *et al*), pp. 1–29. New York: Springer-Verlag.

Bryson, S. E. & Smith, I. M. (1998) Epidemiology of autism: prevalence, associated characteristics, and implications from research and service delivery. *Mental Retardation and Developmental Disabilities Research Reviews*, **4**, 97–103.

Collacott, R. A., Cooper, S. A., & McGrother, C. (1992) Differential rates of psychiatric disorders in adults with Down's syndrome compared with other mentally handicapped adults. *British Journal of Psychiatry*, **161**, 671–674.

Coulter, D. (1993) Epilepsy and mental retardation. *American Journal on Mental Retardation*, **98** (suppl.), 1–11.

Davis, J. P., Judd, F. K. & Herrman, H. (1997) Depression in adults with intellectual disability. *Australian and New Zealand Journal of Psychiatry*, **31**, 243–251.

Dykens, E. M. & Cassidy, S. B. (1995) Correlates of maladaptive behaviour in children and adults with Prader–Willi syndrome. *American Journal of Medical Genetics (Neuropsychiatric Genetics)*, **69**, 546–549.

Einfeld, S. L. & Aman, M. (1995) Issues in the taxonomy of psychopathology in mental retardation. *Journal of Autism and Developmental Disorders*, **25**, 143–167.

Einfeld, S. L. & Tonge, B. J. (1992) *Manual for the Developmental Behaviour Checklist.* Clayton, Melbourne & Sydney: Monash University Centre for Developmental Psychiatry and School of Psychiatry, University of New South Wales.

—— & —— (1996a) Population prevalence of psychopathology in children and adolescents with intellectual disability. I: Rationale and methods. *Journal of Intellectual Disability Research*, **40**, 91–98.

—— & —— (1996b) Population prevalence of psychopathology in children and adolescents with intellectual disability. II: Epidemiological findings. *Journal of Intellectual Disability Research*, **40**, 99–109.

—— & —— (1999) Observations on the use of the ICD–10 Guide for Mental Retardation. *Journal of Intellectual Disability Research*, **43**, 408–412.

——, Tonge, B. J. & Florio, T. (1994) Behavioural and emotional disturbance in fragile-X syndrome. *American Journal of Medical Genetics*, **51**, 386–391.

——, —— & —— (1997) Behavioural and emotional disturbance in individuals with Williams Syndrome. *American Journal on Mental Retardation*, **102**, 45–53.

——, Smith, A., Durvasula, S., *et al* (1999) Behavioural and emotional disturbance in Prader–Willi Syndrome. *American Journal of Medical Genetics*, **82**, 123–127.

Gillberg, C. & Coleman, M. (1992) *The Biology of the Autistic Syndromes* (2nd edn). London: MacKeith Press.

Greenbaum, C. W. & Auerbach, J. G. (1998) The environment of the child with mental retardation: risk, vulnerability and resilience. In *Handbook of Mental Retardation and Development* (eds J. A. Burrack, R. M. Hodapp & E. Ziggler), pp. 583–605. Cambridge: Cambridge University Press.

Gullone, E., Cummins, R. A. & King, N. J. (1995) Adaptive behaviour in children and adolescents with and without an intellectual disability: relationships with fear and anxiety. *Behaviour Change*, **12**, 227–237.

—— , —— & —— (1996) Self-reported fears: a comparison study of youths with and without an intellectual disability. *Journal of Intellectual Disability Research*, **40**, 227–240.

Harrington, R., Whitaker, J., Shoebridge, P., *et al* (1998) Systematic review of efficacy of cognitive behavioural therapies in childhood and adolescent depressive disorder. *BMJ*, **316**, 1559–1563.

Harris, S. L. (1994) Treatment of family problems in autism. In *Behavioral Issues in Autism* (eds E. Schopler & G. B. Mesibov), pp. 161–175. New York : Plenum Press.

Jacobson, J. W. (1990) Do some mental disorders occur less frequently among persons with mental retardation? *American Journal on Mental Retardation*, **94**, 596–602.

King, B. H. (1993) Self-injury by people with mental retardation: A compulsive behavior hypothesis. *American Journal on Mental Retardation*, **98**, 93–112.

King, N. J., Josephs, A., Gullone, E., *et al* (1994) Assessing the fears of children with disability using the Revised Fear Survey Schedule for Children. A comparative study. *British Journal of Medical Psychology*, **67**, 377–386.

Larcharite, C., Boutet, M. & Proulx, R. (1995) Intellectual disability and psychopathology: developmental perspective. *Canada's Mental Health*, **43**, 2–8.

Lewis, J. N., Tonge, B. J., Mowat, D. R., *et al* (2000) Epilepsy and associated psychopathology in young people with intellectual disability. *Journal of Paediatrics and Child Health*, **36**, 172–175.

Lindsay, W. R., Howells, L. & Pitcaithly, D. (1993) Cognitive therapy for depression with individuals with intellectual disabilities. *British Journal of Medical Psychology*, **66**, 135–141.

Lord, C., Rutter, M. L., Goode, S., *et al* (1989) Autism Diagnostic Observation Schedule. A standardized observation of communicative and social behavior. *Journal of Autism and Developmental Disorders*, **19**, 185–212.

——, —— & Le Couteur, A. (1994) Autism Diagnostic Interview – Revised. A revised version of a diagnostic interview for caregivers of individuals with possible pervasive developmental disorders. *Journal of Autism and Developmental Disorders*, **24**, 659–685.

Luscre, D. M. & Center, D. B. (1996) Procedures for reducing dental fear in children with autism. *Journal of Autism and Developmental Disorders*, **26**, 547–556.

Marcus, L., Kunce, L. & Schopler, E. (1997) Working with families. In *Handbook of Autism and Pervasive Developmental Disorders* (eds D. J. Cohen & F. R. Volkmar), pp. 631–649. New York: John Wiley & Sons.

Marfo, K., Dedrick, C. F. & Barbour, N. (1998) Mother–child interactions and the development of children with mental retardation. In *Handbook of Mental Retardation and Development* (ed. J. Burack), pp. 637–668. New York: Cambridge University Press.

Matson, J. L. (1981) Assessment and treatment of clinical fears in mentally retarded children. *Journal of Applied Behaviour Analysis*, **14**, 287–294.

McCracken, J. T. & Diamond, R. P. (1988) Bipolar disorder in mentally retarded adolescents. *Journal of the American Academy of Child and Adolescent Psychiatry*, **27**, 494–499.

McNally, R. J. (1993) Stressors that produce post traumatic stress disorder in children. *Journal of Consulting and Clinical Psychology*, **3**, 531–537.

Ollendick, T. H., Oswald, D. P. & Ollendick, D. G. (1993) Anxiety disorders in mentally retarded persons. In *Psychopathology in the Mentally Retarded* (eds J. L. Matson & R. P. Barrett), pp. 41–85. Boston, MA: Allyn and Bacon.

Parmenter, T., Einfeld, S. & Tonge, B. (1998) Behavioural and emotional problems in the classroom of children and adolescents with intellectual disability. *Journal of Intellectual and Developmental Disability*, **23**, 71–78.

Pisterman, S., Firestone, P., McGrath, P., *et al* (1992) The effects of parent training on parenting stress and sense of competence. *Canadian Journal of Behavioural Science*, **24**, 41–58.

Poindexter, A. R., Cain, N. N., Clarke, D. J., *et al* (1998) Psychotropic medication and developmental disabilities: the international consensus handbook. In *Psychotropic Medication and Developmental Disabilities: The International Consensus Handbook* (eds S. Reiss & M. G. Aman), pp. 215–228. Columbus, OH: Ohio State University.

Quine, L. & Pahl, J. (1985) Examining the causes of stress in families with severely mentally handicapped children. *British Journal of Social Work*, **15**, 501–517.

Reiss, A. L. & Freund, L. (1990) Fragile-X chromosome, DSM–III–R, and autism. *Journal of the American Academy of Child and Adolescent Psychiatry*, **29**, 885–891.

Reiss, S. (1994) Psychopathology in mental retardation. In *Mental Health in Mental Retardation: Recent Advances and Practices* (ed. N. Bouras), pp. 67–78. Cambridge: Cambridge University Press.

—— & Aman, M. G. (1998) *Psychotropic Medication and Developmental Disabilities: The International Consensus Handbook*. Columbus, OH: Ohio State University.

—— & Rojahn, J. (1993) Joint occurrence of depression and aggression in children and adults with mental retardation. *Journal of Intellectual Disability Research*, **37**, 287–294.

Rinck, C. (1998) Epidemiology and psychoactive medication. In *Psychotropic Medication and Developmental Disabilities: The International Consensus Handbook* (eds S. Reiss & M. G. Aman), pp. 31–44. Columbus, OH: Ohio State University.

Roach, E. S. (1988) Diagnosis and management of neurocutaneous syndromes. *Seminars in Neurology*, **8**, 83–86.

Rogers, S. J. (1996) Brief report: Early intervention in autism. *Journal of Autism and Developmental Disorders*, **26**, 243–246.

Rutter, M. (1989) Isle of Wight revisited: twenty-five years of child psychiatric epidemiology. *Journal of the American Academy of Child and Adolescent Psychiatry*, **28**, 633–653.

Sameroff, A., Seifer, R., Barocas, R., *et al* (1987) IQ scores of four year old children: social environmental risk factors. *Pediatrics*, **79**, 343–350.

Sanders, M. R. & Plant, K. (1989) Programming for generalization to high and low risk parenting situations in families with oppositional developmentally disabled pre-schoolers. *Behavior Modification*, **13**, 283–305.

Schloss, P. J., Epstein, M. H. & Cullinan, D. (1988) Depression characteristics among mildly handicapped students. *Journal of the Multihandicapped Person*, **1**, 293–302.

Schonfeld, I. S., Schoffer, D., O'Connor, P., *et al* (1988) Conduct disorder and cognitive functioning: testing three causal hypotheses. *Child Development*, **59**, 993–1007.

Shearn, J. & Todd, S. (1996) Identities at risk: the relationships parents and their adult offspring with learning disabilities have with each other and their social world. *European Journal of Mental Disability*, **3**, 47–60.

Sherrard, J. (1999) *The Epidemiology of Injury in Young People with Intellectual Disability: A Behavioural Perspective*. PhD thesis. Melbourne: Monash University.

Sigafoos, J., & Meikle, B. (1996) Functional communication training for the treatment of multiply determined challenging behavior in two boys with autism. *Behavior Modification*, **20**, 60–84.

Silverman, W. K. & Nelles, W. B. (1988) The anxiety disorders interview schedule for children. *Journal of the American Academy of Child and Adolescent Psychiatry*, **27**, 772–778.

Sloman, L. & Konstantereas, M. (1990) Why families with biological deficits require a systems approach. *Family Process*, **29**, 417–429.

Smalley, S. L., McCracken, J. & Tanguay, P. (1995) Autism, affective disorders, and social phobia. *American Journal of Medical Genetics*, **60**, 19–26.

Szymanski, L., King, B., Goldberg, B., *et al* (1998) Diagnosis of mental disorders in people with mental retardation. In *Psychotropic Medication and Developmental Disabilities: The International Consensus Handbook* (eds S. Reiss & M. G. Aman), pp. 3–17. Columbus, OH: Ohio State University.

Tonge, B. J. (1988) Anxiety in adolescents. In *Handbook of Anxiety* (eds R. Noyes, M. Roth & G Burrows), pp. 269–288. Amsterdam: Elsevier.

— & Einfeld, S. L. (2000) The trajectory of psychiatric disorders in young people with intellectual disabilities. *Australian and New Zealand Journal of Psychiatry*, **34**, 80–84.

—, Dissanayake, C. & Brereton, A. V. (1994) Autism: fifty years on from Kanner. *Journal of Paediatrics and Child Health*, **30**, 102–107.

—, Einfeld, S. L., Krupinski, J., *et al* (1996) The use of factor analysis for ascertaining patterns of psychopathology in children with intellectual disability. *Journal of Intellectual Disability Research*, **40**, 198–207.

Udwin, O. & Yule, W. (1991) A cognitive and behavioural phenotype in Williams syndrome. *Journal of Clinical and Experimental Neuropsychology*, **2**, 232–244.

Wacker, D. P., Berg, W. K., Harding, J. W., *et al* (1998) Evaluation and long-term treatment of aberrant behavior displayed by young children with disabilities. *Journal of Developmental and Behavioral Pediatrics*, **19**, 260–266.

Werry, J. S. A., Aman, M. G. (eds) (1999) *A Practitioner's Guide to Psychoactive Drugs in Children and Adolescents (2nd edn)*. New York: Plenum Press.

World Health Organization (1992) *The ICD–10 Classification of Mental and Behavioural Disorders. Clinical Description and Diagnostic Guidelines*. Geneva: WHO.

— (1996) *The ICD–10 Guide for Mental Retardation*. Geneva: WHO.

# CHAPTER 6

# Autism

Craig Melville and John Cameron

There has been a recent increase in awareness of autistic-spectrum disorders, particularly among the general public, who are concerned about progressively rising rates and a possible link with the mumps, measles and rubella (MMR) vaccine. Furthermore, improved education of professionals working in health, education and social services has contributed to greater understanding. However, as will be highlighted in this chapter, current knowledge of the autistic-spectrum disorders is at an early stage. Therefore, it is important that rigorous research examines their fundamental aspects, addresses some of the ongoing controversies and ultimately helps in the development of improved services.

There is scope for considerable debate and confusion over the use of terminology when describing these disorders. Although many individuals with autism have associated learning disabilities, in recent years there has been an explosion of interest in those disorders that are usually not described as coexisting with a learning disability, for example Asperger syndrome and high-functioning autism. These are included in this chapter as there is a degree of overlap and many individuals exhibiting them will present to professionals working within learning disability services. Therefore, we use the phrase 'autistic-spectrum disorders' (Wing, 1996) as an umbrella term that includes the categories of childhood autism, Asperger syndrome, atypical autism and childhood disintegrative disorder listed in ICD–10 (World Health Organization, 1992).

## Assessment and diagnostic criteria

Over the past 20 years, the development of reliable and valid diagnostic criteria for the autistic-spectrum disorders has been a primary concern for clinicians and researchers. For complex neurodevelopmental disorders such as these, such criteria facilitate reliable clinical diagnosis and are fundamental to the identification of a homogeneous cohort for research. A brief outline of the assessment and diagnosis of autistic-spectrum disorders is provided below (see Volkmar *et al*, 1997).

## The assessment process

A study by Howlin & Moore (1997) showed that, although the majority of families had concerns about their child at a very early age, there was generally a delay of between 2 and 5 years before a definitive diagnosis was made. From this survey, the average age of diagnosis was around 6 years. The evidence accumulating for the effectiveness of intensive early intervention during the pre-school years (Smith *et al*, 2000) has raised concerns that many children are being diagnosed too late. This has highlighted the importance of effective systems and methods for screening, assessment and diagnosis, and has been specifically addressed by several consensus documents (Filipek *et al*, 2000; Sandler *et al*, 2001). Although authors differ in the importance they attach to specific physical investigations such as blood tests or neuroimaging, each of these documents endorses the view that a multi-disciplinary assessment and diagnosis is an essential first step towards provision of appropriate information, support and interventions for children with autistic-spectrum disorders and their families.

Table 6.1 gives an outline of the assessment process (for more detailed information, see Filipek *et al*, 2000).

---

**Box 6.1**  Key areas of assessment

*Clinical history*
Current functioning and problems
Developmental history
Family history
Medical history

*Speech and language assessment, with or without audiology*
Both assessments are necessary in any child with delayed development of language

*Neuropsychological assessment*
Of adaptive functioning, e.g. using Vineland's Adaptive Behaviour Scales (Sparrow *et al*, 1984)
Of IQ, e.g. using the Weschler Intelligence Scale for Children (1991)

*Physical examination and investigations*
To exclude possible medical conditions such as tuberous sclerosis or epilepsy

*Specific interviews or observations for autism*
Autism Diagnostic Interview – Revised (Lord *et al*, 1994)
Autism Diagnostic Observation Schedule – Generic (Lord *et al*, 2000)
Childhood Autism Rating Scale (Schopler *et al*, 1988)
Diagnostic Interview for Social and Communicative Disorders (Wing, 1993)

---

## Diagnostic criteria

All classification systems for autistic-spectrum disorders are based to some extent on the 'triad of social impairment' (Wing & Gould, 1979). In ICD–10, this consists of (1) qualitative abnormalities in reciprocal social interaction; (2) qualitative abnormalities in communication; and (3) a restricted, stereotyped and repetitive repertoire of interests and activities. The criteria given in DSM–IV (American Psychiatric Association, 1994), although not identical, are very similar.

## Childhood autism

Both ICD–10 and DSM–IV have adopted similar criteria for childhood autism (autistic disorder in DSM–IV). These include the triad of social impairments and a specification that onset should be before the age of 3 years. As part of the extensive field trial of the draft DSM–IV criteria, considerable empirical data were collected and the current criteria were proven to have adequate interrater reliability (Volkmar *et al*, 1994).

## Asperger syndrome, atypical autism and childhood disintegrative disorder

According to ICD–10 and DSM–IV, for a diagnosis of Asperger syndrome there should be clinically significant qualitative abnormalities in reciprocal social interaction and a restricted, stereotyped and repetitive repertoire of interests and activities. However, it is differentiated from childhood autism by the absence of any general delay in language or cognitive development. A diagnosis of atypical autism is appropriate if one of the triad of impairments is not evident. This is most often diagnosed in an individual whose more severe level of learning disability affects the presentation of the triad of impairments. Childhood disintegrative disorder is characterised by normal development over at least the first 2 years of life, after which there is a abnormal social functioning and loss of acquired skills.

One key aspect of the clinical validity of a diagnostic category is the ability to delineate it from other categories. Therefore, it is important that several studies have found difficulties in differentiating between childhood autism and the other autistic-spectrum disorders (Allen *et al*, 2001). In the case of Asperger syndrome, these difficulties have led authors to devise their own criteria, modify existing criteria or use alternative approaches to diagnosis (Table 6.2).

In summary, the balance of current evidence suggests that although the category of childhood autism has adequate reliability, existing criteria for the other autistic spectrum disorder subtypes require further study.

---

**Box 6.2** Alternative approaches to the diagnosis of autistic-spectrum disorders

- The dimensional model (Tanguay *et al*, 1998; Leekam *et al*, 2000; Beglinger & Smith, 2001)
- The developmental model (Gillham *et al*, 2000; Szatmari, 2000)
- Statistical techniques to identify valid subtypes, e.g. cluster analysis (Prior *et al*, 1998; Stevens *et al*, 2000)

---

# Epidemiology

Until recently, the prevalence of childhood autism was thought to be between 2 and 5 per 10 000 of the population. However, there has been considerable debate as to whether the rates of autistic-spectrum disorders are increasing (Gillberg & Wing, 1999; Fombonne, 2001), leading to several rigorous, large-scale studies.

## Studies of incidence

Although it is recognised that the limitations of previous study design make comparison between successive cohorts difficult (Fombonne, 2001), several studies have concluded that there is a genuine increase in the incidence of autistic-spectrum disorders. Powell *et al* (2000) concluded that there was an 18% per year increase in the incidence of childhood autism but a 55% per year increase in the incidence of other autistic-spectrum disorders. Kaye *et al* (2001) found a sevenfold increase in the incidence of autism between 1988 and 1999. Whereas the report of California's Department of Developmental Services (1999) also reported an increased incidence, this has been criticised for its flawed design and misuse of data (Fombonne, 2001).

## Prevalence studies

There is considerable variation in the reported prevalence of autistic-spectrum disorders. One possible reason for this is that between-study differences in methodology have affected the results. In a review of prevalence studies of childhood autism, Gillberg & Wing (1999) found that there was a trend for more-recent studies to report higher prevalence rates, but could not determine whether this represented a real increase or greater awareness leading to improved recognition and diagnosis. A second review (Fombonne, 1999) also concluded that the prevalence of childhood autism was higher than originally estimated, but there was no robust evidence of an increased incidence.

It is encouraging that three further studies (Baird *et al*, 2000; Centers for Disease Control and Prevention, 2000; Chakrabati & Fombonne, 2001) have reported broadly similar figures, suggesting that the application of rigorous methodology may improve the reproducibility of results. These have reported prevalence figures of about 60/10 000 for all autistic-spectrum disorders, with a prevalence of 20/10 000 for childhood autism and of 40/10 000 for the other autistic-spectrum disorders. However, the most recent study, using data collected by the British Nationwide Survey of Child Mental Health, reported a prevalence of autistic-spectrum disorders of 26.1/10 000 (Fombonne *et al*, 2001).

Despite the dispute over the exact figures, it is now accepted that the original prevalence figures were an underestimate. Although many unanswered questions surround this area, there are clearly significant implications for service provision.

## Gender

Autistic-spectrum disorders are more common in males, with an accepted male:female ratio of 4:1 (Fombonne, 1999). Ehlers & Gillberg (1993) described a similar ratio for Asperger syndrome in a total population study. The reasons for the increased rates in males are still unknown.

# Aetiology

There is an emerging consensus that childhood autism, or any of the other autistic spectrum disorder subtypes, does not represent a single disorder. Rather, contained within each of the subtypes is a hetero-geneous group of disorders with a complex multifactorial aetiology. This is clearly illustrated by the highly variable clinical presentations and the conflicting evidence from studies that have tried to investigate the aetiology of these disorders.

## Family and genetic studies

There is now strong evidence of the role that genetic factors play in the development of autistic-spectrum disorders. Several useful reviews of this area have been published (Cook, 2001; Lauritsen & Ewald, 2001) and a brief mention of the key findings is given below.

## Twin studies

These consistently show an increased concordance of autistic-spectrum disorders in monozygotic compared with dizygotic twins (Bailey *et al*, 1995). A high concordance rate for less severe communication and social impairments than are found in autistic-spectrum disorders has also been described (Constantino & Todd, 2000).

## Family studies

Among the relatives of individuals with autistic-spectrum disorders, there is an increased prevalence of such disorders, with a recurrence risk in siblings of 4.5%. There is also a greater prevalence of subtle deficits in the domains of communication and social interaction (Piven & Palmer, 1999) and a clustering of personality traits among first-degree relatives (Murphy *et al*, 2000).

These findings add weight to the importance of genetic factors and to the concept of a broader phenotype of autism (Bailey *et al*, 1995).

## Molecular genetics

In light of this clear evidence of a genetic component to the autistic-spectrum disorders, it is interesting that four full-genome scans looking for susceptibility regions have not produced more-conclusive findings (Gutknecht, 2001). It is thought that 15 different loci may interact to play a role in the pathogenesis (Risch *et al*, 1999), and unravelling the genetics of complex neuropsychiatric disorders such as autistic-spectrum disorders remains a significant challenge.

## Neuroimaging

As it is important to have a heterogeneous study cohort and an appropriately matched comparison group, scanning studies involving individuals with autistic-spectrum disorders are problematic and have important ethical implications. Despite this, many studies have been carried out involving mostly individuals with high-functioning autism or Asperger syndrome (Chugani, 2000).

### Structural neuroimaging

To date, studies have tended to focus on the cerebellum and limbic structures. Courchesne *et al* (1994) reported significant cerebellar abnormalities, but these results have not been confirmed at other centres. It is suggested that the differences described by Courchesne *et al* (1994) are accounted for by a failure to compare the autism group with a control group matched for IQ as well as for gender and age (Filipek, 1995). Interestingly, a more recent study (Hardan *et al*, 2001) did find an increase in the size of the cerebellum in children with childhood autism, compared with appropriately matched controls.

Aylward *et al* (1999) described abnormalities of the amygdala and hippocampus in individuals with autism, but other studies found no differences in hippocampal volume. One consistent finding is abnormalities in the posterior regions of the corpus callosum (Hardan *et al*, 2000).

Although results to date are inconclusive and variable, this is attributable to the heterogeneous nature of individuals meeting diagnostic criteria for the autistic-spectrum disorders. It could be that longitudinal studies of normal and abnormally developing brains will provide important clues. For example, a longitudinal magnetic resonance imaging study of males with childhood autism describes significant abnormalities in neuroanatomical development of the cerebellum and cerebrum (Courchesne *et al*, 2001).

### Functional neuroimaging

Although functional neuroimaging studies have enormous potential for investigating autistic-spectrum disorders, they are at an early stage (for a review, see Rumsey & Ernst, 2000). Perhaps what is most exciting is the possibility of studying different levels of functioning of the central nervous system. This includes general brain metabolism or activation studies to investigate the neurocognitive impairments of autistic-spectrum disorders such as 'theory of mind' deficits (Happe *et al*, 1995). At an even more detailed level, neurotransmitter studies looking for abnormalities of the serotonergic (Chugani *et al*, 1999) or dopaminergic systems (Ernst *et al*, 1997) may provide useful insights. Such studies have implicated several regions of the brain (Chugani, 2000) and provide an opportunity to attempt to integrate new information about neurodevelopmental processes, neurocognitive psychology and clinical science.

## Neuropathology

There is little relevant data from neuropathological studies (Bailey *et al*, 1998; Kemper & Bauman, 1998). As found in neuroimaging, the limbic and cerebellar regions of the brain are implicated. More-detailed studies have implicated abnormalities in glutamate receptors and transporters in the cerebellum (Purcell *et al*, 2001), but there is clearly a need for more research in this area.

## Neurochemistry

There is evidence that the serotonergic system of the central nervous system is involved in autistic-spectrum disorders. Consistent abnormalities in measures of serotonin have been described in individuals with autistic-spectrum disorders and in their first-degree relatives (Leboyer *et al*, 1999). These include abnormalities in platelet serotonin levels and a worsening of some symptoms upon tryptophan depletion (McDougle *et al*, 1996*b*); functional neuroimaging studies have demonstrated abnormalities in serotonin synthesis compared with control groups (Chugani, 2000). Further work has attempted to link these findings to the molecular biology of serotonin (Tordjman *et al*, 2001).

These results are of interest in light of the associations described below of autistic-spectrum disorders with a family history of affective disorders and of preliminary findings with regard to the effectiveness of risperidone and antidepressants that act on serotonin receptors in the brain. As information about the role of serotonin in early development of the central nervous system increases, it will be possible to explore the relevance of these findings in more detail.

Various theoretical models of the involvement of neuropeptides such as opioids (Panksepp, 1989) or glutamate (Purcell *et al*, 2001) are at a preliminary stage of investigation.

## Neuropsychology

Over the past decade, important work has been carried out on the neuropsychology of autistic-spectrum disorders (Happe, 1996). This work has evolved into three distinct theories, each of which provides interesting accounts of the problems experienced by individuals with autistic-spectrum disorders.

## Theory of mind hypothesis

Work looking at the concept of theory of mind has provided many useful insights into the autistic-spectrum disorders (interested readers should refer to Baron-Cohen *et al*, 2000). 'Theory of mind' refers to the ability to think about other people in terms of their mental states. As the majority of social interaction involves using these mentalistic skills, it is proposed that deficits in this domain may account for some of the impairments in social interaction seen in individuals with autistic-spectrum disorders. The development of these abilities is linked to early social behaviours such as eye gaze, joint attention and pointing, which have become important indicators in screening and early identification of children with autistic-spectrum disorders. Thereafter, children start to gain some awareness of the thoughts and emotions that are related to the actions and behaviours of other people and continue to develop more-subtle abilities into adolescence. Therapeutic programmes that try to to help the development and use of skills such as joint attention or eye gaze are often part of early intervention programmes. For older children, studies teaching theory of mind have shown that individuals can make significant gains in specific areas of functioning. More recently, investigators have used neuroimaging studies to examine the biological underpinnings of the theory of mind (Frith & Frith, 2000).

## Central coherence

As an alternative starting point, Frith (1989) suggested considering both strengths and deficits in cognitive functioning. It is proposed that individuals with autistic-spectrum disorders have relative strengths in focusing on details of perceptions, but find it more difficult to assimilate individual pieces of information into a more coherent, ordered whole, from which a deeper understanding can be construed. Again in terms of social interaction, focusing on a piece of verbal communication without integrating additional information from a person's facial expressions, tone of voice and body language can lead to misinterpretation and confusion. Frith (1989) hoped that this concept of weak central coherence would, in part, account for both the cognitive strengths and the weaknesses commonly associated with autistic-spectrum disorders (Happe, 2000). As in the theory of mind hypothesis, it has been possible empirically to test these ideas, and many of the predictions seem to be borne out. More recent work has looked at the style of information processing used by relatives of individuals with autistic-spectrum disorders (Happe *et al*, 2001). In keeping with some of the ideas about a broader phenotype of autism, it was found that fathers of children with childhood autism were more likely to have a weak central coherence relative to comparison groups.

## Executive function

Although less studied and influential, the similarity between the planning and sequencing problems experienced by some individuals with autistic-spectrum disorders and by individuals following traumatic brain injury has led some authors to propose executive dysfunction as a central part of the neuropsychological profile (Russell, 1998).

# Prognosis and outcome

From several studies, it is now clear that an individual's measured IQ and language abilities are important predictors of outcome. However, relatively few longitudinal studies have followed children diagnosed in early life as they move into adulthood. Therefore, planning for the provision of appropriate and specific life-span services is difficult.

One longitudinal study (Howlin *et al*, 2001) followed up children with childhood autism and compared them with a group with receptive language disorders. Social functioning in adulthood was significantly related to early language functioning in the autism group. It is important to note that, when followed longitudinally, the group with autism did make significant gains in language functioning. However, overall the autism group was consistently functioning at a lower level and was less independent than the group with language disorders.

Szatmari (2000) studied the developmental trajectories of children diagnosed with childhood autism or Asperger syndrome. For most individuals, differences seen between groups in early childhood were maintained several years later. However, a subset of the group with childhood autism made significant gains in language functioning, such that they appeared to shift onto a developmental trajectory closer to that of the group diagnosed with Asperger syndrome.

The finding from these two studies that some individuals made a significant developmental shift emphasises the importance and potential effectiveness of early, intensive interventions in improving long-term outcome.

# Conditions associated with autistic-spectrum disorders

Studies suggest that between 10% and 30% of cases of autistic-spectrum disorders are associated with recognised syndromes or medical conditions such as tuberous sclerosis, fragile-X syndrome, herpes simplex encephalitis or congenital rubella (for a comprehensive discussion, see Gillberg & Coleman, 2000). By studying such associations, researchers hope to find a starting point towards understanding the aetiology of the autistic-spectrum disorders. However, in the vast majority of cases no identifiable syndromes or conditions are found.

## Learning disability

In studies, as the level of learning disability increases, so does the prevalence of autism. Information from epidemiological work suggests that intellectual functioning is within the normal range in only 20% of persons with childhood autism (Fombonne, 1999). However, the evidence of a broader phenotype and the interest in Asperger syndrome and high-functioning autism has highlighted the fact that the majority of individuals with autistic-spectrum disorders do not have an associated learning disability.

## Epilepsy

It is thought that approximately 30% of individuals with autistic-spectrum disorders experience seizures. The prevalence of epilepsy varies with the level of learning disability (Airaksinen *et al*, 2000). Thus, among individuals with mild learning disability 5% have epilepsy, but this increases to 50% in those with a profound learning disability.

As many individuals with autistic-spectrum disorders have difficulties with communication, seizures may go unrecognised and should be considered in the differential diagnosis of any new behaviours or problems. Recent studies report that 15–20% of children with autistic-spectrum disorders but no history of seizures have an epileptiform electro-encephalogram (EEG). Tuchman (2000) suggests that children with an autistic spectrum disorder but no history of clinical seizures, who develop language regression and have an abnormal EEG, should be considered for treatment with anti-epileptic drugs such as those used in Landau–Kleffner syndrome.

## Comorbid psychiatric disorders

There have been relatively few studies of psychiatric disorders in individuals with autistic-spectrum disorders. Part of the reason seems to be that both DSM–IV and ICD–10 suggest that certain forms of psychopathology, for example hyperactivity or deficits in attention, should always be attributed to an individual's autistic spectrum disorder. However, some evidence suggests that a significant proportion of children, adolescents and adults with autistic-spectrum disorders do experience comorbid psychiatric disorders.

## Attention-deficit hyperactivity disorder

Despite a reluctance to diagnose attention-deficit hyperactivity disorder (ADHD), several studies have suggested that psychopathology similar to that found in ADHD does occur in individuals with autistic-spectrum disorders (Ehlers et al, 1997; Ghaziuddin et al, 1998). It is not surprising, considering the difficulties of symptom quantification, that there have been very few adequate trials of interventions. Even though it is suggested that antipsychotics, psychostimulants and naltrexone may have significant benefits, the small numbers of participants, inadequate study design and concern about adverse effects necessitates caution (Aman & Langworthy, 2000).

## Tourette syndrome

Tourette syndrome occurs in individuals already diagnosed with child-hood autism or Asperger syndrome (Baron-Cohen et al, 1999). The suggested prevalence of Tourette syndrome in children with autistic-spectrum disorders, 4.3–6.5%, greatly exceeds that found in the general population. However, without a matched comparison group it is unclear whether this is specifically related to the autistic spectrum disorder or to other factors such as learning disabilities.

## Affective disorders

There are reports of affective disorders occurring in individuals with childhood autism, and depressive disorders are said to be common in individuals with Asperger syndrome (Ghaziuddin et al, 1998). As the presentation of depressive disorders may be different in comparison to the general population (Perry *et al*, 2001), clinicians should exclude affective disorders as causal factors with any changes in behaviour or functioning. In addition, there are reports of individuals with autistic-spectrum disorders experiencing severe anxiety disorders (Tantum, 2000).

The finding that autistic-spectrum disorders are more frequent in families with a history of affective disorders has led to speculation that autistic-spectrum disorders represent an early-life phenotype of affective disorders (DeLong, 1999). Certainly, as in the case of the affective disorders, there is evidence that serotonin may be implicated in the pathogenesis of autistic-spectrum disorders (see above).

## Schizophrenia

Although childhood autism was previously classified as a form of childhood psychosis, studies from the early 1970s (Kolvin, 1971) clearly delineated autistic-spectrum disorders from schizophrenia and other psychoses. Individuals with pre-existing autistic-spectrum disorders can go on to develop schizophrenia, but, unlike with the affective disorders, family studies have not suggested a specific link. However, the finding that adults with autistic-spectrum disorders experience problems similar to the negative symptoms of schizophrenia (Konstantareas & Hewitt, 2001) raises interesting areas for future research.

## Sleep problems

Children with autistic-spectrum disorders experience significant sleep problems (Richdale, 1999; Schreck & Mulick, 2000) and it is likely that many adults with autistic-spectrum disorders also experience such problems. Although there is evidence for the effectiveness of interventions for sleep problems in populations of children and adults with various developmental disorders, studies specific to autistic-spectrum disorders are lacking.

# Interventions

There is a consensus about the importance of early diagnosis, to allow children in the pre-school period to benefit from early, intensive interventions that require a multi-disciplinary team to address the problems with communication, socialisation and adaptive behaviour. In addition, there is increasing interest in the use of biological and psychological interventions to help with some of the problematic symptoms that are commonly experienced by individuals with autistic-spectrum disorders.

## Early, intensive interventions

There is a significant body of evidence on the effectiveness of early interventions in autistic-spectrum disorders (Smith *et al*, 2000). It is suggested that children of pre-school age gain particular benefits from such interventions (Filipek *et al*, 2000), making significant progress in communication, standardised measures of IQ and other domains of development. There are many different intervention programmes, but reviewing eight established ones, Dawson & Osterling (1997) described certain common elements that are essential to the success of such work. More-targeted interventions aim to address specific impairments in motivation (Koegel *et al*, 2001) or in domains at the core of autistic-spectrum disorders such as communication or socialisation (Koegel, 2000; Rogers, 2000).

Educationally based programmes such as the Treatment and Education of Autistic and other Communication-handicapped Children (TEACCH, Lord & Schopler, 1994) are also of value. Interested readers should refer to recent reviews by Howlin (1998) and Erba (2000).

Despite the extensive literature on early interventions, there is still concern over the lack of empirical evidence from controlled trials (Schreibman, 2000). In addition, given the heterogeneous nature of individuals with autistic-spectrum disorders, it is possible that certain intervention models are effective for certain subgroups but not for others.

## Biological interventions

The use of medication by individuals with autistic-spectrum disorders represents a relatively small but important subject. There have been several reports of the dramatic responses of some individuals to novel biological interventions, but, as is described below, the evidence for the effectiveness of most drugs and other treatments is limited. Arnold *et al* (2000) comment that problems with communication present difficulties in the use of medication, for clinicians and researchers alike. In particular, it is important to consider that many individuals will be unable to complain directly of any adverse effects that might occur.

## Management of symptoms commonly associated with autistic-spectrum disorders

There have been several studies of the effectiveness of medication on symptoms thought of as being part of an autistic-spectrum disorder. With the emergence of new symptoms, behaviours or changes in functioning, a psychiatric disorder should be considered and appropriate treatments offered.

The evidence for the effectiveness of the major classes of psychotropic medication and some novel treatments are discussed briefly below.

There have been two relatively recent reviews of this topic (Tsai, 1999; Posey & McDougle, 2000), to which interested readers should refer.

## Atypical antipsychotics

Although the typical antipsychotics, and in particular haloperidol, demonstrated some efficacy in controlled trials, the unacceptable rates of side-effects such as dyskinesias (Posey & McDougle, 2000) led to interest in the use of atypical antipsychotics.

Risperidone has been the most studied. Trials have generally involved children and adolescents, used an open-label design and demonstrated a significant response in a proportion of participants, with sedation and weight gain the most common side-effects. The one randomised controlled trial of risperidone was in adults with autistic-spectrum disorders (McDougle et al, 1998). Compared with individuals receiving placebo, a proportion of the individuals receiving risperidone demonstrated significant improvements in measured symptoms. A recent open-label trial of risperidone in younger children (3.6–6.6 years old) with autistic-spectrum disorders demonstrated some positive benefits, but reported weight gain as a side effect in 10% of participants (Masi et al, 2001). It is noteworthy that across these studies the dose of risperidone used has been relatively low, ranging from 0.5 mg in the youngest children (Masi et al, 2001) to a mean dose of 2.9 mg in adults. These initial encouraging results have led to a larger controlled trial (McDougle et al, 2000).

There are fewer reports in the literature of the use of the other atypical antipsychotics, although two open trials of olanzapine suggest some efficacy (Potenza et al, 1999; Malone et al, 2001).

## Antidepressants

On the basis that the serotonergic system has been implicated in the aetiology of autistic-spectrum disorders, there have been several trials of antidepressants that act on serotonin. Small controlled trials of clomipramine (Gordon et al, 1993) and fluvoxamine (McDougle et al, 1996a) showed some improvements in symptoms. Posey & McDougle (2000) discuss case reports and open-label studies of the selective serotonin reuptake inhibitors fluoxetine, sertraline and paroxetine. As with any medications, there are concerns about potential adverse effects.

## Naltrexone

There have been several randomised, controlled trials of naltrexone that have followed on from case reports of its effectiveness (Posey & McDougle, 2000). Results have been variable, with descriptions of consistent improvements in overactivity and restlessness but no clear improvements in socialisation or communication.

## Clonidine

Clonidine is used for the management of ADHD and Tourette syndrome. Two controlled trials involving very small numbers found significant improvements in symptoms, but concerns were expressed over side-effects and the durability of these improvements (Fankhauser *et al*, 1992; Jaselskis *et al*, 1992).

## Secretin

After it was reported that three children with childhood autism improved markedly when given secretin during endoscopy, there was great hope that it would prove an effective and safe treatment. However, several randomised, controlled trials have not found any benefits (Lightdale *et al*, 2001; Roberts *et al*, 2001).

## Other medications

In light of the theory that the glutamatergic system in the brain may be involved in the pathogenesis of autistic-spectrum disorders, small double-blind, randomised controlled trials of lamotrigine (Belsito *et al*, 2001) and amantadine (King *et al*, 2001) in children and adolescents have been carried out. Belsito *et al* did not find any significant differences between the groups that received lamotrigine and placebo. However, King *et al* report modest improvements in hyperactivity with amantadine treatment, compared with placebo, and suggest that further studies are warranted.

One common finding in both of these studies is the high response rate reported by the parents of children receiving placebo. This issue has been mentioned in connection with the use of secretin (Sandler & Bodfish, 2000) and emphasises the importance of trial designs that are double-blind and randomised.

# Conclusions

Awareness and knowledge of the autistic-spectrum disorders is growing steadily. Psychiatrists have a potentially important role in the multi-disciplinary work that is required to further our understanding of the nature of these complex disorders. The greater prevalence reported in recent studies has implications for the provision of appropriate services to individuals of all ages.

# References

Airaksinen, E. M., Matilainen, R., Mononen, T., *et al* (2000) A population-based study on epilepsy in mentally retarded children. *Epilepsia*, **41**, 1214–1220.

Allen, D. A., Steinberg, M., Dunn, M., et al (2001) Autistic disorder versus other pervasive developmental disorders in young children: same or different? *European Child and Adolescent Psychiatry*, **10**, 67–78.

Aman, M. G. & Langworthy, K. S. (2000) Pharmacotherapy for hyperactivity in children with autism and other pervasive developmental disorders. *Journal of Autism and Developmental Disorders*, **30**, 451–459.

American Pyschiatric Association (1994) *Diagnostic and Statistical Manual of Mental Disorders* (4th edn) (DSM–IV). Washington, DC: APA.

Arnold, L. E., Aman, M. G., Martin, A., et al (2000) Assessment in multisite randomised clinical trials of patients with autistic disorder. The Autism RUPP Network. *Journal of Autism and Developmental Disorders*, **30**, 99–111.

Aylward, E. H., Minshew, N. J., Goldstein, G., et al (1999) MRI volumes of amygdala and hippocampus in non-mentally retarded autistic adolescents and adults. *Neurology*, **53**, 2145–2150.

Bailey, A., Le Couteur, A., Gottesman, I., et al (1995) Autism as a strongly genetic disorder: evidence from a British twin study. *Psychological Medicine*, **25**, 63–77.

—, Luthert, P., Dean, A., et al (1998) A clinicopathological study of autism. *Brain*, **121**, 889–905.

Baird, G., Charman, T., Baron-Cohen, S., et al (2000) A screening instrument for autism at 18 months of age: a six-year follow-up study. *Journal of the American Academy of Child and Adolescent Psychiatry*, **39**, 694–702.

Baron-Cohen, S., Scahill, V. L., Izaguirre, J., et al (1999) The prevalence of Gilles de la Tourette syndrome in children and adolescents with autism: a large scale study. *Psychological Medicine*, **29**, 1151–1159.

—, Tager-Flusberg, H. & Cohen, D. J. (2000) *Understanding Other Minds* (2nd edn). Oxford: Oxford University Press.

Beglinger, L. J. & Smith, T. H. (2001) A review of subtyping in autism and proposed dimensional classification model. *Journal of Autism and Developmental Disorders*, **31**, 411–422.

Belsito, K. M., Law, P. A., Kirk, K. S., et al (2001) Lamotrigine therapy for autistic disorder: a randomized, double-blind, placebo-controlled trial. *Journal of Autism and Developmental Disorders*, **31**, 175–181.

Centers for Disease Control and Prevention (2000) *Prevalence of Autism in Brick Township, New Jersey 1998: Community Report*. Atlanta, GA: Centers for Disease Control and Prevention.

Chakrabati, S. & Fombonne, E. (2001) Pervasive developmental disorders in preschool children. *Journal of American Medical Association*, **285**, 3093–3099.

Chugani, D. C. (2000) Autism. In *Functional Neuroimaging in Child Psychiatry* (eds M. Ernst & J. M. Rumsey), pp. 171-188. Cambridge: Cambridge University Press.

—, Muzik, O., Behen, M., et al (1999) Developmental changes in brain serotonin synthesis capacity in autistic and nonautistic children. *Annals of Neurology*, **45**, 287–295.

Constantino, J. N. & Todd, R. D. (2000) Genetic structure of reciprocal social behaviour. *American Journal of Psychiatry*, **157**, 2043–2045.

Cook, E. H. (2001) Genetics of autism. *Child and Adolescent Psychiatric Clinics of North America*, **10**, 333–350.

Courchesne, E., Saitoh, O., Yeung-Courchesne, R., et al (1994) Abnormality of cerebellar vermian lobules VI and VII in patients with infantile autism: identification of hypoplastic and hyperplastic subgroups with MR imaging. *American Journal of Roentgenology*, **162**, 123–130.

—, Karns, C., Davis, H. R., et al (2001) Unusual brain growth patterns in early life in patients with autistic disorder: an MRI study. *Neurology*, **57**, 245–254.

Dawson, G. & Osterling J. (1997) Early intervention in autism. In *The Effectiveness of Early Intervention* (ed. M. J. Guralnick), pp. 301–326. Baltimore, MD: Paul H. Brookes.

DeLong, G. R. (1999) Autism: new data suggest a new hypothesis. *Neurology*, **52**, 911–916.

Department of Developmental Services (1999) *Changes in the Population of Persons with Autism and Pervasive Developmental Disorders in California's Developmental Services System: 1987 Through 1998.* Report to the Legislature. (http://www.dds.ca.gov).

Ehlers, S. & Gillberg, C. (1993) The epidemiology of Asperger syndrome. A total population study. *Journal of Child Psychology and Psychiatry*, **34**, 1327–1350.

—, Nyden, A., Gillberg, C., *et al* (1997) Asperger syndrome, autism and attention disorders: a comparative study of the cognitive profiles of 120 children. *Journal of Child Psychology and Psychiatry and Allied Disciplines*, **38**, 207–217.

Erba, H. W. (2000) Early intervention programs for children with autism: conceptual frameworks for implementation. *American Journal of Orthopsychiatry*, **70**, 82–94.

Ernst, M., Zametkin, A. J., Maltochik, J. A., *et al* (1997) Low medial prefrontal dopaminergic activity in autistic children. *Lancet*, **350**, 638–641.

Fankhauser, M. P., Karumanchi, V. C., German, M. L., *et al* (1992) A double-blind placebo-controlled study of the efficacy of transdermal clonidine in autism. *Journal of Clinical Psychiatry*, **53**, 77–82.

Filipek, P. A. (1995) Quantitative magnetic resonance imaging in autism: the cerebellar vermis. *Current Opinion in Neurology*, **8**, 134–138.

—, Accardo, P. J., Ashwal, S., *et al* (2000) Practice parameter: screening and diagnosis of autism. Report of the Quality Standards Subcommittee of the American Academy of Neurology and the Child Neurology Society. *Neurology*, **55**, 468–479.

Fombonne, E. (1999) The epidemiology of autism: a review. *Psychological Medicine*, **29**, 769–786.

— (2001) Is there an epidemic of autism? *Pediatrics*, **107**, 411–412.

—, Du, M. C., Cans, C., *et al* (1997) Autism and associated medical disorders in a French epidemiological survey. *Journal of American Academy of Child and Adolescent Psychiatry*, **36**, 1561–1569.

—, Simmons, H., Ford, T., *et al* (2001) Prevalence of pervasive developmental disorders in the British nationwide survey of child mental health. *Journal of the American Academy of Child and Adolescent Psychiatry*, **40**, 820–827.

Frith, U. (1989) *Autism: Explaining the Enigma.* Oxford: Blackwell.

— & Frith, C. (2000) The physiological basis of theory of mind: functional neuro-imaging studies. In *Understanding Other Minds* (2nd edn) (eds S. Baron-Cohen, H. Tager-Flusberg & D. J. Cohen), pp. 334–356. Oxford: Oxford University Press.

Ghaziuddin, M., Weidmer-Mikhail, E. & Ghaziuddin, N. (1998) Comorbidity of Asperger syndrome: a preliminary report. *Journal of Intellectual Disability Research*, **42**, 279–283.

Gillberg, C. & Coleman, M. (2000) *The Biology of the Autistic Syndromes.* London: MacKeith Press.

— & Wing, L. (1999) Autism: not an extremely rare disorder. *Acta Psychiatrica Scandinavica*, **99**, 399–406.

Gillham, J. E., Carter, A. S., Volkmar, F. R., *et al* (2000) Toward a developmental operational definition of autism. *Journal of Autism and Developmental Disorders*, **30**, 269–278.

Gordon, C. T., State, R. C., Nelson, J. E., *et al* (1993) A double-blind comparison of clomipramine, desipramine and placebo in the treatment of autistic disorder. *Archives of General Psychiatry*, **50**, 441–447.

Gutknecht, L. (2001) Full-genome scans with autistic disorder: a review. *Behavior Genetics*, **31**, 113–123.

Happe, F. (1996) The neuropsychology of autism. *Brain*, **119**, 1377–1400.

— (2000) Parts and wholes, meaning and minds: central coherence and its relation to theory of mind. In *Understanding Other Minds* (2nd edn) (eds S. Baron-Cohen, H. Tager-Flusberg & D. J. Cohen), pp. 222–252. Oxford: Oxford University Press.

**131**

—, Ehlers, S. & Fletcher, P. (1995) Theory of mind in the brain. Evidence from a PET scan in Asperger syndrome. *Neuroreport*, **8**, 197–201.

—, Briskman, J. & Frith, U. (2001) Exploring the cognitive phenotype of autism: weak 'central coherence' in parents and siblings of children with autism: I. Experimental tests. *Journal of Child Psychology and Psychiatry*, **42**, 299–307.

Hardan, A. Y., Minshew, N. J. & Keshavan, M. S. (2000) Corpus callosum size in autism. *Neurology*, **55**, 1033–1036.

—, —, Harenski, K., *et al* (2001) Posterior fossa magnetic resonance imaging in autism. *Journal of the American Academy of Child and Adolescent Psychiatry*, **40**, 666–672.

Howlin, P. (1998) Practitioner review: psychological and educational treatments for autism. *Journal of Child Psychology and Psychiatry and Allied Disciplines*, **39**, 307–322.

— & Moore, A. (1997) Diagnosis in autism – a survey of over 1200 patients in the UK. *Autism*, **1**, 135–162.

—, Mawhood, L. & Rutter, M. (2001) Autism and developmental receptive language disorder – a follow-up comparison in early adult life. II: Social, behavioural, and psychiatric outcomes. *Journal of Child Psychology and Psychiatry and Allied Disciplines*, **41**, 561–578.

Jaselskis, C. A., Cook, E. H., Fletcher, K. E., *et al* (1992) Clonidine treatment of hyperactive and impulsive children with autistic disorder. *Journal of Clinical Psychopharmacology*, **12**, 322–327.

Kaye, J. A., del Mar Melero-Montes, M. & Jick, H. (2001) Mumps, measles and rubella vaccine and the incidence of autism recorded by general practitioners: a time trend analysis. *BMJ*, **322**, 460–463.

Kemper, T. & Bauman, M. (1998) Neuropathology of infantile autism. *Journal of Neuropathology and Experimental Neurology*, **57**, 645–652.

King, B. H., Wright, D. M., Handen, B. L., *et al* (2001) Double-blind, placebo-controlled study of amantadine hydrochloride in the treatment of children with autistic disorder. *Journal of the American Academy of Child and Adolescent Psychiatry*, **40**, 658–665.

Koegel, L. K. (2000) Interventions to facilitate communication in autism. *Journal of Autism and Developmental Disorders*, **30**, 383–391.

—, Koegel, R. L. & McNerney, E. K. (2001) Pivotal areas in intervention for autism. *Journal of Clinical Child Psychology*, **30**, 19–32.

Kolvin, I. (1971) Studies in the childhood psychoses. I: Diagnostic criteria and classification. *British Journal of Psychiatry*, **118**, 381–384.

Konstantareas, M. M. & Hewitt, T. (2001) Autistic disorder and schizophrenia: diagnostic overlaps. *Journal of Autism and Developmental Disorders*, **31**, 19–28.

Lauritsen, M. & Ewald, H. (2001) The genetics of autism. *Acta Psychiatrica Scandinavica*, **103**, 411–427.

Leboyer, M., Phillipe, A., Bouvard, M. P., *et al* (1999) Whole blood serotonin and plasma beta endorphin in autistic probands and their first degree relatives. *Biological Psychiatry*, **45**, 158–163.

Leekam, S., Libby, S., Wing, L., *et al* (2000) Comparison of ICD–10 and Gillberg's criteria for Asperger syndrome. *Autism*, **4**, 11–28.

Lightdale, J. R., Hayer, C. D., Adam Lind-White, C. J., *et al* (2001) Effects of intravenous secretin on language and behavior of children with autism and gastrointestinal symptoms: a single-blinded, open-label pilot study. *Pediatrics*, **108**, e90.

Lord, C. & Schopler, E. (1994) TEACCH services for preschool children. In *Preschool Education Programs for Children with Autism* (eds S. Harris & J. Handleman), pp. 87–106. Austin, TX: Pro-Ed.

—, Rutter, M. & Le Couteur, A. (1994), Autism Diagnostic Interview – Revised: a revised version of a diagnostic interview for caregivers of individuals with possible pervasive developmental disorders. *Journal of Autism and Developmental Disorders*, **24**, 659–685.

—, Risi, S., Lambrecht, L., *et al* (2000) The Autism Diagnostic Observation Schedule – Generic: a standard measure of social and communication deficits associated with the spectrum of autism. *Journal of Autism and Developmental Disorders*, **30**, 205–223.

Malone, R. P., Cater, J., Sheikh, R. M., *et al* (2001) Olanzapine versus haloperidol in children with autistic disorder. An open pilot study. *Jouranl of the American Academy of Child and Adolescent Psychiatry*, **40**, 887–894.

Masi, G., Cosenza, A., Mucci, M., *et al* (2001) Open trial of risperidone in 24 young children with pervasive developmental disorders. *Journal of the American Academy of Child and Adolescent Psychiatry*, **40**, 1206–1214.

McDougle, C. J., Naylor, S. T., Cohen, D. J., *et al* (1996*a*) A double-blind, placebo-controlled study of fluvoxamine in adults with autistic disorder. *Archives of General Psychiatry*, **53**, 1001–1008.

—, Naylor, S. T., Cohen, D. J., *et al* (1996*b*) Effects of tryptophan depletion in drug-free adults with autistic disorder. *Archives of General Psychiatry*, **53**, 993–1000.

—, Holmes, J. P., Carlson, D. C., *et al* (1998) A double-blind, placebo-controlled study of risperidone in adults with autistic disorder and other pervasive developmental disorders. *Archives of General Psychiatry*, **55**, 633–641.

—, Scahill, L., McCracken, J. T., *et al* (2000) Research Units on Pediatric Psychopharmacology (RUPP) autism network. Background and rationale for an initial controlled study of risperidone. *Child and Adolescent Psychiatric Clinics of North America*, **9**, 201–224.

Murphy, M., Bolton, P. F., Pickles, A., *et al* (2000) Personality traits of the relatives of autistic probands. *Psychological Medicine*, **30**, 1411–1424.

Panksepp, J. (1989) A neurochemical theory of autism. *Trends in Neuroscience*, **2**, 174–177.

Perry, D. W., Marston, G. M., Hinder, S. A. J., *et al* (2001) The phenomenology of depressive illness in people with a learning disability and autism. *Autism*, **5**, 265–275.

Piven, J. & Palmer, P. (1999) Psychiatric disorder and the broad autism phenotype: evidence from a family study of multiple-incidence autism families. *American Journal of Psychiatry*, **156**, 557–563.

Posey, D. J. & McDougle, C. J. (2000) The pharmacotherapy of target symptoms associated with autistic disorder and other pervasive developmental disorders. *Harvard Review of Psychiatry*, **8**, 45–63.

Potenza, M. N., Holmes, J. P., Kanes, S. J., *et al* (1999) Olanzapine treatment of children, adolescents and adults with pervasive developmental disorders: an open-label pilot study. *Journal of Clinical Psychopharmacology*, **19**, 37–44.

Powell, J. E., Edwards, A., Edwards, M., *et al* (2000) Changes in the incidence of childhood autism and others in preschool children from two areas of the West Midlands, UK. *Developmental Medicine and Child Neurology*, **42**, 624–628.

Prior, M., Leekam, S., Ong, B., *et al* (1998) Are there subgroups within the autistic spectrum? A cluster analysis of a group of children with autistic spectrum disorders. *Journal of Child Psychology and Psychiatry*, **39**, 893–902.

Purcell, A. E., Jeon, O. H., Zimmerman, A. W., *et al* (2001) Postmortem brain abnormalities of the glutamate neurotransmitter system in autism. *Neurology*, **57**, 1618–1628.

Richdale, A. L. (1999) Sleep problems in autism: prevalence, cause and intervention. *Developmental Medicine and Child Neurology*, **41**, 60–66.

Risch, N., Spiker, D., Lotspeich, L., *et al* (1999) A genomic screen of autism: evidence for a multilocus etiology. *American Journal of Human Genetics*, **65**, 493–507.

Roberts, W., Weaver, L., Brian, J., *et al* (2001) Repeated doses of porcine secretin in the treatment of autism: a randomized, placebo-controlled trial. *Pediatrics*, **107**, e71.

Rogers, S. J. (2000) Interventions that facilitate socialization in children with autism. *Journal of Autism and Developmental Disorders*, **30**, 399–409.

Rumsey, J. M. & Ernst, M. (2000) Functional neuroimaging of autistic disorders. *Mental Retardation and Developmental Disabilities*, **6**, 171–179.

Russell, J. (1998) *Autism as an Executive Disorder*. Oxford: Oxford University Press.

Sandler, A. D. & Bodfish, J. W. (2000) Placebo effects in autism: lessons from secretin. *Journal of Developmental and Behavioral Pediatrics*, **21**, 347–350.

—, Brazdziunas, D., Cooley, W. C., *et al* (2001) Technical report: the pediatrician's role in the diagnosis and management of autistic spectrum disorder in children. *Pediatrics*, **107**, e85.

Schopler, E., Reichler, R. & Renner, B. R. (1988) *The Childhood Autism Rating Scale (CARS)*. Los Angeles, CA: Western Psychological Services.

Schreck, K. A. & Mulick, J. A. (2000) Parental report of sleep problems in children with autism. *Journal of Autism and Developmental Disorders*, **30**, 127–135.

Schreibman, L. (2000) Intensive behavioral/psychoeducational treatments for autism: research and future directions. *Journal of Autism and Developmental Disorders*, **30**, 373–381.

Smith, T., Groen, A. D. & Wynn, J. W. (2000) Randomized trial of intensive early intervention for children with pervasive developmental disorder. *American Journal of Mental Retardation*, **105**, 269–285.

Sparrow, S. S., Balla, D. A. & Cicchetti, D. V. (1984) *Vineland Adaptive Behaviour Scales*. Circle Pines, MN: American Guidance Service.

Stevens, M. C., Fein, D. A., Dunn, M., *et al* (2000) Subgroups of children with autism by cluster analysis: a longitudinal examination. *Journal of the American Academy of Child and Adolescent Psychiatry*, **39**, 346–352.

Szatmari, P. (2000) The classification of autism, Asperger's syndrome, and pervasive developmental disorder. *Canadian Journal of Psychiatry – Revue Canadienne de Psychiatrie*, **45**, 731–738.

Tanguay, P. E., Robertson, J., Derrick, A. (1998) A dimensional classification of autism spectrum disorder by social communication domains. *Journal of the American Academy of Child and Adolescent Psychiatry*, **37**, 271–277.

Tantam, D. (2000) Psychological disorders in adolescents and adults with Asperger syndrome. *Autism*, **4**, 47–62.

Tordjman, S., Gutknecht, L., Carlier, M., *et al* (2001) Role of the serotonin transporter gene in the behavioural expression of autism. *Molecular Psychiatry*, **6**, 434–439.

Tsai, L. Y. (1999) Psychopharmacology in autism. *Psychosomatic Medicine*, **61**, 651–656.

Tuchman, R. (2000) Treatment of seizure disorders and EEG abnormalities in children with autism spectrum disorders. *Journal of Autism and Developmental Disorders*, **30**, 484–489.

Volkmar, F. R., Klin, A., Siegel, B., *et al* (1994) Field trial for autistic disorder in DSM–IV. *American Journal of Psychiatry*, **151**, 1361–1367.

—, — & Cohen, D. J. (1997) Diagnosis and classification of autism and related conditions: consensus and issues. In *Handbook of Autism and Pervasive Developmental Disorders* (2nd edn) (eds J. Cohen & F. R. Volkmar), pp. 5–40. New York: John Wiley & Sons.

Wechsler, D. (1991) *Wechsler Intelligence Scale for Children – Third Edition (WISC–III)*. San Antonio, TX: Psychological Corporation.

Wing, L. (1993) *The Diagnostic Interview for Social and Communicative Disorders* (3rd edn). Bromley: Centre for Social and Communicative Disorders/Elliot House.

— (1996) Autistic spectrum disorders. *BMJ*, **312**, 327–328.

— & Gould, J. (1979) Severe impairments of social interaction and associated abnormalities in children: epidemiology and classification. *Journal of Autism and Developmental Disorders*, **9**, 11–29.

World Health Organization (1992) *The Tenth Revision of the International Classification of Diseases and Related Health Problems* (ICD–10). Geneva: WHO.

# CHAPTER 7

# Communicating with people with learning disability

Julia Scotland and W. Fraser

## Early infant communication

Skilled dialogue with people who have learning disabilities requires an understanding of how infants typically learn interaction and communication skills as speech and language develop. Alongside the acknowledged developmental milestones in the acquisition of speech and language, non-verbal behaviour has an important role in learning communication skills from birth and throughout life. The acquisition of language follows distinct milestones (Table 7.1).

The child with a learning disability progresses through these stages at a slower rate. In some disabling conditions, there is only delay in language development, owing to cognitive impairment and a relatively unrewarding language environment. However, in most syndromes language development is also asynchronous with other aspects of

**Table 7.1**  Average ages for the milestones of speech and language acquisition

| Age | Vocalisation |
| --- | --- |
| 6 months | Babbles |
| 10 months | Reduplications appear: 'ma-ma', 'da-da' |
| 1 year | One-word sentences |
| 18 months | Two-word utterances |
| 20 months | Telegrammatic speech |
| 2 years | Pre-sleep monologues |
| 2.5 years | 50-word lexicon, 5-word sentences; uses personal pronoun |
| 3 years | Plurals established, 250 words |
| 3.5 years | Pronounces 'p' and 'b', 'm' and 'w', 'h'; asks how and why questions |
| 4 years | Tells story; still produces many morphological errors |
| 4.5 years | Pronounces 't', 'k', d', 'ng', 'y'; asks what words mean |
| 5.5 years | Pronounces 'f', 'z', 's', 'v' |
| 6.5 years | Pronounces 'sh', 'zh', 'th'; adult morphology is complete; listens to another's view point in conversation |
| 8 years | Pronounces 'ch,' 'r', 'wh' |

development. For example, in Down's syndrome there is disproportionate delay and in Asperger syndrome there is a qualitative difference in language acquisition.

From birth, a child interacts with others and is conveying information about states of mind. In the early months, vocalisations communicate feelings of pain and distress or surprise, and gain the attention of adults. After 6 months, gestures such as pointing are combined with vocalisations to influence other people. At 10 months, 'protolanguage' emerges. In protolanguage, 'interpersonal functions' influence what others do, and 'ideational functions' convey the child's state of mind. These are conveyed by gestures with vocalisation and by vocalisations alone respectively. Halliday (1973) rejected the idea that the child is acquiring things such as sounds, words or grammar; rather, he or she is actively learning to convey meaning. It is therefore necessary to study how the child expresses intentions.

Austin (1962) mapped the infant's acquisition of semiotics. Early infant behaviours such as cries, gazes and short reaches that have communicative effects on adults, even if there is no evidence that infants understand their ability to have such effects, are assigned to what Austin terms the 'perlocutionary' stage. As caregivers respond with an assigned meaning to these early infant actions, children gradually discover the ability to evoke responses from others. The 'illocutionary' stage follows, which is characterised by the child's coordinated actions on objects and people, related to the development of a small set of gestures directed at receivers – give, show, request and point – by which the child indicates an intention in order to have an effect on a receiver. Finally, the 'locutionary' stage arrives when the child produces actual linguistic forms to carry his or her intentions.

## Language acquisition

Linguists continue to debate how language is acquired, but the consensus from studies indicates three factors. First, there is a consistent order of acquisition, recognised as distinct milestones in the development of speech and language (see Table 7.1) and as identifiable levels of language. Table 7.2 gives an overview of those levels and shows the distinction between receptive and expressive language. Both are interdependent, but there is a danger of focusing on the expressive aspects at the expense of comprehension, which provides the basis for expression. Second, there is a variable rate of acquisition. Third, there is individual variation between children in the way that language is acquired: some children initially use more social phrases, for example 'more biscuit', whereas others prefer referential language that labels things, for example 'daddy book'. Ingram (1989) provides in-depth discussion of language acquisition.

It is generally acknowledged that it is important to the development of communication skills that individuals have something to say, a way of expressing this and a reason to do so.

## Something to say about needs, concepts or interests

Individuals may have such global brain damage or delay in the maturation of the 'wiring up' of the nervous system that they are unable to identify their own bodily needs such as hunger and toileting.

**Table 7.2** Levels of language

| Perception/comprehension | Production/expression | Channel |
|---|---|---|
| | **Pragmatics (use)** | |
| *Knowing that someone is:* | *Functions such as:* | *May be any or all of:* |
| Giving information | Giving information | Extralinguistic, e.g dress |
| Requesting information | Requesting information | Paralinguistic, e.g prosody |
| Telling you off | | Body language, proxemics, eye gaze |
| Teasing you | Teasing | Linguistic |
| Thanking you | Expressing feelings | Timing and turn-taking |
| | **Semantics (meaning)** | |
| *Knowing that someone is telling you:* | *Informing about:* | *Conveyed by:* |
| Where an object is | Communicating position of object | Gesture |
| What a person is doing | Possession | Topic selection |
| That something has disappeared | Action on object | Lexical selection |
| What something looks like | Past events | Appropriateness of information |
| | **Syntax (grammar)** | |
| *Understanding grammar:* | *Structuring sentences:* | *Rules such as:* |
| Understanding that plurality is often signalled by a final /s/ and that the past may be signalled by /ed/ | Using different forms to indicate different verb tenses; using /and/ to link ideas; using /because/ to signal cause and effect | Word order; grammatical rules; contingency of responses |
| | **Phonology (sound contrasts)** | |
| *Discriminating sounds:* | *Contrasting sounds:* | |
| Knowing that the difference between /t/ and /k/ causes a change in meaning | Changing sounds to change meaning, e.g. car/tar/far | Speech sound system |
| | **Phonetics (sounds)** | |
| Hearing and listening to sounds regardless of their meaning | Producing speech sounds regardless of their meaning | Hearing; listening; articulation |

Until they are aware of their needs, they are unlikely to try to communicate about them. Anecdotal information from adults with autistic-spectrum disorder describes difficulties in interpreting sensory information. Grandin and Scariano (1986), Carlton (1993) and Williams (1992) suggest that it is this area of perceptual confusion where communication first begins to break down in children with autistic-spectrum disorders.

Before concepts can be learned, perception must enable individuals to make sense of their immediate surroundings. A prerequisite for the development of perceptual skills is a level of attention control that can be selective and sustained (Kindlon, 1998). As children relate perceptions to the range of contexts in which they are experienced, they map groups of objects onto concepts, which are then expressed via words, for example objects that the child drinks out of are mapped onto the word 'cup'.

Play has a very important role in concept development and the learning of essential prerequisites for speech and language development. Visuo-motor play involving looking and manipulating emerges as children first begin to play with their own fingers and grasp objects. Exploration by watching, touching, mouthing or sorting next emerges as they begin to imitate, interpret and rehearse what to do with familiar objects. Thus, functional play develops, with children relating to toys, for example brushing a doll's hair, in preparation for symbolic representation. This is essential for verbal language and leads to pretend play, where children re-enact events and learn that a system can represent reality.

Interests usually provide an individual with the motivation to communicate with others. The first words of typically developing children usually draw an adult's attention to things that interest them. In contrast, the first words of a child with autistic-spectrum disorder are more likely to be 'demand' words, and are often idiosyncratic (Weatherby, 1986).

## A way of saying it

In typically developing children, pointing emerges towards the end of the first 12 months as an early mode of communication. Proto-imperative pointing communicates 'I want', and proto-declarative pointing shares experiences with an adult. These usually develop simultaneously. It is well documented that children with autism do not generally follow this pattern of development. It has been shown that teaching pointing skills can facilitate the use of spontaneous communication in pupils with autistic-spectrum disorder and severe learning disability (Potter & Whittaker, 1997).

Spoken language develops during the second year, supported by prosody, gesture, body language, eye gaze and facial expression. There are, however, those who will never learn spoken language. Evidence suggests that 75% of individuals with autistic-spectrum disorder have an additional learning disability and that between 30% and 50% of these fail to develop speech. Experience suggests that if children are using words before the age of 6 years and phrases before 12 years, they may develop useful spoken phrase speech. If they are attempting words before 13 years, then they may develop useful speech at a single-word level. If they are using few words before 6 years of age and not many more before the age of 13, they are likely to remain mute.

For many of these individuals who fail to develop speech, challenging behaviour becomes an effective but unacceptable mode of communicating need and of drawing attention to themselves. In such cases, it is necessary to enable, where feasible, an acceptable way of communicating by offering an alternative and augmentative system of communication. Makaton (Walker, 1973) is often introduced as a basic language development programme and manual signing system. Teaching signs, however, is not enough unless these are associated with communicative intent. Some signing and symbol systems can demand a level of sophistication similar to that of spoken language. It may be more helpful to introduce something much more rudimentary, as in the following examples.

- *Objects of reference* These are associated with actual events and objects that are meaningful to the child, for example the child's cup to request a drink or the home/school bag to signify home time. The simplest and most helpful starting point for individuals who are at a pre-intentional stage of communication is probably the use of objects of reference to indicate needs (Park, 1997). Some individuals may be able to use a more iconic representation of the object or event such as photographs, miniature objects or part of the object. Park provides a helpful review of the literature on objects of reference and the hierarchical progression from objects of reference as indices to the use of much more arbitrary picture symbols.
- *The Picture Exchange Communication System* Described by Bondy & Frost (1998), this system requires interaction with others from the outset. The aim is for individuals to acquire the key communication skill of requesting by initiating interaction in a social exchange. Thus, those who have no functional communication skills are trained to give a picture of a desired object or event to another person in exchange for that object or event. The request is not pre-empted by asking 'what do you want?'; rather, the individual is tempted by a highly desirable object and, as they reach for this, a facilitator moulds the child to hand a picture of the object over in exchange for what is wanted. So, using behavioural principles, the child learns to initiate communication (Baker, 2000).

Providing those who have communication difficulties with an augmentative mode of communication has many positive benefits. It helps them to understand what has been said to them, provides them with a means of expressing needs, enables them to initiate interaction and communication (thus fostering independence), supports their attempts to respond appropriately to communicative initiatives, enhances interaction with those who are familiar with the augmentative system and may provide a mode of functional communication in the absence of verbal comprehension and expression. See Wilson (2000) for an overview of current approaches to alternative and augmentative communication.

Those who have speech may still have difficulties with the social aspects of language usage such as body language, facial expression, eye gaze and prosodic features. They may rely on echolalia and/or fail to respond to the social markers given by others, lacking strategies for conversation and lacking an awareness of what knowledge is shared with their conversational partner.

The goal of language intervention must be to assist children in acquiring the most effective, adaptable, generalisable and acceptable communication skills possible. Thus, no longer is it assumed that an infant, child, young person or adult must have speech before he or she can benefit from communication skills training. Programmes to enhance effective communication may be implemented for people with every level of disability. The professional who works with people with learning disabilities must now have some familiarity with alternative and augmentative communication systems and appreciate the importance of 'total communication' (Hollins, 2000).

## A reason for saying it

The presence of spoken language does not necessarily mean that the person is able or willing to communicate (Rutter, 1996). Attempts at communication must be rewarded. Consistent relevant responses to speech attempts are an important way of helping a child to map words to meaning. There must be a need to communicate: if every need is automatically met, then there is little incentive to struggle to ask for things. In the case of a person for whom independence has been enabled by placing everything within reach, it may be necessary to engineer the environment to create situations where it is necessary to communicate with another in order to satisfy need.

## Early intervention

Professionals involved in facilitating communication skills in children with learning disabilities believe that early intervention is essential. Parents testify to the value of early support and intervention in helping them to make a positive contribution to the development of their child's communication skills. Common sense suggests the importance of avoiding the adverse effects for parents and children of experiencing failure, and of preparing early for augmentative modes of communication and effective functional communication. Those who design such programmes claim success. Independent reviewers are less convinced. Guralnick (1997) describes the current debate surrounding the efficacy and cost-effectiveness of early intervention.

Studies do lack rigour, but specifically defined situations and strictly controlled variables are unlikely to reflect the true situation of the communication difficulties of those with learning disabilities (Robson 1993). Recent early intervention programmes have focused on developing social interaction strategies within the family and among peers, i.e. ecologically driven models of intervention (Spiker & Hopmann, 1997).

## Role of speech and language therapist

The Royal College of Speech and Language Therapists (1996) recommends that all people with learning disabilities should have access to specialist speech and language therapy provided in a location appropriate to their communication needs, and where they spend a significant amount of time. Before intervention, assessment is important. Assessment will include information on the locations where the client is situated, with particular reference to the way these influence and support an individual's communicative competence. The emphasis of speech and language therapy, particularly for adults with learning disabilities, has shifted towards an advisory role providing support and training for carers who implement individualised programmes of intervention (Dobson & Worrall, 2001).

### Assessment

Assessment remains significant in the use of speech and language therapy time. The diverse nature of learning disability requires that the assessment of communicative competence be measured in a variety of ways (Dormandy & Van der Gaag, 1989). Speech and language therapists rely heavily upon observation and upon information from carers and clients to inform their assessment. Appropriate materials, particularly for the assessment of adults, remain very limited. Assessment should inform about a range of factors, in particular the communicative repertoire, the mode, function and success of communication, the carer's skills in enabling communication, and the appropriateness of the environment for encouraging exchange. Each of these is discussed below.

### Communicative repertoire

This includes the range of functions, frequency of use, locations of use, and communicative partners.

### Mode of communication

Communication can be perlocutionary or illocutionary, verbal or non-verbal, formal or informal.

*Crying* is the typical infant's earliest perlocutionary mode of communication. Mothers of typical children are made aware of their offspring's subjective states from the child's crying. There are three main aspects that influence the cry signal: the internal state of the infant, his or her age and the situation in which it is involved. A fourth factor, relevant to children with disabilities, is any clinical disorder, for example children with Cri du Chat syndrome typically have a high-pitched voice.

Parents use the child's cry as an alerting device, detecting a change in its causal characteristics. The child and the setting in which the crying is occurring are observed and examined to decide whether the infant is in pain and why. In people with learning disability, the rough order of likely causes of pain are: locomotor discomfort; eyelash in eye; sore throat; sore ear; colic; oesophagitis; sphincter spasm; voluntary muscle spasm; joint pain, etc.

*Non-verbal behaviour* Cultural rules about the meanings of non-verbal behaviours vary significantly. It is important to provide those learning to communicate with opportunities to learn the rules as soon as possible. Timing is important in communication, which can rapidly break down if this is disrupted. Posture, movement, gesture, facial expression, the space kept from others, touch, reaction to touch, looks and eye contact are all integral to human interaction, and are as important to communication as are the words we use, although we are often unaware of the non-verbal cues we are giving. Some non-verbal cues have the same meaning for all, for example a smile usually communicates friendly feelings. Eye contact, although not essential to communication, does help to differentiate speaker/listener roles and gives signals about whose turn it is to speak. Gestures can also fill in for words (Burford, 1988). Interactions are two-way and it is therefore important that practitioners are aware of the effect and influence of their own non-verbal behaviours. Touch is a fundamental form of early communication, but in the UK touching those we do not know, apart from a formal handshake, is not acceptable. People with intellectual disabilities enjoy the rudimentary communication of touching and being close and this may lead to misunderstandings or make them vulnerable to abuse. However, touch can be a very effective mode of communication (Burford, 1988). Children with Down's syndrome use non-verbal strengths to compensate for their limited language (Franco & Wishart, 1995).

*Speech* typically becomes evident by the end of the first year, when duplicated syllables such as 'mama' and 'dada' appear: this stage is universal to most languages. These single, though duplicated, words are really one-word sentences. Typical children at around 18 months cross a language watershed. They start to link objects and ideas together and, when they have developed the idea of the permanency of objects, they are able to label things. Children develop a two-word stage when they employ only a small number of semantic operations (8–15). The types of meaning that are usually grammatically encoded are, in order of frequency: naming; recurrence; non-existence; agent and action; agent and object; agent and action and object; action and location; entity and location; possessor and possession; and entity and demonstration.

At about 2 years of age, personal pronouns start to be used, usually in the order of 'my', 'me', 'you' and 'I'. 'We' starts at about 3 years. The 2-year-old learns words, and the 3-year-old starts to use them. At this stage, typical children are pattern learners. They tend at first to over-regularise rules, for example one sheep, two sheeps, but these mistakes tend to vanish by the age of 7 years. 'Normal' children extend control over the prosodic system, the grammatical system and the phonological system in a piecemeal fashion, bringing one aspect under control at a time. Prosody is under control early, normally by 1 year, but it may be 8 or 9 years before children can cope with the more complex consonant clusters. Individuals with learning disabilities may continue to make mistakes, for example in the use of plurals, pronouns and past tenses. When you press them, you realise that they often know the rules, yet, showing impulsiveness in language, they seek the easy way out. Normal adult competence (in some aspects of language) may never be reached.

## Function of communication

Communication has many fuctions, for example to seek attention, to meet needs, to reject and refuse to interact socially, to give information, to ask questions, to express feelings and opinions, to respond to communicative initiatives, to negotiate, to repair and clarify misunderstandings, and to direct others.

## Success of communication

Communicative successs relates to attending, understanding and expressing. Beveridge & Conti-Ramsden (1987) consider that children who have learning disabilities are non-assertive and deferential with their 'normal' peers. They are also particularly likely to experience problems in using language in social interactions with peers both with and without disabilities. The experience of situations that present uncontrolled or aversive outcomes induces a psychological state of learned helplessness and a general disposition to avoid participation in certain types of problem situations.

The current policies of inclusion do not guarantee that full social integration will follow. The social world is, to quote Beveridge & Conti-Ramsden (1987), 'a baffling and problem-strewn battleground, even for many non-handicapped adults', and social integration requires skills in a large number of methods and strategies for solving many of the problems. Unless people with learning disabilities can do this, they will remain on the fringe of society.

### Skills of carers

Carers can play a major role in enabling meaningful communication exchanges. Professionals must be aware of and practice a variety of techniques in order to communicate with people who have severe learning disabilities (Box 7.1).

The ENABLE package (Hurst-Brown & Keens, 1990) provides a useful framework from which to draw up a profile of communication

---

**Box 7.1**  Communication with people with severe learning disability

- Make it enjoyable – practise in those situations where the person is most communicative
- Teach new concepts in meaningful contexts
- Teach pointing and exchange skills; enable the making of choices
- Use every relevant opportunity for communication and ensure that each is a rewarding experience
- Do not cramp your style by too much formality
- Be an opportunist: sing, act, whistle, change the pitch of your voice or the rate of your speech
- Use consistent labels
- Take small steps, and do not reach for a level far beyond the person's development
- Remember to signal vigorously with your face and do not forget that the person may not signal back
- Remember that an individual who is not looking may not be listening
- Give the person time to answer
- Cue the person by his or her name
- The onus is on you to ensure you are understood
- Establish routines that enable situational understanding if verbal comprehension is limited
- The behaviour of the person with a learning disability is the starting point. Difficulties in being able to understand language and/or to communicate effectively may result in challenging behaviour
- Focusing on functional communication and the social and pragmatic aspects of communication is effective
- Relate to the person's understanding and interests rather than to chronological age. (Note that this does fit the normalisation philosophy of Wolfensberger, 1983.)
- Always assume intentionality – that the behaviour, however strange, means something

---

skills, interactions and the environment of individuals with learning disabilities, in both one-to-one and group situations.

Mitchell (1987), in a review of parents' interactions with infants who are at risk or have developmental disabilities, noted that mothers of premature infants tend to be more active and intrusive and less responsive than are mothers of full-term infants in joint activities such as playing or feeding. Infants with learning disabilities present similarly as problematic interactive partners for their parents.

As individuals with learning disabilities are exposed to parent-dominated interventions, they come to develop feelings of ineffectiveness or learned helplessness. The parents similarly 'turn off' as competent interactive partners. There is now considerable literature on room and group management and caregiver variables for facilitating infant development. As Mitchell (1987) pointed out, 'Parent/infant interaction is no place for parents to dance to a different drummer. For the most part, the infant should call the tune'.

Awareness of the subtleties of the developmental sequences mentioned above is a necessary prerequisite for skilled consultations with people who have profound disabilities. The professional must be able to apply the approaches of mother/infant interaction dialogue to people stuck in the first-year (perlocutionary or early illocutionary) phases.

### Appropriateness of the environment

The environment should provide motivation and reward for communication. Noise levels should be such that conversation is possible. Furniture should be arranged to ensure comfort and positioning that encourage interaction. Communication aids should also be accessible (Bartlett & Bunning, 1997).

### Additional factors affecting language development

Any intervention must acknowledge all factors that, in addition to intellectual disability, may influence the learning of communication skills. These include neurological and sensory impairment such as epilepsy, cerebral palsy, visual and/or hearing impairment and tactile defensiveness. Mental health problems may also influence the effectiveness of intervention (Stansfield, 1998).

## Intervention

There is variation among speech and language therapists and health trusts in the type of intervention provided. Most speech and language therapists deliver indirect therapy, either addressing the needs of individuals or groups by concentrating on developing opportunities for communication or working to effect change to make the environment more conducive to good communication for the client, through teaching and training carers (Money, 2000).

Some therapists believe it appropriate to provide direct therapy where they concentrate on the client's communication abilities on a one-on-one basis or in group sessions.

Many therapists use a combination of the two approaches. Money (1997) concluded that direct and indirect therapy need to be combined to maximise the communication skills of both the client and their communicative partner.

Communication can be a key factor in understanding challenging behaviour. Traditionally, the emphasis of intervention has been on improving expressive skills. Less interest has been focused on the strategies used to communicate with people with learning disabilities and on how far they have understood what has been said to them, although it is widely acknowledged that communication is a two-way process, involving a receiver and a sender. Training carers to give them the skills to communicate within the level of understanding of their client has been shown to increase the quantity and quality of communication with individuals with intellectual disabilities, enhance their independence and reduce the level of challenging behaviours (Dormandy, 1993; Bradshaw, 1998; Chatterton, 1999).

## Range of intervention strategies

Recent approaches have been based on observation of infants' and mothers' interactions, where mothers respond to what their infants are doing to develop a sequence of interactions and enabling the babies to participate. The carer is thus building on what the child is able to do rather than trying to teach the child a skill that he or she does not have. An increasing range of professionals are acknowledging that the typical development of carer–infant interactions provides guidelines for developing communication in people with intellectual disability.

Intensive interaction approaches have been shown to be effective in developing sociability and communication in people with severe and complex learning difficulties and are based on the process of carer–infant interaction (Burford, 1988; Nind, 1996). The approach recognises the preverbal developmental stage of the individual and suggests that behavioural difficulties may in fact be difficulties with communication and sociability (Nind & Hewett, 1994; Nind, 1996). Intensive interaction exploits and gives structure to the range of interactive and intuitive games that are part of typical carer–infant interaction. This creates reciprocal enjoyment, through which the 'teachers' adapt their own communicative behaviours in response to that of their 'pupils' in order to be engaging and meaningful and to attribute intent to the pupils' behaviours. Mothers and infants have what appear to be universals of pace of interactions, depending on the occasion and purpose. Nigerian and Scottish mothers, for instance, have been found to share precisely the same 'mother song rhythms' (Trevarthen, 1986), as do skilled interlocutors with people with profound handicaps. Burford (1988) identified five categories according to rate of 'action cycles', each cycle having its own communicative purpose.

Musical interaction, based on interactive play, has also been shown to be helpful with children who were considered unable to benefit from conventional speech and language therapy (Wimpory & Nash, 1998). Research lends support to the value of music therapy with children and adults with learning disabilities (Bunt, 1994). Art therapy also offers a way for people to express and explore thoughts, needs and feelings (Willoughby-Booth, 1998).

Any intervention should enhance the independent living skills of the client and reduce dependence on therapists and carers. It should facilitate choice and active participation in the community.

## Autistic-spectrum disorders

Most children with autistic disorders show delayed language development. However, some children with high-functioning autism or Asperger syndrome may develop mature language with rather pedantic grammar. People with an autistic-spectrum disorder often break phonological, syntactic and semantic constraints (pragmatic and situational rules are also often broken). Baltaxe (1980) showed this most noticeably in higher-functioning autism, for example in switching from an inappropriate 'formal' code to an inappropriate 'informal' code. When children with autistic-spectrum disorder of normal or near-normal IQ acquire adult speech, deviance is still noticeable. In addition to continuously breaking situational constraints and conventions of discourse, their prosody (stress, rhythm and intonation) still remains quaint. Baltaxe (1980) has commented that their speech is often improperly modulated, produced with overprecision, flat and colourless. The communicative failure of a person with Asperger syndrome is largely due to a cognitive deficit rather than a primary linguistic defect; that is, the problem is likely to be in a lack of appreciation of the other person's perspective in the social use of language (see Chapter 6).

The poorly developed theory of mind of people with high-functioning autism means that in spite of their apparantly fluent language, they may not be able to transmit their intentions clearly and they might make little or no self-repair of incomplete or 'fuzzy' unclear utterances. Sensitive help from a professional to clarify these obscure utterances may be necessary.

An extensive range of interventions has been proposed for children with autistic-spectrum disorders over recent years. A number of approaches have some evidence of effectiveness, but this is variable in quality. There is no study with rigorous control of variables such as intensity of intervention. Thus, the effectiveness of any single approach cannot be precisely isolated (Jordan *et al*, 1998).

## Educational issues

The Salamenca statement (UNESCO, 1994) affirmed the rights of all those with disabilities to have their special educational needs met within the regular education system. The 'inclusion debate' continues to reflect the anxieties of many about the implications of inclusive education (Farrell, 2001; Garner & Gains, 2001). There is a risk that if integration is viewed merely as curricular access and fails to address individual needs, exclusion rather than inclusion will result (Jordan & Powell, 1994). In our experience, the availability of effective inclusive education is dependent on attitudes, on how provision is resourced and on the availability of skilled teachers with the appropriate experience and/or training.

The Draft Special Educational Needs Code of Practice 2001 produced by the Department for Education and Skills strengthens the rights of all to be educated in a mainstream school. The code also recommends that, as communication is fundamental to learning, speech and language therapy should be normally recorded on a child's statement of educational need as an educational provision. Where the NHS is unable to provide such therapy for a child whose statement specifies it as an educational need, the responsibility rests on the local education authority to provide it unless the parents have made appropriate alternative arrangements.

## Mild learning disabilities

People with mild learning disabilities are recognised as unusual by the manner of their speech, but the causes are harder to pinpoint. Individuals with mild learning disabilities are impaired in a variety of cognitive abilities and in their knowledge of the world. Accordingly, their mastery of pragmatics may be patchy. They may have problems, for example, in taking turns: normally one speaker gives way to the next, without marked overlap or noticeable hesitation. They may be unable to produce or understand illocutionary acts, having difficulty inferring from the information available what the intention of an utterance is. People with learning disabilities may have difficulty with conversational obligations: a participant in a communicative interaction often has the option to speak or not to speak, but after a question, the listener is usually obliged to speak. They may have problems in selecting the content of their utterances. As a communicative exchange is more than a series of unrelated speaking turns, there is a logical progression and a competent listener keeps track of the topic to make an appropriate contribution. It is also important to establish reference: the listener must determine what an expression refers to and the speaker must ensure that the reference identification is possible. There must be an appropriate use of ties, i.e. linguistic devices such as 'this' and 'that', which make sentences coherent. Speakers must also ensure that when they are not understood, they repair the situation and correct any errors in their utterances. The cognitive abilities involved in such actions as repair are commonly referred to as metacognitive, i.e. they involve the ability to reflect on one's cognitive processes. Reflection is not a strength of people with learning disabilities.

During communicative interactions, the inability of some individuals with learning disabilities to provide organised texts and to design information adequately in extended discourse can cause distress, anxiety and even phobic states. This failure to take into account the listener's state of mind is at its worst in people with Wing & Gould's (1979) triad of social impairment (qualitative abnormalities in reciprocal social interaction and in communication, and a restricted, stereotyped and repetitive repertoire of interests and activities), but all who have learning disabilities are affected to some extent.

Leudar (1989) provides a useful framework for problems of pragmatics in the discourse of people with learning disabilities, describing problems of intention, of convention and of face. In problems of discernment of intention, it is difficult or impossible to discover, even in people with learning disabilities who have good syntax, what the point is. Leudar describes the conventions of conversation as the communicative 'maxims' that audiences assume speakers are abiding by. Leudar's research identified 'maxims of conversation' (originally desribed by Grice, 1975) that people who have mild learning disabilities are more likely to violate than are members of the general population. These are: the 'maxims' of quality (whether what they say is backed by evidence); relevance (whether they pick up the topic and say what is relevant); manner (whether they explain themselves in enough detail or tend to say more than is needed to be informative); disclosure (e.g. whether they talk to strangers as if they know them well); communality (whether they pay attention to the needs and interests of others).

Although unable to reflect on the causes of their communicative incompetence, people with learning disabilities may be only too aware of their conversational limitations and inappropriateness, and will take steps to avoid situations in which these might be revealed. They may become fussed when conversations are too quick or they are out of their depth, so that action must be taken by both themselves and their audience to maintain face. Leudar has also pointed out that violations of certain 'maxims' are characteristic of certain behavioural disturbances, and has shown a strong relationship between behavioural disturbance and the communicative environment. The onset of a psychiatric illness such as schizophrenia may be heralded by loss of coherence on topics. Then, as the illness progresses, syntax may also be lost, although this loss may be reduced by antipsychotic medication. The Communicative Assessment Profile (CASP; Van der Gaag, 1989), evaluates both the individual's linguistic ability and the communicative environment.

## Consultation skills

The principles of communicating with people with more-severe learning disabilities apply equally to those who have a mild learning disability. It is important to make all consultations interesting and enjoyable for people with learning disabilities. An important prerequesite is to have become well-versed regarding the interests, likes and dislikes of clients. This should enable consultants to respond sensitively as they look and listen for cues from their clients, thus making it possible to maintain a conversation. Most psychiatric interview techniques need to be modified, as they are designed for people of normal ability. Flynn (1986) provides examples of interviewing techniques and guidelines appropriate for use in learning disability.

## Advocacy issues

Intervention should always be client-centred, respecting individuals' needs and opinions and promoting their active participation in any intervention and the decision-making process associated with it. Research literature that includes the views of those with intellectual disability is sparse. Atkinson (2000) reminds us of a long history of people with learning disabilities giving up in the struggle to speak out and instead remaining silent. It is important that we are open to hear what our clients are trying to tell us, and that we provide them with a mode of communication that enables self-advocacy. This may mean at times that there should be an advocate to interpret affective and emotional communication on behalf of those with profound and multiple disabilities. Unfortunately, reliable measures of such behaviour have yet to be achieved (Hogg, 1996). Minkes *et al* (1994) describe a project in which a wide range of media (photographs, pictures and simplified questionnaires) was used to establish the views of children with intellectual disabilities regarding their experience of respite care. Some schools, to enable pupils to contribute to their own annual review advice (Department for Education and Skills, 2001), are using similar strategies. McCall *et al* (1997) and Clarke *et al* (2001) highlight the importance of consulting alternative and augmentative communication users in priorities based on their user experience.

## Collaborative/multi-agency work

Community teams working with adults with learning disabilities are not new and many have established good practice in working collaboratively, integrating speech and language therapy into care plans.

For some children, a language programme that is an integral part of the whole school day is more appropriate than being withdrawn from the classroom for a speech therapy session. Such language programmes will be delivered by school staff, but may require regular monitoring and evaluation by a speech and language therapist. It is good practice for education professionals who have received sufficient and appropriate professional development in the field of speech and language difficulties to support and assist the work of therapists in educational settings. Collaborative practice is essential for successful intervention with children and young people with speech and language difficulties. The operational flexibilities introduced under the Health Act 1999 for health services and local authorities should help to promote greater collaboration. McConnachie & Pennington (1997) discuss the requirements for setting up successful multi-disciplinary training.

Many schools have already established good collaborative practice; others are still working to achieve this. In integrated services, it is appropriate for different disciplines to take a lead on different aspects of support. A key professional in secondary and tertiary services will be a speech and language therapist. However, communication skills and a sound understanding of language development and disorder are essential for the general psychiatrist (Hollins, 2000).

The overall message of this chapter is that even those with most profound disabilities do produce communicative acts, and that parents and care staff can be very skilled in reacting to often opaque communications. The professional ought to be at least as skilled.

## References

Atkinson, J. L. (2000) Bringing lives into focus: the disabled person's perspective. In *Transition and Change in the Lives of People with Intellectual Disabilities* (ed. D. May). London: Jessica Kingsley.

Austin, J. L. (1962) *How to Do Things with Words*. London: Oxford University Press.

Baker, S. (2000) Learning through pictures. *Communication*, Spring, **34**, 15–17.

Baltaxe, C. (1980) Prosodic abnormalities in autism. In *Frontiers of Research: Proceedings of the Vth IASSMD Conference* (ed. P. Mittler). Baltimore, MD: University Park Press.

Bartlett, C. & Bunning, K. (1997) The importance of communication partnerships: a study to investigate the communicative exchanges between staff and adults with learning disabilities. *British Journal of Learning Disabilities*, **25**, 148–153.

Beveridge, M. & Conti-Ramsden, G. (1987) Social cognition and problem solving in persons with mental retardation. *Australia and New Zealand Journal of Developmental Disabilities*, **13**, 99–106.

Bondy, A. S, & Frost, L. A. (1998) The Picture Exchange Communication System. *Seminars in Speech and Language*, **19**, 373–388.

Bradshaw, J. (1998) Assessing and Intervening in the Communication Environment. *British Journal of Learning Disabilities*, **26**, 62–66.

Bunt, L. (1994) Research in music therapy in Great Britain: outcome research with handicapped children. *British Journal of Music Therapy*, **15**, 15–21.

Burford, B. (1988) Action cycles: rhythmic actions for engagement with children and young adults with profound mental handicap. *European Journal of Special Needs Education*, **3**, 189–206.

Carlton, S. (1993) *The Other Side of Autism.* Worcester: Self Publishing Association.

Chatterton, S. (1999) Communication skills workshops in learning disability nursing. *British Journal of Nursing*, **28**, 90–96.

Clarke, M., McConnachie, H., Price, K., *et al* (2001) Views of young people using augmentative and alternative communication systems. *International Journal of Language and Communication Disorders*, **36**, 107–115.

Department for Education and Skills (2001) *Special Educational Needs Code of Practice.* London: Department for Education and Skills.

Dobson, S. & Worrall, N. (2001) The way we were … a comparison of two surveys to find out how service delivery to adults with learning disabilities has changed over the past ten years. *Royal College of Speech and Language Therapists Bulletin*, **589**, 7–9.

Dormandy, K. (1993) Developments in communication assessment and intervention. In *Communication and Adults in Learning Disabilities* (eds K. Dormandy & A. Van Der Gaag). London: Whurr.

—— & Van Der Gaag, A. (1989). What colour are the alligators? A critical look at methods used to assess communication skills in adults with learning difficulties. *British Journal of Disorders of Communication*, **24**, 265–281.

Farrell, P. (2001) Special education in the last twenty years: have things really got better? *British Journal of Special Education*, **28**, 3–9.

Flynn, M. (1986) Adults who are mentally handicapped as consumers: issues and guidelines for interviewing. *Journal of Mental Deficiency Research*, **30**, 369–377.

Franco, F. & Wishart, J. (1995) Use of pointing and other gestures by young Down syndrome. *American Journal on Mental Retardation*, 100, 160–182.

Garner, P. & Gains, C. (2001) The debate begins… *Special*, 20–23.

Grandin, T. & Scariano, M. (1986) *Emergence Labelled Autism.* London: Arena Press.

Grice, H. P. (1975) Logic and conversation. In *Syntax and Semantics 3: Speech Acts* (eds P. Cole & J. L. Morgan), pp. 41–58. New York: Academic Press.

Guralnick, M. (1997) (ed.) *The Effectiveness of Early Intervention.* Baltimore, MD: Brooks.

Halliday, M. A. K. (1973) *Explorations in the Functions of Language.* London: Edward Arnold.

Hogg, J. (1996) Communication and learning disability: briefing and update on development. *Journal of the Royal Society of Medicine*, **89**, 414–415.

Hollins, S. (2000) Developmental psychiatry – insights from learning disability. *British Journal of Psychiatry*, **177**, 201–206.

Hurst-Brown, L. & Keens, A. (1990) *ENABLE: Encouraging a Natural and Better Life Experience.* London: Forum Consultancy.

Ingram, D. (1989) *First Language Acquisition: Method, Description and Explanation.* Cambridge: Cambridge University Press.

Jordan, R. & Powell, S. (1994) Critical notes on integration and entitlement. *European Journal of Special Needs Education*, **9**, 27–37.

Jordan, R., Jones, G. & Murray, D. (1998) *Educational Interventions for Children with Autism: A Literature Review of Recent and Current Research*. Sudbury: Department for Education and Employment.

Kindlon, D. J. (1998) The measurement of attention. *Child Psychology and Psychiatry Review*, **3**, 772–780.

Leudar, I. (1989) Communicative environments for mentally handicapped people. In *Language and Communication in Mentally Handicapped People* (eds M. Beveridge, G. Conti-Ramsden & I. Leudar), pp. 274–299. London: Chapman and Hall.

McCall, F., Markova, I., Murphy, J., *et al* (1997) Perspectives on AAC systems by the users and by their communication partners. *European Journal of Disorders of Communication*, **32**, 235–257.

McConnachie, H. & Pennington, L. (1997) In-service training for schools on augmentative and alternative communication. *European Journal of Disorders of Communication*, **32**, 277–289.

Minkes, J., Robinson, C. & Weston, C. (1994) Consulting the children: interviews with children using residential respite care services. *Disability Society*, **9**, 47–57.

Mitchell, D. R. (1987) Parents' interactions with their developmentally disabled or autistic infants: a focus for intervention. *Australia and New Zealand Journal of Developmental Disabilities*, **13**, 73–82.

Money, D. (1997) A comparison of three approaches to delivering a speech and language therapy service to people with learning disabilities. *European Journal of Disorders of Communication*, **32**, 449–466.

—— (2000) Delivering quality. *Royal College of Speech and Language Therapists Bulletin*, **573**, 9–10.

Nind, M. (1996) Efficiency of intensive interaction: developing sociability and communication in people with severe and complex learning difficulties using an approach based on caregiver–infant interaction. *European Journal of Special Education*, **11**, 48–66.

—— & Hewett, D. (1994) *Access to Communication: Developing the Basics of Communication with People with Severe Learning Difficulties through Intensive Interaction*. London: Fulton.

Park, K. (1997) How do objects become objects of reference? A review of the literature on objects of reference and a proposed model for the use of objects in communication. *British Journal of Special Education*, **24**, 108–114.

Potter, C. A. & Whittaker, C. A. (1997) Teaching the spontaneous use of semantic relations through multipointing to a child with autism and severe learning disability. *Child Language Teaching and Therapy*, **13**, 177–193.

Robson, C. (1993) *Real World Research. A Resource for Social Scientists and Practitioner Researchers*. Oxford: Blackwell.

Royal College of Speech and Language Therapists (1996) *Communicating Quality 2*. London: Royal College of Speech and Language Therapists.

Rutter, M. (1996) Autism research: prospects and priorities. *Journal of Autism and Developmental Disorders*, **26**, 257–275.

Spiker, D. & Hopmann, M. R. (1997) The effectiveness of early intervention for children with Down syndrome. In *The Effectiveness of Early Intervention* (ed. M. Guralnick), pp. 271–306. Baltimore, MD: Brooks.

Stansfield, J. (1998) Communication in adults with severe learning disabilities. In *Hallas' The Care of People with Intellectual Disabilities* (eds W. Fraser, D. Sines & M. Kerr). Oxford: Butterworth Heinemann.

Trevarthern, C. (1986) Development of intersubjective motor control in infants. In *Motor Development in Children: Aspects of Coordination and Control* (eds M. G. Wade & H. T. A. Whiting), pp. 209–283. Dordrecht: Martinus Nijhoff.

UNESCO (1994) *The Salamanca Statement and Framework for Action on Special Needs Education*. Paris: UNESCO.

Van Der Gaag, A. (1989) *The Communication Assessment Profile for Adults with Learning Difficulties (CASP)*. London: Speech Profiles.

Walker, M. (1973) *An Experimental Evaluation of the Success of a System of Ccommunication for the Deaf Mentally Handicapped* (MSc thesis). Available for reference from author or from following libraries: RNID, Gower Street, London; The Hilliard Collection, John Ryland's Library, Manchester University.

Weatherby, A. (1986) Ontogeny of communicative functions in autism. *Journal of Autism and Developmental Disorders*, 16, 295–315.

Williams, D. (1992) *Nobody Nowhere*. London: Doubleday.

Willoughby-Booth, S. (1998) Art therapy. In *Hallas' The Care of People with Intellectual Disabilities* (eds W. Fraser, D. Sines & M. Kerr). Oxford: Butterworth Heinemann.

Wilson, A. (2000) *AAC 2000: Practical Approaches to Augmentative and Alternative Communication*. Edinburgh: CALL Centre, University of Edinburgh.

Wimpory, D. & Nash, S. (1998) Musical interactive therapy – therapeutic play for children with autism. *Child Language Teaching and Therapy*, 152, 17–27.

Wing, L. & Gould, J. (1979) Severe impairments of social interaction and associated abnormalities in children: epidemiology and classification. *Journal of Autism and Developmental Disorders*, 9, 11–29.

Wolfsenburger, W (1983) Social role valorisation: a proposed new term for the principle of normalisation. *Mental Retardation*, 21, 234–239.

# CHAPTER 8

# Adults with learning disabilities and psychiatric problems

Mike Vanstraelen, Geraldine Holt and Nick Bouras

The co-occurrence of psychiatric illness with a learning disability has been well established, and people with learning disabilities are more likely to suffer from mental ill health (including behavioural disorders, personality disorders, autistic-spectrum disorders and attention-deficit hyperactivity disorder) (Deb *et al*, 2001*b*). The arrival of effective medical and psychosocial treatments for psychiatric disorders makes their diagnosis in those with learning disabilities all the more pressing.

In this chapter, we discuss the relationship between psychiatric problems and challenging behaviour, give an outline of aspects of assessment and diagnosis in those with learning disabilities and describe common psychiatric disorders, including schizophrenia, mood disorders, anxiety disorders, obsessive–compulsive disorder and eating disorders. Delirium and dementia are discussed in Chapters 9 and 15. The chapter concludes with an update on the planning and provision of psychiatric services.

## Psychiatric problems *v*. challenging behaviour

Emerson (1995) describes challenging behaviour as a social construct defined by social impact, without any implication about the underlying processes (Emerson *et al*, 1999). Nevertheless, challenging behaviour is the most common reason for referral to a psychiatrist in those with learning disabilities (Day, 1985).

Two large-scale studies reported by Emerson *et al* (1999), both with methodological weaknesses, found no compelling correlation between psychiatric illness and challenging behaviour. They suggest that there are at least four types of relationship of clinical significance between challenging behaviour and psychiatric disorder:

(1)   family factors associated with the development of challenging behaviour appear to be similar to those associated with the development of conduct disorder;

(2)  challenging behaviours may represent the atypical presentation of an underlying psychiatric disorder; some forms of self-injurious behaviour may represent an obsessive–compulsive disorder (see below);

(3)  challenging behaviours may occur as secondary features of psychiatric disorders among those with severe learning disabilities;

(4)  psychiatric disorders may establish a motivational basis for the expression of challenging behaviours, maintained by operant behavioural processes.

## Assessment and diagnosis

The principles of psychiatric assessment of those with learning disabilities are similar to those in general adult and child psychiatry. Particular attention, however, must be given to:

- the patient's level of understanding and ability to communicate;
- details from informants and direct observation by the clinician;
- the history of the presenting complaint over time;
- the patient's developmental history (Holland, 2000);
- physical disabilities (including sensory impairments) and medical history.

Assessment aims not only to detect the presence of mental health problems, but also to identify the features that make a person vulnerable to them. Any therapeutic interventions must take into account a number of factors, including the client's wishes, the diagnosis and these vulnerability factors. Only by addressing the last of these will the risk of relapse be reduced. They can be considered under three headings: psychological (for instance characteristic ways of thinking), biological (such as genetic predisposition or medication) and social (including environmental factors). Some of these vulnerability factors, such as brain damage, cannot be changed, but others, such as better control of epilepsy, can and should form part of the care plan. Recent guidelines on the assessment of mental health in those with learning disabilities, based on published evidence and the opinions of experts (Deb *et al*, 2001*b*), will help the clinician.

The introduction of operational criteria in ICD–10 (World Health Organization, 1992) and DSM–IV (American Psychiatric Association, 1994) and the use of structured and semi-structured interviews, such as the Psychiatric Assessment Schedule for Adults with Developmental Disability (PAS–ADD; Moss *et al*, 1993), have significantly increased the reliability of the diagnostic process in psychiatry. However, whether symptom definitions have the same validity in those with and without learning disabilities is more difficult to establish. The use of clinical judgement as an ultimate validity criterion is limited, possibly more so when applied to those with learning disabilities (Moss, 1999).

For those with moderate to severe learning disability, the *Diagnostic Criteria for Psychiatric Disorders for Use with Adults with Learning Disabilities/Mental Retardation* (DC–LD; Royal College of Psychiatrists, 2001) describes criteria for the diagnostic classification of mental health problems based on a consensus of current practice and opinion among psychiatrists working in learning disability. The aim is to complement the use of ICD–10 for those with milder or no learning disabilities.

# Schizophrenia and schizotypal and delusional disorders

## Schizophrenia

The estimated point prevalence of schizophrenia in people with learning disabilities is 3% (Fraser & Nolan, 1994), compared with 0.4% in the general population (Meltzer *et al*, 1995). The highest rates are reported in those with mild and borderline learning disability (Lund, 1985). Schizophrenia has an earlier onset in learning disability (35.4 years) than in the general population(43.8 years) (Meadows *et al*, 1991).

### Presentation

In those with mild learning disabilities and good verbal skills, the presentation of schizophrenia is similar to that in individuals without learning disabilities. There is a tendency for those with learning disabilities to show less psychopathology, especially persecutory delusions and formal thought disorder (Meadows *et al*, 1991). Paranoid symptoms and catatonia are the hallmarks of schizophrenia in the group with more-severe learning disabilities (Eaton & Menolascino, 1982). Turner (1989) reported that disturbed and aggressive behaviour, bizarre rituals and 'hysterical' behaviours are frequent atypical symptoms.

In view of the limitations in identifying psychopathology in people with more-severe learning disabilities, the DC–LD suggests that the non-affective psychotic disorders should not be sub-classified to the extent of ICD–10 (Royal College of Psychiatrists, 2001). Increased rates of schizophrenia have been reported in adults with velo-cardo-facial syndrome (Murphy *et al*, 1999).

### Treatment as a multi-professional modality

After a thorough assessment (including of risk) and diagnosis, deciding on the most appropriate place of treatment and the use of medication are important in the acute phase of the illness.

Evidence for the effectiveness of antipsychotic medication in people with these disorders and learning disabilities rests mainly on case reports and small series of patients in uncontrolled studies (Duggan & Brylewski, 1999). Nevertheless, antipsychotics are in widespread clinical use, mainly on the basis of the extrapolation of findings from general adult psychiatry. Treatments should be tailored to the individual, and so take into account any co-existing medical conditions such as epilepsy, other drugs being taken and any other particular requirements.

Other interventions such as cognitive–behavioural therapy (Dickerson, 2000) do deserve attention in those with mild or borderline learning disability, but have seldom been formally researched in this population.

Staff training in the recognition of symptoms will help to detect early relapse. Assessment and management of expressed emotion in families (Anderson & Adams, 1996) and professional carers (Clarke, 1999) can also be beneficial. Respite care and rehabilitation for those with more-chronic illnesses, including the use of day services, should be part of a comprehensive long-term management plan.

The UK700 trial outcome study of those with a severe psychotic illness reported that those with borderline intellectual disability benefit from intensive as compared with standard case management (Tyrer *et al*, 1999). Research is being undertaken to establish if this is also the case for the whole spectrum of people with learning disabilities.

## Schizoaffective disorder and atypical psychosis

The literature on schizoaffective disorder in learning disability is very sparse. Cycloid psychosis as a descriptive term has recently re-emerged with regard to atypical psychotic symptoms (ICD–10 acute polymorphic psychotic disorder without symptoms of schizophrenia) in those with Prader–Willi syndrome (Verhoeven *et al*, 1998).

# Affective disorders

## Mood disorders

People with learning disabilities can develop the full range of affective disorders. Impaired social functioning and intelligence influence the clinical presentation (Sovner & Hurley, 1983)

## Depressive disorder

Reported estimates of the point prevalence of depression in those with and without learning disabilities vary between 2% and 3% (Bouras & Drummond, 1992; Collacott *et al*, 1992; Patel *et al*, 1993; Meltzer *et al*, 1995; Cooper, 1997). Adults with mild learning disabilities living in the community may experience depression at a higher rate than non-disabled persons (Prout & Schaefer, 1985). People with Down's syndrome are possibly more likely to be diagnosed as having a depressive disorder than those with learning disabilities due to other causes (Collacott *et al*, 1992).

## Presentation

The clinical features of depression in adults with learning disabilities vary with the level of disability (Davis *et al*, 1997*b*). Those with mild learning disability show the same symptoms as their non-disabled peers, but with somewhat more prominence of loss of confidence and tearfulness (Marston *et al*, 1997).

In those with more-severe forms of learning disability, somatic symptoms and their behavioural correlates, such as changes in energy and activity levels, sleep and appetite changes, and social withdrawal (Laman & Reis 1987; Davis *et al*, 1997*b*; Clarke & Gomez, 1999; Evans *et al*, 1999; Matson *et al*, 1999), are suggestive of affective disorders. Regression to increased dependency, psychomotor agitation, increased irritability, worsening of already existing behavioural problems (Meins, 1995), aggressive (Reiss & Rojahn 1993) and self-injurious behaviours, reduced communication and social isolation (Sovner *et al*, 1993; Marston *et al*, 1997), catatonic features and visual hallucinations are more common in this group.

Suicidal thoughts and behaviours are thought to occur less frequently in those with depression and learning disability, but even in severe disability people are not unable to form such an intention (Walters, 1990; Patja *et al*, 2001).

High levels of depressed mood are associated with self- and informant-rated measures of poor social skills and low levels of social support in those with learning disabilities (Reiss & Benson, 1985; Laman & Reiss, 1987). Informant- and self-report ratings of self-concept are significantly negatively correlated with depression (Benson & Ivins, 1992). Social comparison is thought to be associated with self-esteem and depression in people with learning disabilities in the same way as it is for people without such disabilities (Dagnan & Sandhu, 1999).

Depression is also correlated with the frequency of negative automatic thoughts and feelings of hopelessness in people with mild learning disabilities (Nezu *et al*, 1995). As with schizophrenia, depression may be part of the psychiatric phenotype of genetic syndromes associated with learning disability, such as fragile X syndrome (Tranebjaerg & Orum, 1991; see Chapter 3).

## Treatment as a multi-professional modality

For those with the most severe forms of depression and those with suicidal intent, hospital admission needs to be considered. The full range of bio-psychosocial treatments should be available for people with learning disabilities.

A small number of uncontrolled case and small-series studies suggest that antidepressants can be effective in those with a learning disability combined with depressive disorder (Howland, 1992; Jawed *et al*, 1993;

Sovner *et al*, 1993; Masi *et al*, 1997; Verhoeven *et al*, 2001), but may have considerable side-effects, including increased irritability and acting out (Aman *et al*, 1986).

The literature on the use of psychological therapies for depression in this population is limited (Gaedt, 1995; Lindsay *et al*, 1993; Lindauer *et al*, 1999). Hollins & Sinason (2000) and Davis *et al* (1997*a*) highlighted the lack of available psychological therapies, of trained therapists and of research into efficacy in this area.

Electroconvulsive therapy might be effective as an adjunct to treatment in the acute phase of the most severe acute and otherwise non-responsive episodes of depression in those with learning disabilities (Cutajar & Wilson, 1999).

## Bipolar affective disorder

Deb & Hunter (1991) recorded cyclical changes in behaviour and mood in 4% of adults with learning disabilities, with and without epilepsy. The lifetime prevalence rate of manic–depressive (bipolar) disorder is 1% in those without a learning disability (Weissman *et al*, 1988).

### Similarities to and differences from people without learning disabilities

Cyclical changes in affect and activity level can be observed in and reported by people with mild to even very severe learning disabilities and their carers. These suggest a diagnosis of manic–depressive disorder (Reid, 1972). A daily record of mood and activity level can be kept. The mania rating scale items of the DASH–II screening instrument for those with learning disabilities ('restless or agitated', 'decreased need for sleep', 'irritable', 'easily distracted', 'extremely happy or cheerful for no obvious reason', 'talks loudly and quickly') show good internal correlation and specificity with the mania DSM–IV diagnosis (Matson & Smiroldo, 1997). This confirms earlier descriptions by Reid (1972), Heaton-Ward (1977) and Hucker *et al* (1979). Hassan & Mooney (1979) described pressure of speech rather than flight of ideas, increased and decreased appetite, echolalia, crying and over-activity. Mixed affective states and rapid cycling forms (more than four episodes a year) of bipolar affective disorder might be more common in those with learning disabilities (Berney & Jones, 1988). In Down's syndrome, mania is very uncommon among women, whereas in the general population the male : female ratio is equal. Those with Down's syndrome also less frequently have a positive family history (Cooper & Collacott, 1993).

In the general population, rapid cycling forms are seen more commonly in women, but in those with learning disabilities, the gender ratio is equal (Vanstraelen & Tyrer, 1999).

### Treatment as a multi-professional modality

In the acute phase of treatment, antipsychotics have been used with success (Vanstraelen & Tyrer, 1999). There is some evidence that lithium (Rivinus & Harmatz, 1979), sodium valproate and possibly carbamazepine are effective in the prophylaxis of rapid-cycling bipolar affective disorder in those with learning disabilities (Vanstraelen & Tyrer, 1999).

People with learning disabilities should have access to the full range of medical (Howland, 1992; Sovner et al, 1993; Masi et al, 1999; Clarke & Gomez, 1999), psychological (Lindsay et al, 1993) and social treatments for affective disorders.

## Persistent mood disorders

There are few studies of dysthymia, which is probably underdiagnosed, in those with learning disabilities (Jancar & Gunaratne, 1994; Masi et al, 1999). Similarly, cyclothymia (persistent mood swings not meeting severity criteria for affective disorders) has as yet received little attention in this population.

# Neurotic, stress-related and somatoform disorders

## Anxiety disorder

Stavrakaki & Mintsioulis (1997) recorded that 27% of individuals with learning disabilities had anxiety disorders. Generalised anxiety disorder is thought to be at least as common as in the general adult population (Deb et al, 2001a).

### Presentation

Gostason (1987) showed that those with mild learning disabilities have a higher degree of neuroticism than controls without learning disabilities and those with more-severe learning disabilities. Common symptoms are over-activity, panic attacks, agoraphobia, sexual dysfunction, mood changes, depersonalisation and derealisation, disruptive behaviours (including aggression and self-mutilation), somatic complaints, and sleep and appetite disturbance (Stavrakaki & Mintsioulis, 1997). In mild learning disability, symptoms of generalised anxiety disorder are similar to those in the general population, with increased 'brooding', somatic complaints and sleep disorder (Masi et al, 2000).

In more-severe learning disability, only the behavioural symptoms associated with anxiety can be reliably assessed, ruling out many core psychological symptoms of the disorder (Matson et al, 1997).

Comorbidity with other psychiatric illnesses such as depression (Stavrakaki & Mintsioulis, 1997) is common. High levels of anxiety are

**161**

thought to be part of the behavioural psychiatric phenotype in Williams syndrome (Stavrakaki & Mintsioulis, 1997).

**Treatment as a multi-professional modality:**

Treatment methods include pharmacotherapy, behavioural therapies, environmental adaptation and staff training. There is some evidence that anxiolytic drugs such as buspirone are effective in treating those with learning disabilities with anxiety (Ratey *et al*, 1989).

## Obsessive–compulsive disorder

Compulsive behaviours have reported frequencies of between 3.5% in adults with mild to profound learning disabilities (Vitiello *et al*, 1989) and 40% in those individuals with severe to profound disabilities (Bodfish *et al*, 1995). Ordering compulsions are reported to be the most prevalent.

### Presentation

The diagnostic criteria for obsessive–compulsive disorder in the general population include complex cognitive experiences such as the recognition that the thoughts or acts are under self-control. Such experiences may be impossible to identify or clarify in a person with learning disabilities.

Vitiello *et al* (1989) and Bodfish *et al* (1995) reported that compulsions were significantly associated with stereotypies and self-injurious behaviour. There are arguments for self-injurious behaviours (King, 1993), compulsions and stereotypies to be considered atypical presentations of obsessive–compulsive disorders. Both are thought to be mediated in part by the basal ganglia, they share part of their phenomenology (compulsions without obsessions have been reported in adults (Weissman *et al*, 1994)), and there is some evidence that compulsions, stereotypies and obsessive–compulsive disorder respond to drugs that cause serotonin reuptake inhibition. The nature of the relationship between such stereotyped movements or rituals and obsessive–compulsive disorders needs further clarification. The various diagnostic manuals rate them as separate disorders at present.

Obsessions and compulsions can arise in a number of disorders other than obsessive–compulsive disorder, such as depression and pervasive developmental disorder (Deb *et al*, 2001).

Obsessions and compulsions have also been associated with specific syndromes such as Prader–Willi syndrome (Dykens & Hodapp, 1999). Some specific stereotyped movements have been associated with disorders such as Rett syndrome (hand-wringing movements in front of the body) and Smith–Magenis syndrome (body self-hugging, self-biting). These are included in the behavioural phenotypes of these disorders. Although obsessions and compulsions may need pharmacological treatment in individuals with Prader–Willi syndrome, the need for and effectiveness of serotonin reuptake inhibitors in the treatment of stereotyped movements in Rett syndrome and Smith–Magenis syndrome is less established.

**Treatment as a multi-professional modality:**

If the obsessions or compulsions are symptoms of another disorder, this latter should be the initial focus of treatment. As noted above, treatment with selective serotonin reuptake inhibitors may be beneficial in obsessive–compulsive disorder, as may various behavioural techniques. These are discussed in more depth in Chapters 10, 11 and 12.

## Adjustment disorder and post-traumatic stress disorder

Children and adults with learning disability are vulnerable to emotional, physical and sexual abuse (Turk & Brown, 1993). The risk of post-traumatic stress disorder and adjustment disorder is therefore likely to be significantly increased.

# Behavioural syndromes

## Eating disorders

Gravestock (2000) suggested that 1–19% of adults with learning disabilities living in the community and 3–42% of those living in institutions have a diagnosable eating disorder, with higher rates in those with more-severe learning disabilities.

### Presentation

Eating disorder research in those with learning disabilities has covered pica, rumination and regurgitation, psychogenic vomiting, food faddiness or refusal, psychogenic loss of appetite, binge eating disorders and anorexia nervosa. In individuals with learning disabilities living in the community, deviant eating behaviour is more likely to occur in those with a comorbid psychiatric disorder (Jawed et al, 1993) and to be associated with considerable physical and social comorbidity (Gravestock, 2000). However, the impact of diagnosable eating disorders on weight, physical and mental health and social functioning has not been adequately addressed. Appropriate diagnostic criteria, multimodal assessment and clinically effective treatment approaches need to be developed.

# Planning and provision of psychiatric services

The publication of the Mansell Report (1993) on Services for People with Learning Disabilities and Challenging Behaviour or Mental Health Needs in the United Kingdom and the Royal College of Psychiatrists (1996/1997) Council Report 'Meeting the Mental Health Needs of People with Learning Disability' delivered the impetus and recommendation for the development of specialist mental health teams with expertise in both learning disability and mental health (Bouras & Holt, 2000). The White Paper *Valuing People: A New Strategy for Learning Disability for the 21st Century* (Department of Health, 2001) acknowledges this, but states that people with learning disabilities should be enabled to access general psychiatric services whenever possible.

However, generic psychiatric services often do not meet the needs of this client group, either in community settings or in hospitals (Bouras & Holt, 2001). This reflects a number of issues, including staff training (general psychiatric teams may feel that they do not have the necessary skills), resources (pressure on services, so that people with learning disabilities can be viewed as taking scarce resources from the general psychiatric population) and the vulnerability of those with learning disabilities (general psychiatric environments can be volatile and potentially violent).

The White Paper proposes clear protocols for collaboration between specialist learning disability services, specialist mental health services and generic mental health services. These will need to be agreed and in place if the assertion that the National Service Framework for Mental Health (Department of Health, 1999a) applies to all adults of working age (including those with learning disabilities) is to become a reality. The White Paper does not offer any clarification of the organisational and funding implications of achieving this.

If alternatives to in-patient treatment are to be sought whenever possible for people with learning disabilities and psychiatric disorders, the skills of staff supporting them in residential settings, whether family members or paid carers, will need to be increased. At present, many such people have no expertise in care of people with learning disabilities and psychiatric disorders. This is reflected in the difficulty of discharging people with learning disabilities and mental health needs from in-patient general psychiatric wards (Shepherd *et al*, 1997) and from specialist learning disability psychiatric beds (Watts *et al*, 2000) to suitable community placements.

For specialist services to be able to work with people in the community, the knowledge base of direct carers will need to be improved. Carers must feel confident in carrying through and monitoring interventions in collaboration with specialist services.

The White Paper proposes that if in-patient assessment and treatment are necessary, local services will have access to a specialist resource for those who cannot appropriately be admitted to general psychiatric services, even with specialist support. There is a scarcity of such resources at present within the NHS (Department of Health, 1999*b*), particularly for those requiring secure or medium-secure provision. This has led to a flourishing private industry, with people being placed sometimes at significant distances from families and friends. This makes monitoring of placement and reintegration into the local community more complicated. Financial resources are diverted from local services, making it more difficult for them to develop.

With the introduction of primary care trusts, it will be vital that the needs of those with learning disabilities and psychiatric disorders are recognised and provided for. The interface issues between the various services already highlighted will need to be clarified and resolved. This is a specialist area and primary care trusts will need appropriate advice in working within it.

# References

Aman, M. G., White, A. J., Vaithianathan, C., *et al* (1986) Preliminary study of imipramine in profoundly retarded residents. *Journal of Autism and Developmental Disorders*, **16**, 263–273.

American Psychiatric Association (1994) *Diagnostic and Statistical Manual of Mental Disorders* (4th edn) (DSM–IV). Washington, DC: APA.

Anderson, J. & Adams, C. (1996) Family interventions in schizophrenia: an effective but underused treatment. *BMJ*, **313**, 505–506.

Benson, B. A. & Ivins, J. (1992) Anger, depression and self-concept in adults with mental retardation. *Journal of Intellectual Disability Research*, **36**, 169–175.

Berney, T. & Jones, P. M. (1988) Manic–depressive disorder in mental handicap. *Australia and New Zealand Journal of Developmental Disabilities*, **14**, 219–225.

Bodfish, J. W., Crawford, T. W., Powell, S. B., *et al* (1995) Compulsions in adults with mental retardation: prevalence, phenomenology and comorbidity with stereotypy and self-injury. *American Journal of Mental Retardation*, **100**, 183–192.

Bouras, N. & Drummond, C. (1992) Behaviour and psychiatric disorders of people with mental handicaps living in the community. *Journal of Intellectual Disability Research*, **36**, 349–357.

—— & Holt, G. (2000) The planning and provision of psychiatric services for people with mental retardation. In *New Oxford Textbook of Psychiatry* (eds M. G. Gelder, J. J. Lopez-Ibor & N. C. Andreasen), pp. 2007–2012. Oxford: Oxford University Press.

—— & —— (2001) Community mental health service for adults with learning disabilities. In *Textbook of Community Psychiatry* (eds G. Thornicroft & G. Smukler), pp. 397–407. Oxford: Oxford University Press.

Clarke, D. (1999) Functional psychosis in people with mental retardation. In *Psychiatric and Behavioural Disorders in Developmental Disabilities and Mental Retardation* (ed. N. Bouras), pp.188–199. Cambridge: Cambridge University Press.

—— & Gomez, G. A. (1999) Utility of modified DCR–10 criteria in the diagnosis of depression associated with intellectual disability. *Journal of Intellectual Disability Research*, **43**, 413–420.

**165**

Collacott, R. A., Cooper, S. A. & McGrother, C. (1992) Differential rates of psychiatric disorders in adults with Down's syndrome compared with other mentally handicapped adults. *British Journal of Psychiatry*, **161**, 671–674.

Cooper S. A. (1997) Psychiatry of elderly compared to younger adults with intellectual disability. *Journal of Applied Research in Intellectual Disability*, **10**, 303–311.

— & Collacott, R. J. (1993) Mania and Down's syndrome. *British Journal of Psychiatry*, **161**, 739–743.

Cutajar, P. & Wilson, D. (1999) The use of ECT in intellectual disability. *Journal of Intellectual Disability Research*, **4**, 421–427.

Dagnan, D. & Sandhu, S. (1999) Social comparison, self-esteem and depression in people with intellectual disability. *Journal of Intellectual Disability Research*, **43**, 372–379.

Davis, J. P., Judd, F. K. & Herrman, H. (1997a) Depression in adults with intellectual disability. Part 1: A review. *Australian and New Zealand Journal of Psychiatry*, **31**, 243–251.

—, — & — (1997b) Depression in adults with intellectual disability. Part 2: A pilot study. *Australian and New Zealand Journal of Psychiatry*, **31**, 232–242.

Day, K. (1985) Psychiatric disorder in the middle-aged and the elderly mentally handicapped. *British Journal of Psychiatry*, **147**, 660–667.

Deb, S. & Hunter, D. (1991) Psychopathology of people with mental handicap and epilepsy. II: Psychiatric illness. *British Journal of Psychiatry*, **159**, 826–830.

—, Thomas, M. & Bright, C. (2001a) Mental disorder in adults who have a learning disability. 1: Prevalence of functional psychiatric illness among a 16–64 years old community-based population. *Journal of Intellectual Disability Research*, **5**, 495–505.

—, Matthews, T., Holt, G., *et al* (2001b) *Practice Guidelines for Assessment and Diagnosis of Mental Health Problems in Adults with Intellectual Disability*. Brighton: Pavilion Publishing.

Department of Health (1999a) *Modern Standards and Service Models: Mental Health National Service Framework*. London: Stationery Office.

— (1999b) *Facing the Facts. Services for People with Learning Disabilities. A Policy Impact Study of Social Care and Health Services*. London: Stationery Office.

— (2001) *Valuing People: A New Strategy for Learning Disability for the 21st Century* (CM5086). London: Stationery Office.

Dickerson, F. B. (2000) Cognitive behavioural psychotherapy for schizophrenia: a review of recent empirical studies. *Schizophrenia Research*, **43**, 71–90.

Duggan, L. & Brylewski, J. (1999) Effectiveness of antipsychotic medication in people with intellectual disability and schizophrenia: a systematic review. *Journal of Intellectual Disability Research*, **43**, 94–104.

Dykens, E. M. & Hodapp, R. M (1999) Behavioural phenotypes towards new understandings of people with developmental disabilities. In *Psychiatric and Behavioural Disorders in Developmental Disabilities and Mental Retardation* (ed. N. Bouras), pp. 96–108. Cambridge: Cambridge University Press.

Eaton, L. F. & Menolascino, F. J. (1982) Psychiatric disorders in the mentally retarded: types, problems, and challenges. *American Journal of Psychiatry*, **139**, 1297–1303.

Emerson, E. (1995) *Challenging Behaviour: Analysis and Intervention in People with Learning Difficulties*. Cambridge: Cambridge University Press.

—, Moss, S. & Kiernan, C. (1999) The relationship between challenging behaviour and psychiatric disorders in people with severe developmental disabilities. In *Psychiatric and Behavioural Disorders in Developmental Disabilities and Mental Retardation* (ed. N. Bouras), pp. 38–48. Cambridge: Cambridge University Press.

Evans, K. M., Cotton, M. M., Einfield, S. L., *et al* (1999) Assessment of depression in adults with severe or profound intellectual disability. *Journal of Intellectual Disability Research*, **24**, 147–160.

Fraser, W. & Nolan, M. (1994) Psychiatric disorders in mental retardation. In *Mental Health in Mental Retardation: Recent Advances and Practices* (ed. N. Bouras), pp. 79–92. Cambridge: Cambridge University Press.

Gaedt, C. (1995) Psychotherapeutic approaches in the treatment of mental illness and behaviour disorders in mentally retarded people: the significance of a psychoanalytical perspective. *Journal of Intellectual Disability Research*, **39**, 233–239.

Gostason, R. (1987) Psychiatric illness among the mild mentally retarded. *Upsala Journal of Medical Sciences*, **92** (suppl. 44), 115–124.

Gravestock, S. (2000) Eating disorders in adults with intellectual disability. *Journal of Intellectual Disability Research*, **44**, 625–637.

Hassan, M. K. & Mooney, R. P. (1979) Three cases of manic depressive illness in mentally retarded adults. *American Journal of Psychiatry*, **136**, 1069–1071.

Heaton-Ward, A. (1977) Psychosis in mental handicap (the Blake Marsh Lecture 1976). *British Journal of Psychiatry*, **130**, 525–533.

Holland, A. J. (2000) Classification, diagnosis, psychiatric assessment and needs assessment. In *New Oxford Textbook of Psychiatry* (eds M. G. Gelder, J. J. Lopez-Ibor & N. C. Andreasen), pp. 1935–1939. Oxford: Oxford University Press.

Hollins, S. A. & Sinason, V. (2000) Psychotherapy, learning disabilities and trauma: new perspectives. *British Journal of Psychiatry*, **176**, 32–36.

Howland, R. H. (1992) Fluoxetine treatment of depression in mentally retarded adults. *Journal of Nervous & Mental Disease*, **180**, 202–205.

Hucker, S. J., Day, K. E., George, S., *et al* (1979) Psychosis in mentally handicapped adults. In *Psychiatric Illness and Mental Handicap* (eds P. E. Snaith), pp. 52–76. London: Gaskell.

Jancar, J. & Gunaratne, I. J. (1994) Dysthymia and mental handicap. *British Journal of Psychiatry*, **164**, 691–693.

Jawed, S. H., Krishnan, V. H., Prasher, V. P., *et al* (1993) Worsening of pica as a symptom of depressive illness in a person with severe mental handicap. *British Journal of Psychiatry*, **162**, 835–837.

King, B. H. (1993) Self injury by people with mental retardation: a compulsive behaviour hypothesis. *American Journal on Mental Retardation*, **98**, 93–112.

Laman, D. S. & Reiss, S. (1987) Social skill deficiencies associated with depressed mood of mentally retarded adults. *American Journal on Mental Deficiency*, **92**, 224–229.

Lindauer, S. E., DeLeon, I. G. & Fisher, W. W. (1999) Decreasing signs of negative affect and correlated self-injury in an individual with mental retardation and mood disturbances. *Journal of Applied Behavioural Analysis*, **32**, 103–106.

Lindsay, W. R., Howells, L. & Pitcaithly, D. (1993) Cognitive therapy for depression with individual with intellectual disabilities. *British Journal of Medical Psychology*, **66**, 135–141.

Lund, J. (1985) The prevalence of psychiatric morbidity in mentally retarded adults. *Acta Psychiatrica Scandinavica*, **72**, 563–570.

Mansell, J. L. (Chairman) (1993) *Services for People with Learning Disabilities and Challenging Behaviour or Mental Health Needs: Report of a Project Group*. London: HMSO.

Marston, G. M., Perry, D. W. & Roy, A. (1997) Manifestations of depression in people with intellectual disability. *Journal of Intellectual Disability Research*, **41**, 476–480.

Masi, G., Marcheschi, M. & Pfanner, P. (1997) Paroxetine in depressed adolescents with intellectual disability: an open label study. *Journal of Intellectual Disability Research*, **41**, 268–272.

——, Murri, M., Favilla, L., *et al* (1999) Dysthymic disorders in adolescents with intellectual disability. *Journal of Intellectual Disabiliy Research*, **43**, 80–87.

——, Favilla, L. & Mucci, M. (2000) Generalised anxiety disorder in adolescents and young adults with mental retardation. *Psychiatry*, **63**, 54–64.

Matson, J. L. & Smiroldo, B. B. (1997) Validity of the Mania Subscale of the Diagnostic Assessment for the Severely Handicapped – II (DASH–II). *Research in Developmental Disabilities*, **18**, 221–225.

—, Smiroldo, B. B., Hamilton, M., *et al* (1997) Do anxiety disorders exist in persons with severe and profound mental retardation? *Research in Developmental Disabilities*, **18**, 39–44.

—, Rush, K. S., Hamilton, M., *et al* (1999) Characteristics of depression as assessed by the Diagnostic Assessment for the Severely Handicapped – II (DASH–II). *Research in Developmental Disabilities*, **20**, 305–313.

Meadows, G., Turner, T., Campbell, L., *et al* (1991) Assessing schizophrenia in adults with mental retardation: a comparative study. *British Journal of Psychiatry*, **158**, 103–105.

Meins W. (1995) Symptoms of major depression in mentally retarded adults. *Journal of Intellectual Disability Research*, **39**, 41–45.

Meltzer, H., Gill, B., Petticrew, M., *et al* (1995) *The Prevalence of Psychiatric Morbidity among Adults Living in Private Households: OPCS Survey of Psychiatric Morbidity in Great Britain. Report.* London: Stationery Office.

Moss, S. C. (1999) Assessment: conceptual issues. In *Psychiatric and Behavioural Disorders in Developmental Disabilities and Mental Retardation* (ed. N. Bouras), pp. 18–37. Cambridge: Cambridge University Press.

—, Patel, P., Prosser H., *et al* (1993) Psychiatric morbidity in older people with moderate and severe learning disability (mental retardation). Part I: Development and reliability of the patient interview (PAS–ADD). *British Journal of Psychiatry*, **163**, 471–480.

Murphy, K. C., Jones, L. A. & Owen, M. J. (1999) High rates of schizophrenia in adults with velo cardio facial syndrome. *Archives of General Psychiatry*, **56**, 940–945.

Nezu, C. M., Nezu, A. M., Rotherburg, J. L., *et al* (1995) Depression in adults with mild mental retardation: are cognitive variables involved? *Cognitive Therapy and Research*, **19**, 227–239.

Patel P., Goldberg D. & Moss S. (1993) Psychiatric morbidity in older people with moderate and severe learning disability (mental retardation). Part II: The prevalence study. *British Journal of Psychiatry*, **163**, 481–491.

Patja, K., Ivanainen, M., Raitasuo, S., *et al* (2001) Suicide mortality in mental retardation: a 35 year follow up study. *Acta Psychiatrica Scandinavica*, **103**, 307–311.

Prout, H. T. & Schaefer, B. M. (1985) Self-reports of depression by community-based mildly mentally retarded adults. *American Journal of Mental Deficiency*, **90**, 220–222.

Ratey, J. J., Sovner, R., Mikkelsen, E., *et al* (1989) Buspirone therapy for maladaptive behavior and anxiety in developmentally disabled persons. *Journal of Clinical Psychiatry*, **50**, 382–384.

Reid, A. H. (1972) Psychosis in adult mental defectives. I: Manic depressive psychosis. *British Journal of Psychiatry*, **120**, 205–212.

Reiss, S. & Benson, B. A. (1985) Psychosocial correlates of depression in mentally retarded adults. I: Minimal social support and stigamatization. *American Journal of Mental Deficiency*, **89**, 331–337.

— & Rojahn, J. (1993) Joint occurrence of depression and aggression in children and adults with mental retardation. *Journal of Intellectual Disability Research*, **37**, 287–294.

Rivinus, T. M. & Harmatz, J. S. (1979) Diagnosis and lithium treatment of affective disorder in the retarded: five case studies. *American Journal of Psychiatry*, **136**, 551–554.

Royal College of Psychiatrists (1996/1997) *Meeting the Mental Health Needs of People with Learning Disability* (Council Report CR56). London: Royal College of Psychiatrists.

— (2001) *DC–LD [Diagnostic Criteria for Psychiatric Disorders for Use with Adults with Learning Disabilities/Mental Retardation]* (Occasional Paper OP48). London: Gaskell.

Shepherd, G., Beadsmoore, A., Moore, C., *et al* (1997) Relation between bed use, social deprivation, and overall bed availability in acute adult psychiatric units, and alternative residential options: a cross sectional survey, one day census data, and staff interviews. *British Medical Journal*, **314**, 262–266.

Sovner, R., & Hurley, A. D. (1983) Do the mentally retarded suffer from affective illness? *Archives of General Psychiatry*, **40**, 61–67.

——, Fox, C. J., Lowry, M. J., *et al* (1993) Fluoxetine treatment of depression and associated self-injury in two adults with mental retardation. *Journal of Intellectual Disability Research*, **37**, 301–311.

Stavrakaki, C. & Mintsioulis, G. (1997) Implications of clinical study of anxiety disorders in persons with mental retardation. *Psychiatric Annals*, **27**, 182–189.

Tranebjaerg, L. & Orum, A. (1991) Major depressive disorder as a prominent but underestimated feature of fragile X syndrome. *Comprehensive Psychiatry*, **32**, 83–87.

Turk, V. & Brown, H. (1993) The sexual abuse of adults with learning disabilities: results of a two year incidence survey. *Mental Handicap Research*, **6**, 193–216.

Turner, T. H. (1989) Schizophrenia and mental handicap: a historical review, with implications for further research. *Psychological Medicine*, **19**, 301–314.

Tyrer P., Hassiotis, A., Ukoumunne, O., *et al* (1999) UK 700 Group. Intensive case management for patients with borderline intelligence. *Lancet*, **354**, 999–1000.

Vanstraelen, M. & Tyrer, S. P. (1999) Rapid cycling bipolar affective disorder in people with intellectual disability. A systematic review. *Journal of Intellectual Disability Research*, **43**, 349–359.

Verhoeven, W. M., Curfs, L. M. & Tuinier, S. (1998) Prader–Willi syndrome and cycloid psychosis. *Journal of Intellectual Disability Research*, **42**, 455–462.

——, Veendrik-Meekes, M. J., Jacobs, G. A., *et al* (2001) Citalopram in mentally retarded patients with depression: a long-term clinical investigation. *European Psychiatry*, **16**, 104–108.

Vitiello, B., Spreat, S. & Behar, D. (1989) Obsessive–compulsive disorder in mentally retarded patients. *Journal of Nervous and Mental Disease*, **177**, 232–236.

Walters, R. M. (1990) Suicidal behaviour in severely mentally handicapped patients. *British Journal of Psychiatry*, **157**, 444–446.

Watts, R. V., Richold, P. & Berney, T. P. (2000) Delay in the discharge of psychiatric in-patients with learning disabilities. *Psychiatric Bulletin*, **24**, 179–181.

Weissman, M. M., Leaf, P. J., Tischler, G. L., *et al* (1988) Affective disorders in five United States communities. *Psychological Medicine*, **18**, 141–153.

——, Bland, R. C., Canino, G. J., *et al* (1994) The cross national epidemiology of obsessive–compulsive disorder. The cross national collaborative group. *Journal of Clinical Psychiatry*, **55** (suppl. 3), 5–10.

World Health Organization (1992) *The ICD–10 Classification of Mental and Behavioural Disorders*. Geneva: WHO.

# CHAPTER 9

# Psychiatry of learning disability in older people

Sally-Ann Cooper

This chapter focuses on the psychiatry of learning disability in older people. It should be read in conjunction with other chapters in this book, in particular Chapter 15, regarding the psychiatry of Down's syndrome, as the specific association between Down's syndrome and dementia will not be detailed here.

The latter part of the 20th century saw a growing awareness of the importance of recognising and meeting the needs of older people with learning disabilities. The key factor for such a change was the increasing lifespan of all people with learning disabilities. Although the population as a whole is living longer, the rate of increase in lifespan is greater for people with learning disabilities than it is for the rest of the general population. In other words, the lifespan of people with learning disabilities is starting to catch up with that of the rest of the population. This change was demonstrated by Puri *et al* (1995). They compared the mean age at death for people with learning disabilities living in institutions during different periods of time. During the period 1931–1935, it was 14.9 years for men and 22.0 years for women. Twenty years later, during the period 1951–1955, mean age at death had increased to 29.2 years for men and 36.3 years for women, and during 1976–1980 (at the same UK institution), it had increased to 58.3 years for men and 59.8 years for women.

Other similar studies have shown the same trend, although later studies may not be representative of all people with learning disabilities, in view of the process of resettlement of individuals from long-stay hospitals, with some resettlement programmes discharging younger individuals in advance of older people. Findings from the community also confirm the trend of increasing lifespan (McCurley *et al*, 1972; Miller & Eyman, 1978; Strauss & Kastner, 1996). Janicki *et al* (1998) reported mean age at death for all people with learning disabilities aged 40 years or over living in New York State during the period 1984–1993 according to the New York State database of people with learning disabilities. They found that the oldest person with learning disabilities lived to the age of 102 years, and that the average age at death was 66.1 years. This compared with 70.4 years for the mean age at death for the New York State general population. People with Down's syndrome do not, on average, live as long as people with learning disabilities resulting from other causes: Janicki *et al* (1998) reported the mean age at death to be 55.8 years, with the oldest person living to be 77 years. Previous research has also highlighted that the individuals with learning disabilities who live the longest are women who do not have Down's syndrome, have milder rather that more severe levels of learning disabilities and have good mobility (Jacobson *et al*, 1985). Among people with profound learning disabilities, life expectancy is shorter for those who are immobile and require tube feeding (Eyman *et al*, 1990). The average lifespan of people with learning disabilities in general is showing a marked increase each decade (Richards & Siddiqui, 1980; Carter & Jancar, 1983; Fryers, 1984, 1997; Malone, 1988).

There are many reasons for the lifespan changes. In part, they mirror changes seen in the general population, with factors affecting the general population also affecting people with learning disabilities. There are also some factors that are of greater relevance for people with learning disabilities. These include a move away from institutional care, which may have contributed to the spread of infectious diseases; changing attitudes, bringing better and healthier lifestyles (Carter & Jancar, 1983); and access to medical treatments that used to be denied, such as treatment for respiratory infections and congenital heart disease. Examples of such denial include the proposal that surgical treatment for atrioventricular canal defects should not be offered to children if they had Down's syndrome (Bull *et al*, 1985), although others at the time rejected this notion and advocated an equitable provision of surgery (Menaham & Mee, 1985; Wilson *et al*, 1985). A pivotal case in testing public attitudes was that of *R v Arthur* (1981). The defendant made an entry in the case notes of a baby with Down's syndrome, stating 'parents do not wish it to survive. Nursing care only'. Food was withheld and DF118 5 mg prescribed 4-hourly. The baby died after 69 hours and the cause of death was recorded as bronchopneumonia. Although the defendant was acquitted of murder, important ethical issues were highlighted by the trial. Subsequently, provision of medical care has improved for children and adults with learning disabilities, and this is cited as one cause of the increased longevity found in a British study (McLoughlin, 1988).

The trend towards increasing lifespan is expected to continue. The majority of today's adults with learning disabilities will live into middle age and many will live into old age. Consequently, although older people with learning disabilities form only a small proportion of the whole population, of the general population of older people and of the population of all adults with learning disabilities, they are increasing in number. Hence, a knowledge of the mental health needs of older people with learning disabilities is important.

## Comparison with younger adults

It may be useful to consider some of the similarities and differences between younger and older adults with learning disabilities, particularly when considering service provision. There is no internationally agreed definition of whom the term 'older adult' refers to, as in part it relates to individual factors as well as to chronological age. However, if one considers persons over 60 years of age, some differences are seen when compared with younger adults with learning disabilities.

As learning disabilities affect more males than females, there are a greater number of men than women among younger adults with learning disabilities. This gender ratio changes with increasing age, as women with learning disabilities tend to live longer than men (as in the general population). Consequently, for the population aged 60 and over, an equal gender distribution is found, with women starting to outnumber men in extreme old age (Cooper, 1998a).

As people with more-severe learning disabilities do not, on average, live as long as individuals with milder learning disabilities, older adults with learning disabilities tends to have a higher ability level when compared with the younger adult population. For similar reasons, older adults have lower rates of epilepsy, although this is still reported to be present in about 20% of the population aged 65 years or over (Cooper, 1998b). Certain types of learning disability are less common in older than in younger adults. This is due to differences in lifespan; for example, people with Down's syndrome, cerebral palsy or learning disabilities caused by syndromes also associated with multiple physical disabilities usually die at a younger age.

Although these population differences are seen between younger and older adults with learning disabilities, it is important to note that lifespan changes are affecting all people with learning disabilities. Consequently, the current cohort of older adults with learning disabilities includes individuals with a wide ranges of conditions: profound learning and multiple physical disabilities; other complex disabilities; Down's syndrome; cerebral palsy; a variety of other syndromes associated with learning disability; epilepsy; mobility and feeding problems; and developmental disabilities such as autistic-spectrum disorders. Furthermore, the number of such individuals reaching old age will continue to increase.

People with learning disabilities may have additional risk factors that predispose towards or precipitate mental health needs. These include all of the risk factors that affect members of the general population – biological, psychological and social factors – but also additional risk factors associated with having learning disabilities. The latter include: biological factors such as the behavioural phenotypes associated with certain causes of learning disabilities, epilepsy and other neurological disorders; psychological factors such as neglect, exploitation, abuse and disadvantages in early life that affect personality development and development of coping strategies; social factors such as limited social networks, isolation, low income, lack of employment and recreational opportunities, multiple concurrent life events, stigma and being excluded; and developmental factors such as needs related to communication or limited verbal skills. The older person with learning disabilities remains vulnerable to the risk factors for mental health needs that affect both the general population and people with learning disabilities, but additionally acquires risk factors that are associated with ageing. As people age, they experience physical health problems, may become frail, may acquire additional sensory impairments, have changing social networks and social environments and their risk for certain mental health needs increases, particularly in dementia.

Many of today's older adults with learning disabilities have experienced institutional care, often from birth or a very young age. Service provision for people with learning disabilities in the past was largely confined to the institutions, and parents were often advised that it was best to admit their son or daughter to an institution. In some cases, this may have influenced the individual's personality development, as some experienced adverse events damaging to their development, failed to have a special parental figure during their early developmental phase and grew up with a repeated pattern of broken relationships owing to staff changes. Although some of the current cohort of younger adults with learning disabilities will have had similar past experiences, the advent of community care will hopefully bring changes for tomorrow's young adults in terms of enabling personality development, healthy coping styles, confidence, self-esteem and assertiveness that might have beneficial effects on predisposition to mental health needs in adult life (i.e. protective rather than vulnerability factors). This is speculative and requires scientific testing, but the negative aspects of past life experiences appear very real for many older adults with learning disabilities.

Many young adults with learning disabilities live in their family home with parents, or move to their own home but retain regular contact with family members. As individuals with learning disabilities age, they may be bereaved of parents and family contact may diminish. Family and family friends often form a very important part of the social networks of adults with learning disabilities, and this therefore becomes limited for the older person with learning disabilities.

The psychiatric assessment of an older person with learning disabilities has many similarities to that of a younger person with learning disabilities. Whether psychiatric disorders present differently in older compared with younger adults with learning disabilities has not yet been researched. Some disorders, of course, become more prevalent – particularly dementia. The assessment must consider the additional physical problems and frailty that are related to older age and can cause the onset of sensory impairments, pain or mobility problems. These problems can significantly affect mental health. Treatment plans will often be similar to those devised for younger adults with learning disabilities, but additional considerations are required. For example, the context of the person's social networks may be important and specific work regarding bereavement may be required. Drugs should be prescribed in therapeutic doses, as for younger adults, but require careful monitoring as there are theoretical risks of a higher level of drug side-effects (although this has not been scientifically tested). For drugs that are hepatically metabolised and renally excreted, it is important to measure serum urea and electrolytes and to perform liver function tests. The prescriber should also be aware of, and monitor for, the potential risk of psychotropic drugs affecting cognitive skills or inducing confusional states.

A consideration of group differences (as above) is important when trying to identify population needs and plan appropriate services. Many adults, both younger and older, are similar in terms of the things that are important to them: choice, appropriate support for independence, having their own home, occupation, recreation and social opportunities, and having friends and a close relationship. However, individuals also differ from each other and have their particular likes and dislikes, differing life experiences and differing social situations. It is always important to try to understand and respect the perspective of the individual when undertaking psychiatric assessments and developing plans for treatments, interventions and supports.

## Comparison with the older general population

Older people with learning disabilities are at risk of age-related disorders, including physical disorders, becoming frail and acquiring mental health needs such as dementia. In this respect, they share similarities with the older general population. However, many older people with learning disabilities retain their lifelong disabilities into old age, and therefore have biological differences from the general population. These differences have a bearing upon their needs, the most appropriate methods of assessment and their required treatments, interventions and supports. Psychological, social and developmental differences (including communication needs) must also be considered.

Although epilepsy is less common among older compared with younger adults with learning disabilities, about 20% of people with learning disabilities aged 65 years or older have epilepsy (Cooper, 1998*b*). Hence, psychiatric assessments of older adults with learning disabilities often need to consider the differential diagnosis of mental disorder, epilepsy, particularly complex partial seizures, and anti-epileptic drug side-effects (as all can present in a similar way). Treatment plans need to consider the drug interactions that exist between most psychotropic drugs and anti-epileptic drugs. The person undertaking the assessments and implementing the treatment plan will require experience and a knowledge base across all of these areas. This issue is less pertinent when working with older people from the general population.

An understanding of behavioural phenotypes and problem behaviours is just as important when working with older as with younger adults with learning disabilities, whereas it is of lesser importance for the general population. Many syndromes that cause learning disabilities are associated with particular behavioural phenotypes, such as Down's syndrome with dementia and depression, Prader–Willi syndrome with affective psychosis, and autism with depression. Individuals with such syndromes can live into old age and present with these associated mental health needs late in life. A knowledge of the associations of syndromes can also appropriately influence treatment choices in a way that is not of relevance for older adults from the general population. For example, Down's syndrome is associated with a relative brain seroton-ergic deficiency and therefore first-line drug treatment for depressive episodes should be a selective serotonergic reuptake inhibitor.

The level of a person's learning disability has a pathoplastic effect upon clinical presentation of psychiatric disorders. Consequently, clinical presentations differ between the older general population and the older person with a learning disability. For example, when depressed, only the most able persons with learning disabilities will describe worthlessness, hopelessness, suicidal ideation or nihilism. Reporting such symptoms requires the person to have good verbal skills and also to have achieved the intellectual level required to understand such complex concepts. A person with severe learning disabilities is unlikely to achieve this degree of sophisticated reasoning. Conversely, some symptoms seen commonly in psychiatric disorders in older adults with learning disabilities occur rarely in the older general population. Examples of these include aggression, loss of skills, reduced speech and increase in or onset of problem behaviours, all of which are common symptoms of depression in adults with learning disabilities. Differences in symptomatology within the same psychiatric disorder between older and younger adults with learning disabilities have not been scientifically studied. For further details of the pathoplastic effects of ability level on clinical symptomatology within psychiatric disorders, readers are referred to DC–LD (Royal College of Psychiatrists, 2001).

Given the wide ability range found within any group of older adults with learning disabilities, there are both similarities and differences when compared with the general population. For those with only mild learning disabilities, in the absence of other additional lifelong disabilities (for example, syndromes with an associated behavioural phenotype, epilepsy, autistic-spectrum disorders, problem behaviours or specific disabilities such as specific communication needs), mental health needs may be similar to those found in the older general population. Appropriate approaches to assessment and devising the required treatment, intervention and support plans may also be similar. However, this will not be the case for people with more-severe or profound learning disabilities, where particular attention will be required to understand any late-life onset of psychiatric disorder within the context of the person's lifelong disabilities; paying attention to communication needs, appropriate and detailed methods of assessment, and devising developmentally appropriate treatment, intervention and support plans are all necessary.

The past experiences of older people with learning disabilities have both similarities and differences when compared with those of older people of average ability. The more able person with learning disabilities may have memories of the same past events, such as the Second World War, the Queen's coronation and decimalisation. However, the details of their memories may well differ – for example, the war effort of a person with learning disabilities may well have been confined within an institution. This has a bearing when considering psychiatric interventions such as reminiscence groups, and also when considering the aetiologies of psychiatric disorders. Institutional living will have been experienced by many of the current cohort of older people with learning disabilities. This is in marked contrast to the older general population and has a lasting impact on the person throughout life and into old age. Other past experiences are also likely to differ. For example, in the past, people with significant learning disabilities were unlikely to have been occupied in paid employment, unlike the general population. They are more likely to have had restricted life experiences and opportunities.

Family networks are also likely to differ for the older person with learning disabilities compared with the older person from the general population. The majority of persons with learning disabilities do not marry or raise children. Consequently, family networks following the bereavement of parents tend to be limited to siblings and nieces or nephews (who are likely also to have other family commitments). This contrasts with the older general population, the majority of whom will be in contact with their adult children and may still have a living spouse. When an older person with learning disabilities acquires a mental disorder, they are less able to turn to family members for practical or emotional support and are more reliant on services.

Older people of average ability are likely to live at home. When they become frail, in many circumstances it is possible to remain at home with additional community supports. They may start to attend day clubs or centres for additional support. Older people with learning disabilities might have attended a day centre as their main form of occupation during adult life, but be retired from it on reaching old age, despite this often being a time when needs are increasing (Cooper, 1998a). Some older persons with learning disabilities live in their own homes, but others live in group care settings specifically designed for adults with learning disabilities or in care settings designed for older people of average abilities (i.e. nursing homes). In either of these situations, older individuals with learning disabilities are likely to be in the minority, perhaps the only person with special needs and there is a risk that these needs will be overlooked. A similar phenomenon to that for which Reiss *et al* (1982) coined the term 'diagnostic overshadowing' can occur: in learning disability care settings designed for younger adults, newly acquired needs of older adults might be inappropriately attributed to untreatable aspects of ageing. In care settings designed for the older general population, newly acquired needs of older adults with learning disabilities might be inappropriately attributed to untreatable aspects of learning disabilities (Cooper, 1997a).

# Psychiatric disorders

## *Prevalence*

Given that the older person with learning disabilities is vulnerable to acquiring mental health needs due to the risk factors that affect the whole of the general population, the risk factors specific to people with learning disabilities and the risk factors associated with ageing, one would speculate that a high prevalence of mental health needs would be found in this population. Studies have sought to describe the mental health needs of the older population, although the conclusions that can be drawn are limited owing to:

(a)   biased sampling, such as being limited to individuals living within institutions or referred for psychiatric assessment;
(b)   samples that are large and likely to be representative of the population with learning disabilities, but rely on known diagnoses rather than conducting individual assessments;
(c)   samples representative of the population with learning disabilities, all of whom participated in an individual psychiatric assessment for the purpose of the study, but which are limited by small sample size (Corbett, 1979; Lund, 1985; Moss & Patel, 1993; Cooper, 1997b,c).

The further consideration of prevalence in this chapter will focus on this last group.

It can be misleading to talk about the overall prevalence of mental health needs within the population without defining which disorders are included, as most studies differ in this regard. Similarly, studies differ in terms of the age ranges included, the methods of assessment employed and the diagnostic criteria utilised. All of the published studies cited above pre-date the publication of DC–LD (Royal College of Psychiatrists, 2001) and all used different diagnostic criteria, usually modified in a variety of different ways. Despite these differences, the studies do show a high prevalence of mental health needs, as expected, and similarities between studies when comparing findings of prevalences for specific disorders. Cooper (1997b) found an overall prevalence of psychiatric disorders in 68.7% of older adults with learning disabilities aged 65 years and over (n=134) compared with 47.9% for adults with learning disabilities aged 20–64 years (n=73). These figures include problem behaviours, dementia, autism and past history of affective disorder, as well as point prevalence for mental illness.

The studies provide a replicated finding for prevalence of depression: 4.3% for those aged 45 years and over (n=94) (Lund, 1985), 5.7% for those aged 50 years and over (n=105) (Moss and Patel, 1993), 4.5% for those aged 60 years and over (n=110) (Corbett, 1979) and 6.0% for those aged 65 years and over (n=134) (Cooper, 1997b). Schizophrenia, which has previously been noted to occur at least at three times the general population rate (Turner, 1989), is found to continue to be prevalent in older adults with learning disabilities, with a point prevalence of about 3% (Corbett, 1979; Lund, 1985; Cooper, 1997b). Anxiety disorders appear to be common and problem behaviours are found to persist into old age, as was previously highlighted by Reid & Ballinger (1995), as do pervasive developmental disorders. Indeed, the full range of psychiatric disorders occur in older adults with learning disabilities, including high rates of dementia, depressive episodes, anxiety disorders and problem behaviours. The importance of accurate diagnosis has been highlighted, as in many cases carers and non-specialist staff may misinterpret symptoms of potentially treatable mental illness in older people with learning disabilities (as in younger adults with learning disabilities) as being problem behaviours related to environmental or developmental factors, with resultant failure to deliver appropriate treatments and interventions (Cooper, 1998c).

## Dementia

Dementia is particularly prevalent in older people with learning disabilities. It is well recognised that Down's syndrome is associated with dementia (Oliver & Holland, 1986; Holland & Oliver, 1995), with about half of all individuals with Down's syndrome who live long enough eventually acquiring clinical dementia (Prasher, 1995). This contrasts with the near 100% of adults with Down's syndrome over the age of 40 years who are found at post-mortem examination to have the neuropathological changes of Alzheimer's disease (Mann, 1988). The association between Down's syndrome and dementia is discussed in greater depth in Chapter 15. However, most adults with Down's syndrome do not yet live into old age and less than 4% of the population with learning disabilities aged 65 years or over have Down's syndrome. Despite this, about 22% aged 65 years or over have dementia (Lund, 1985; Cooper, 1997c) and about 12% aged 50 years or over (Lund, 1985; Moss & Patel, 1993; Cooper, 1997c). This is four times the prevalence rate for dementia in the age-matched general population. A comparison of these findings with findings for people with Down's syndrome and the pooled European prevalence data for dementia within the general population (Hofman *et al*, 1991) suggests that having Down's syndrome brings forward one's risk for dementia by about 30 years, and having learning disabilities brings forward one's risk by about 15 years. This is illustrated in the Fig. 9.1, which plots data from the general population (Hofman *et al*, 1991), the population with Down's syndrome (Prasher, 1995) and the population with learning disabilities (Cooper, 1997c).

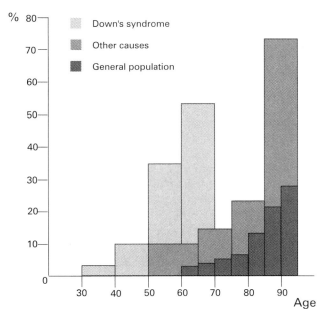

**Fig 9.1** Comparative prevalence rates of dementia at different ages for people with Down's syndrome, people with learning disabilities of different causes and the non-learning-disabled population

Neuropathological studies have also confirmed a high prevalence of Alzheimer's disease during post-mortem examination of adults with learning disabilities from causes other than Down's syndrome: 31% of older adults (Barcikowski *et al*, 1989); 54% of adults aged 50–64 years; and 76% of those aged 66–75 years (Popovitch *et al*, 1990).

Although there has been considerable research effort to gain an understanding of the neuroradiological findings, genetic studies, clinical presentation and progress of dementia in adults with Down's syndrome, little research has been conducted into dementia in people with learning disabilities from causes other than Down's syndrome. The cause of the higher prevalence rate when age-matched with the general population is unknown. Prevalence increases with age, as for the general population. Other possible risk factors for dementia such as oestrogen reduction, oxidative/inflammatory stress, vascular factors (smoking, diabetes, hypertension, cardiac ischaemia), head trauma, educational level, chemicals (iron, aluminium), depression, parental age, alcohol and genetic factors (amyloid precursor protein, presenilin-1, presenilin-2, apolipoprotein-E genotype, $\alpha_1$-antichymotrypsin, cytochrome C oxidase, tau gene mutations, angiotensin converting enzyme) remain unstudied in this population.

Diagnosis of dementia is dependent on a thorough psychiatric assessment and the elimination of the other differential diagnoses by considering the psychopathology of dementia and other mental disorders (notably depressive episodes and psychoses) and the elimination of physical causes for the presentation by direct questioning, physical examination, blood and urine tests and other special investigations as indicated. As for any psychiatric assessments undertaken with younger or older adults with learning disabilities, it is always essential to conduct the assessment with a relative and/or support worker as well as with the individuals themselves. It is important to determine what features have changed, i.e. to distinguish new symptoms from long-standing traits, and to establish the time-scale of events. The information of current support workers, who know the person quite well now but have only limited past information on the individual must be supplemented with that of an informant from the past – a living relative if possible, or a past carer, for example from a day centre that the person used to attend when younger. Even the most able person with learning disabilities will require a collateral history to be taken, perhaps because he or she has difficulties remembering time-scales, sequences of events or detailed information, even when great care is taken to ask open, developmentally appropriate questions and to be alert to the possibility of suggestibility.

Instruments used to screen for dementia in the general population, such as the Mini-Mental State Examination (Folstein *et al*, 1975), are not appropriate for use with people with learning disabilities. This is because the score gained depends on the person's underlying level of learning disability, regardless of the presence or extent of acquired dementia. Diagnosis is essentially a clinical one, with demonstration of skill loss, together with a psychopathological profile of dementia rather than other mental illness, and elimination of other possible physical or environmental causes of skill loss. Aylward *et al* (1997) discuss some of the ratings that might be considered and DC–LD (Royal College of Psychiatrists, 2001) presents diagnostic criteria for dementia, specifically designed for this particular population. Rating scales such as the Vineland Scale (Sparrow *et al*, 1987) and the Adaptive Behaviour Scale (Nihira *et al*, 1993), which measure adaptive behaviour (skills), may be useful for monitoring the progress of dementia or for comparing current performance with an assessment of the previous best functional level. The role of cognitive assessments and screens such as the Severe Impairment Battery (University of Pittsburgh, 1993), the Test for Severe Impairment (Albert & Cohen, 1992) and the Dementia Questionnaire for Persons with Mental Retardation (Evenhuis, 1992) has yet to be determined.

In learning disability, as in Down's syndrome, non-cognitive symptoms are a common feature of dementia. They include psychiatric symptoms such as anxiety, altered mood, persecutory delusions and hallucinations, as well as problem behaviours such as aggression and disturbed sleep (Cooper & Prasher, 1998). These non-cognitive symptoms can often be more distressing to the person and to the person's support worker or carer than are the cognitive or skill changes of dementia, and if present, they warrant direct treatments and interventions to minimise such symptomatology.

The required multi-disciplinary management of dementia will vary from person to person, depending on their individual circumstances. However, the following areas should be considered when treatment, intervention and support plans are devised.

(1)   Maximise functioning by correcting any other identified health or care needs, for example correct anaemias, treat urinary tract infections, adjust hearing aids, prescribe spectacles, buy properly fitting shoes, and provide foot and toenail care.

(2)   Provide information to the people with learning disabilities and to their relative or support worker in a manner that is understandable and sensitive to the potentially high emotional impact that it may have.

(3)   Minimise the cognitive symptoms of dementia. This will require environmental considerations such as: placing pictures on doors to identify rooms; daily timetabling of activities and maintaining a routine, with presentation of diary or timetable information in pictorial form; reminiscence groups and practising of skills as part

of an ordinary daily routine; and treatment of mild to moderate dementia with cognition-enhancing drugs such as donepezil (ensure careful clinical monitoring).

(4)   Minimise the non-cognitive symptoms of dementia, which can be the most distressing and disabling features of the disorder. Identification of the most appropriate interventions will depend on a thorough assessment of cause. For example, physical aggression in dementia may be due to a variety of reasons, for example: psychotic symptoms; extreme anxiety or autonomic arousal; irritability, sometimes in the context of a superimposed depressive episode; 'catastrophic reaction' due to unrealistic demands, perhaps with a carer who has not understood changing needs and adjusted his or her expectations; disorientation such as waking in the night, believing that it is daytime, and being told by the carer to return to bed; and lack of personal space, perhaps if more time is now spent at home if 'retired' from a previously attended day centre. The correct management depends on identifying the cause, and may include drug treatments (antipsychotics and antidepressants can be effective, but require careful monitoring to ensure that they are not impairing cognitive function), anxiety management, snoezelen multi-sensory therapy rooms, aromatherapy, carer education, programming of routines and social activities, respite care and day care.

(5)   Maximise quality of life by ensuring good occupational and recreational activities. As social care needs change, different activities may need to be developed and support packages modified. This will require ongoing monitoring and adjustment by a care manager.

(6)   It is important to offer support for carers. Practical support may be required, such as educational material, additional funded staff, laundry services, advice on daily care and emotional support.

# Conclusions

Older people with learning disabilities are only a small minority of the population, and therefore in many areas there will not be developed supra-specialist services specifically to meet their needs. However, existing services must develop the flexibility and skills to provide suitable support and care. The demand will increase during the 21st century as the increase in lifespan already observed continues. In addition to lifelong developmental disabilities, older people with learning disabilities have a high prevalence of other mental health needs, some of which have onset late in life. Accurate assessments and the development of management plans requires a range of skills, experience and knowledge regarding the psychiatry of adults with learning disabilities and the additional effects of ageing.

# References

Albert, M. & Cohen, C. (1992) The test for severe impairment: an instrument for the assessment of people with severe cognitive dysfunction. *Journal of the American Geriatric Society*, **40**, 449–453.

Aylward, E. H., Burt, D. B., Thorpe, L. U., *et al* (1997) Diagnosis of dementia in individuals with intellectual disability: report of the task force for development of criteria for diagnosis of dementia in individuals with mental retardation. *Journal of Intellectual Disability Research*, **41**, 152–164.

Barcikowski, M., Silverman, W., Zigman, W., *et al* (1989). Alzheimer-type neuropathology and clinical symptoms of dementia in mentally retarded people without Down's syndrome. *American Journal on Mental Retardation*, **93**, 551–557.

Bull, C., Rigby, M. L. & Shinebourne, E. A. (1985) Should management of complete atrioventricular canal defect be influenced by coexistent Down's syndrome? *Lancet, ii*, 1147–1149.

Carter, G. & Jancar, J. (1983) Mortality in the mentally handicapped: a fifty year survey at the Stoke Park Group of hospitals (1930–1980). *Journal of Mental Deficiency Research*, **27**, 143–156.

Cooper, S.-A. (1997a) Deficient health and social services for elderly people with learning disabilities. *Journal of Intellectual Disability Research*, **41**, 331–338.

—— (1997b) Epidemiology of psychiatric disorders in elderly compared with younger adults with learning disabilities. *British Journal of Psychiatry*, **170**, 375–380.

—— (1997c) High prevalence of dementia among people with learning disabilities not attributable to Down's syndrome. *Psychological Medicine*, **27**, 609–616.

—— (1998a) A population-based cross-sectional study of social networks and demography in older compared with younger adults with learning disabilities. *Journal of Intellectual Disabilities for Nursing, Health and Social Care*, **2**, 212–220.

—— (1998b) A clinical study of the effects of age on the physical health of people with intellectual disabilities. *American Journal on Mental Retardation*, **102**, 582–589.

—— (1998c) Behaviour disorders in adults with learning disabilities. Effect of age and differentiation from other psychiatric disorders. *Irish Journal of Psychological Medicine*, **15**, 13–18.

—— & Prasher, V. P. (1998) Maladaptive behaviours and symptoms of dementia in adults with Down's syndrome compared with adults with learning disabilities of other aetiologies. *Journal of Intellectual Disability Research*, **42**, 293–300.

Corbett, J. A. (1979) Psychiatric morbidity and mental retardation. In *Psychiatric Illness and Mental Handicap* (eds F. E. James & R. P. Snaith), pp. 11–25. London: Gaskell.

Evenhuis, H. M. (1992) Evaluation of a screening instrument for dementia in ageing mentally retarded persons. *Journal of Intellectual Disability Research*, **36**, 337–347.

Eyman, R. K., Grossman, H. J., Chaney, R. H., *et al* (1990) The life expectancy of profoundly handicapped people with mental retardation. *New England Journal of Medicine*, **323**, 584–589.

Folstein, M. F., Folstein, S. E. & McHugh, P. R. (1975) "Mini-Mental State": a practical method for grading the cognitive state of patients for the clinician. *Journal of Psychiatric Research*, **12**, 189–198.

Fryers, T. (1984) *The Epidemiology of Severe Intellectual Impairment: The Dynamics of Prevalence*. London: Academic Press.

—— (1997) Impairment, disability and handicap: categories and classifications. In *Seminars in the Psychiatry of Learning Disabilities* (ed. O. Russell), pp. 16–30. London: Gaskell.

Hofman, A., Rocca, W. A., Brayne, C., *et al* (1991) The prevalence of dementia in Europe: a collaborative study of 1980–1990 findings. *International Journal of Epidemiology*, **20**, 736–748.

Holland, A. J. & Oliver, C. (1995) Down's syndrome and the links with Alzheimer's disease. *Journal of Neurology, Neurosurgery and Psychiatry*, **59**, 111–115.

Jacobson, J. W., Sutton, M. S. & Janicki, M. P. (1985) Demography and characteristics of ageing and aged mentally retarded persons. In *Ageing and Developmental Disabilities: Issues and Approaches* (eds M. P. Janicki & H. M. Wisniewski), pp. 115–141. Baltimore, MD: P. H. Brooks.

Janicki, M. P., Dalton, A. J., Henderson, M., *et al* (1998) Mortality and morbidity among older adults with intellectual disabilities: Health services considerations. *Disability and Rehabilitation*, **21**, 284–294.

Lund, J. (1985) The prevalence of psychiatric disorder in mentally retarded adults. *Acta Psychiatrica Scandinavica*, **72**, 563–570.

Malone, Q. (1988) Mortality and survival of the Down's syndrome population in Western Australia. *Journal of Mental Deficiency Research*, **32**, 59–65.

Mann, D. M. A. (1988) Alzheimer's disease and Down's syndrome. *Histopathology*, **13**, 125–137.

McCurley, R., Mackay, D. N. & Scally, B. G. (1972) The life expectation of the mentally subnormal under community and hospital care. *Journal of Mental Deficiency Research*, **16**, 57–66.

McLoughlin, I. J. (1988) Study of mortality experiences in a mental-handicap hospital. *British Journal of Psychiatry*, **153**, 645–649.

Menahem, S., & Mee, R. B. B. (1985) Complete atrioventricular canal defect in presence of Down's syndrome. *Lancet*, **1**, 834–835.

Miller, C. & Eyman, R. (1978) Hospital and community mortality rates among the retarded. *Journal of Mental Deficiency Research*, **22**, 137–145.

Moss, S. & Patel, P. (1993) The prevalence of mental illness in people with intellectual disability over 50 years of age, and the diagnostic importance of information from carers. *Irish Journal of Psychology*, **14**, 110–129.

Nihira, K., Leland, H. & Lambert, N. (1993) *American Association on Mental Retardation Adaptive Behaviour Scale – Residential and Community* (2nd edn). Austin, TX: Pro-ed.

Oliver, C & Holland, A. J. (1986) Down's syndrome and Alzheimer's disease: a review. *Psychological Medicine*, **16**, 307–322.

Popovitch, E. R., Wisniewski, H. M., Barcikowska, M., *et al* (1990) Alzheimer neuropathology in non-Down's syndrome mentally retarded adults. *Acta Neuropathologica*, **80**, 362–367.

Prasher, V. P. (1995) Age specific prevalence, thyroid dysfunction and depressive symptomatology in adults with Down syndrome and dementia. *International Journal of Geriatric Psychiatry*, **10**, 25–31.

Puri, B. K., Lekh, S. K., Langa, A., *et al* (1995) Mortality in a hospitalised mentally handicapped population: a 10 year survey. *Journal of Intellectual Disability Research*, **39**, 442–449.

R v Arthur (1981) 12 Butterworths medico-legal reports 1.

Reid, A. H. & Ballinger, B. R. (1995) Behaviour symptoms among severely and profoundly mentally retarded patients. A 16–18-year follow-up study. *British Journal of Psychiatry*, **167**, 452–455.

Reiss, S., Levitan, G. W. & Szyszko, J. (1982) Emotional disturbance and mental retardation: diagnostic overshadowing. *American Journal of Mental Deficiency*, **86**, 567–574.

Richards, B. W. & Siddiqui, A. Q. (1980) Age and mortality trends in residents of an institute for the mentally handicapped. *Journal of Mental Deficiency Research*, **24**, 99–105.

Royal College of Psychiatrists (2001) *DC–LD [Diagnostic Criteria for Psychiatric Disorders for use with Adults with Learning Disabilities/Mental Retardation]* (Occasional Paper OP48). London: Gaskell Press.

Sparrow, S. S., Balla, D. A. & Cichetti, D. V. (1987) *A Revision of the Vineland Social Maturity Scale by E.A. Dou.* Circle Pines, MN: American Guidance Services, Inc.

Strauss, D. & Kastner, T. A. (1996) Comparative mortality of people with mental retardation in institutions and community. *American Journal on Mental Retardation*, **101**, 26–40.

Turner, T. H. (1989) Schizophrenia and mental handicap: an historical review. *Psychological Medicine*, **19**, 301–314.

University of Pittsburgh (1993) *The Severe Impairment Battery.* Suffolk: Thames Valley Test Company.

Wilson, N. J., Gavalaki, E. & Newman, C. G. H. (1985) Complete atrioventricular canal defect in presence of Down's syndrome. *Lancet, i*, 834.

# CHAPTER 10

# Counselling and psychotherapy

## Sheila Hollins

Psychodynamic principles underlie the approach used in this chapter. The ideal psychotherapy candidate is said to be young, intelligent, attractive and articulate – not a description that fits the usual image of people with learning disabilities. One of the challenges facing the therapist of such supposedly ideal patients is the need to examine their intellectual defence against feelings. Their skills with language may be used to try and distract and divert the therapist from their real conflicts. But just as psychotherapists working with very young children do not work primarily through language, therapists working with inarticulate adults do not. In all psychodynamic work, from the very first session, therapeutic use is made of the transference and countertransference of feelings in the relationship between therapist and patient, or patients. The therapist has to learn to listen with his or her eyes and feelings as well as ears; to listen to what is not said as well as to what is spoken.

## The evidence base

So far, evidence for the effectiveness of psychological therapies has relied on the assumption that findings from mainstream research will apply equally to people with learning disabilities (Parry, 2000). Methodological and ethical issues have prevented large-scale outcome studies from being designed specifically for this population. Case series have been published that demonstrate good face validity, but do not provide the more stringent levels of evidence requested by commissioners (Frankish, 1989; Hollins & Sinason, 2000).

## Assessment

To engage in therapy, emotional contact between patient and therapist is essential and the therapist will try to establish whether the patient has even a limited ability to make object relationships. A common assumption about people with learning disabilities is that their intellectual impairment will prevent them from meaningful, emotional engagement. It is customary for the therapist to make trial interpretations in the assessment interview, to see how the patient responds. Is the patient going to be able to take any risks? Will he or she give any sign of his or her understanding? Part of the assessment interview must be an honest appraisal by the therapist of his or her own feelings and reactions to the patient. I would like to suggest that the therapist must also take some risks at this first meeting. Other people's, and even one's own, assumptions may need to be confronted (McConachie & Sinason, 1989).

When I met George for the first time after referral for help with his difficult behaviour, his mother advised me not to sit close to him as he would surely hit me. This was said in front of George, who had athetoid cerebral palsy and whose angry movements were rather inaccurate and exhausting. I replied that it was not me he wanted to hit and as I sat on the chair beside his bed, his body stilled and he turned to look at me. Counselling someone without speech who is not responding conventionally, trusting one's intuition and interpreting behaviour as an intentional communicative attempt, especially when other people may not agree with your interpretation (Leudar, 1989), can lead one to feel rather foolish. What is important, however, is the ability to form a relationship with the person who is seeking help and to provide an opportunity for trust to develop so that he or she dares to show something of his or her real self.

If children and adults without good intellect – even without speech – have feelings, including feelings about other people, experience comfort in warm, loving relationships and experience the loss of important people, places and events, then a psychodynamic approach to imagining and understanding such a person's experience of life seems both possible and important.

Assessment for any psychotherapeutic intervention must consider the availability of an appropriate venue. The requirements may be straightforward and simply include a quiet, private place easily accessible to the client. On the other hand, the therapist may require some art or play materials, which cannot be readily transported. For example, I lost my ability to communicate with one young man who had no speech and only rudimentary communication aids when he moved from the hustle and bustle of his parents' home to the quiet and rather sterile environment of a local authority hostel. No longer could he eye-point to the photo of his sister's wedding, to the telephone or to the toys belonging to his nephews. No longer could he strain to hear the content of his parents' conversation in the kitchen. Without these clues, I was lost for a 'way in' to his current concerns.

Careful thought must be given about whether to offer treatment in the patient's own home, where interruptions are more likely, or in a clinic setting where reliance on a third party may interfere with attendance. Well-meaning escorts or carers may unwittingly undermine the patient–therapist relationship by cancelling sessions or arriving late, by trying to talk to the therapist between sessions, by failing to respect confidentiality, or by interrupting the session to see how things are going or to offer the therapist a cup of tea. Establishing clear boundaries for therapy is essential, and it is advisable to ensure that another worker is available and willing to work with the carer, and to deal with any practical arrangements or other needs that emerge for the patient during treatment.

Finally, part of the assessment is to determine the level of psychotherapy that is appropriate, given the needs of the individual and the qualifications and experience of the therapist. This will be explored further in the section on therapeutic aims.

## Communication

Effective counselling is dependent on well-developed and appropriate communication skills in the counsellor. Effective communication involves at least two people, each of whom has two roles. Turn-taking by the participants requires and allows each person to move from one role, such as listening and observing, to another, such as talking or signing.

The members of the partnership must move at the same speed, and thus the counsellor has to judge how long to pause to allow time for the partner to respond. People who have autistic traits or an avoidant personality offer a major challenge to the counsellor. Their discomfort with eye contact and difficulty in making object relationships will interfere with attempts to take turns. To illustrate this, I will tell the story of one middle-aged and institutionalised woman I was asked to assess, shortly before her move from hospital to a group home. The staff were concerned that she showed no apparent understanding of the move and would not engage in the group's preparations for the move. I found her in a corner of the dining room on her own, with a large pile of pieces of paper or card, most of which had been scribbled on with the same symmetrical but meaningless 'writing', and which she was sorting and resorting with her head bowed. My entrance provoked no flicker of acknowledgement that anyone had entered. I paused for a while to see whether a delayed response would emerge and then tried some different ways of making contact. The comment that finally broke the ice was my question about the colour of her eyes. 'With your head down like that I cannot see what colour your eyes are – mine are blue.' This woman, who had never met me before, responded 'Your eyes are grey, not blue!' Engaging with such a person is arduous, and without occasional gems of feedback such as the one described can leave the therapist feeling very unsure about the impact of his or her attempts to communicate.

Therapy is likely to be complicated by conceptual and communication difficulties, and another medium may need to be used as an added or alternative channel for communication, for example therapies including art, music or drama.

Communication does not necessarily involve spoken language, but always includes an awareness of body language (Morris, 1987) and behaviour. Appropriate and full use of communication aids should also be explored, and signed or written language or drawings may be important (Brafman, 2001). Cultural influences on communication roles must be taken into account – an aspect of communicating that is highlighted when working in a multi-racial community.

## Preconceptions and misconceptions

Whereas some adults with learning disabilities may be at an early developmental level emotionally, comparisons with work with children should be used cautiously, and the range of life experiences of the adult must be remembered, even if therapy is focusing on pre-Oedipal relationships. Increasing doubt is now being thrown on previous assumptions about the lack of understanding of people with profound learning disabilities (Sinason, 1992). Participation in infant observation seminars may help to increase our skills in understanding the communicative attempts of some of the people in this group.

Another misconception is that psychoanalytic psychotherapy is about cure. The debate about learning disability and psychoanalysis in the past tended to revolve around the hope that psychoanalytic techniques would cure the child or adult of the primary impairment, for example the cause of the learning disability or the autistic behaviour. If the impairment could not be cured, therefore, it was said that nothing could be done. In this country, psychodynamic theories about the causation of autism have been discredited. More recently, Sinason (1986, 1992, 2000) has written about the way secondary mental handicap can be a defence against trauma experienced by the individual. Sometimes the learning disability turns out to be less severe than originally thought, when emotional conflicts have been resolved and the person has acquired the freedom to think. Usually when organic brain damage is present, such emotional release does not result in major cognitive gains. Considerable effort is now being focused on understanding the nature and remediation of such emotional and communication disorders. Bystanders may wrongly assume either that an inability to express one's thoughts is synonymous with impaired intelligence, or that emotional intelligence is linked to an ability to articulate one's feelings.

In many instances of severe learning disability, the brain is damaged permanently, and a request for therapy may be misunderstood as a denial of the reality of this damage, or as a search for another diagnostic exploration, which might uncover a remediable cause. However, realistic requests for therapy might arise from a wish to come to terms with the internal and external experiences of the individual who has such damage (Hollins, 1999). To understand this further demands knowledge of the features that are often seen in the psychological adjustments of people with such disabilities and their families. This will be explored in more detail in the next section.

## Therapeutic aims

People with learning disabilities will benefit from counselling or psychotherapy in the same way, and for similar reasons, as people without learning disabilities. Relationship or adjustment and personality difficulties are common presenting problems.

Cawley (1977) described several levels of psychotherapy of increasing depth and complexity (see Table 10.1) and the therapist must decide on the appropriate level and aim for each individual.

At the first level, providing relief, support and counselling are all part of the repertoire of any good doctor or social worker. Sharing one's problems with a sympathetic, impartial listener can put things into clearer perspective. Such supportive counselling may include the need to provide information or education, for example on sexual matters. The main aim at this level of intervention is either to restore the status quo in someone whose equilibrium is temporarily impaired by a crisis such

**Table 10.1**  Levels of psychotherapy (from Cawley, 1997)

| 1 | Outer (support and counselling) | 1 | Unburdening of problems to sympathetic listener |
| --- | --- | --- | --- |
| | | 2 | Ventilation of feelings within supportive relationship |
| | | 3 | Discussion of current problems with non-judgemental helper |
| 2 | Intermediate | 4 | Clarification of problems, their nature and origins, within deepening relationship |
| | | 5 | Confrontation of defences |
| | | 6 | Interpretation of unconscious motives and transference phenomena |
| 3 | Deeper | 7 | Repetition, remembering, and exploration and reconstruction of past analysis |
| | | 8 | Regression to less-adult and less-rational functioning |
| | | 9 | Resolution of conflicts by re-experiencing and working them through |

as a bereavement, or to build up the strength of the person with a severe personality disorder in order to achieve the best possible adjustment. Exploring the inner world of such people is unnecessary, and may be contraindicated in someone whose defences are precarious.

Intermediate levels of psychotherapy aim to clarify problems within a deepening relationship, in which the therapist confronts the defence mechanisms used by the patient and interprets the way he or she relates to the therapist.

At deeper levels, more active psychodynamic work explores earlier traumas and conflicts in an attempt to reconstruct an individual's inner world, and allow him or her to relinquish disabling symptoms. At this level, the aim is to achieve change in personality functioning and an increase in maturity. Advice is withheld, and emotional regression within the sessions is encouraged. Anxiety is expected to occur and may be necessary to enable the working-through of past conflicts, and medication to reduce these symptoms is discouraged.

Thus, although support is part and parcel of all psychotherapies, exploration is not and is reserved for the deeper levels, as practised by suitably qualified and experienced clinicians, usually under supervision.

The focus of psychotherapeutic work may depend on the stage reached in the life cycle of an individual or family, and on any recent or unresolved life events. Themes that seem to be common at several different stages have been described elsewhere as the three secrets (Hollins & Grimer, 1988). These are the secrets of disability and dependence, of each person's sexuality and of their own and their parents' mortality. In fact, these are universally difficult issues for us to understand and adjust to, and all three are taboo subjects to a greater or lesser extent in different cultures and age-groups. People with learning disabilities are often subjected to a conspiracy of silence about these areas, over and above any conventional reticence.

## Disability and dependence

When the diagnosis of a disabling medical condition is made, either at birth or after a later traumatic event, the shocked family members experience the loss of their normal, healthy child (Bicknell, 1983). Their reaction may be similar to the reaction of parents whose child has died, albeit compounded by the daily reminder their surviving, damaged child provides for them.

We can only surmise about the experience for such an individual of being a disappointment to parents. Each person will have feelings and attitudes about his or her own limitations and the effect of these upon the family (Hollins, 1999). Vanier (1985) suggests that every human being, with or without a disability, is to some extent a disappointment to his or her parents and to him- or herself.

Attachment relationships in infancy may have been distorted for a number of reasons: perhaps because of the emotional work involved in coming to terms with a child's difference, because of enforced separation from a sickly child or because of a primary impairment in the responsiveness of the child (Bowlby, 1988).

The achievement of satisfactory separation in adulthood depends on these early relationships developing more or less normally. The aim of therapy with young families will be to come to terms with difference, disappointment and confusion. The therapist will be able to share the reality of disability, to feel the hopelessness and even panic that parents may feel. Later, the individual with a learning disability and with some insight may have similar feelings about him- or herself.

People with learning disabilities sometimes comment on their own difficulties, which a carer in attendance might quickly contradict: 'You're not stupid' or 'There's nothing wrong with the way you talk'. Such social convention, which expects one to ignore the person's impairments, may be quite inappropriate (Sinason, 1992). The counsellor or therapist has an opportunity to respond differently by acknowledging the patient's insight. For example, the therapist might say that he or she agrees with him/her and wonders whether it feels upsetting to look or sound different.

The family denial of disability may be an attempt to hide the painful 'secret' of disability from each other and from the affected individual; unfortunately, such confusion often leads to fear and loneliness.

# Sexuality

Physical sexual development is not delayed in people with learning disabilities, although emotional maturity usually is, and the arrival of puberty can be an unwelcome reminder to parents of their child's approaching adulthood. Parental fears about their adolescent child's naïvety and vulnerability may well be justified. Likewise, parents may have fears about their child's inappropriate sexual behaviour, perhaps leading to embarrassing situations in the neighbourhood or even to a conviction for a sexual offence. Infantilising attitudes, which see people with learning disabilities as eternal children, may contribute to a tendency in parents to want to protect their children from the possible consequences of their sexuality. Unfortunately, such attitudes may delay internal awareness for an individual that he or she is changing from a child into an adult. Vulnerability to sexual abuse is high and secondary emotional disabilities caused by such trauma may present with difficult behaviours such as eye-poking or other self-injury (Sinason, 1988, 1992; Cooke & Sinason, 1998).

As is so often the case when counselling people with learning disabilities, there is likely to be an educational aspect to the task.

Personal relationship and sex education classes are not as available for children in special schools as for those in mainstream education. Nothing can be assumed in terms of the extent or accuracy of any factual knowledge about sexual matters, and an apparent familiarity with the vocabulary of sex is never a guide to understanding.

### Case examples

Moses was 18 years old when arrested for indecent exposure. He had mild learning disabilities and a very smart and pleasant appearance. The police officer questioning him asked him if he was responsible for about twenty other minor sexual offences in the area, and because the officer seemed pleased when he answered in the affirmative he repeatedly said 'yes' hoping that he could go home sooner. When I asked him to explain the charges against him, he did not know the meaning of several key words including indecent exposure, guilty and not guilty.

James had been abused by an older male relative when he was 8 or 9 years old, and in his thirties he was charged with indecently assaulting a boy of 15. In therapy, it soon became apparent that his own perception of himself was as a peer of the teenager. He did not recognise himself as an adult, and despite formal knowledge of the law, he had real difficulty understanding that the teenager was under age.

# Bereavement and loss

Loss frequently looms large in the recent history of people with learning disabilities referred for psychiatric assessment (Hollins & Esterhuyzen, 1997). A relative inability to take control of one's own life seems to make one more vulnerable to loss, and contributors to this vulnerability might include withholding of information, or a misattribution of one's behaviour.

For example, a person may not have been told about an important change or loss, or his or her feelings about loss and change may have been difficult to articulate and his or her reaction misunderstood or ignored. Furthermore, the ability to make contact with a peer or carer who has moved may be precluded by an inability to write, telephone or drive a car. After the death of a significant person, the need to look for them, to check whether they have really gone for ever or to visit places that remind someone of that person may be overlooked by carers.

The death of a parent may be the start of a chain of losses. Emergency admission to residential care is commonplace, possibly some distance from home, resulting in a change of daily activities and the loss of friends and familiar staff (Oswin, 1991). The bereaved person may be worried about who has taken on their responsibilities, such as feeding the cats or bringing in the post. None of the old familiar routines will be experienced again, and it is not unknown for the family home to be disposed of without the individual with a disability ever going back. David Cook's novel *Walter* movingly describes a similar sequence of events (Cook, 1978).

Therapeutic aims will focus on the provision of accurate information, including death education, and on supporting the healthy resolution of grief (Conboy-Hill, 1992; Read, 1996; Stroebe & Schut, 1999).

## Different therapeutic approaches

Individual, group and family work all have a place, depending on the identified needs at any particular stage. Counselling or therapy might focus on a life event that has occurred, and on the consequences within the individual or family group. Parent counselling, family therapy and bereavement counselling should all be considered. (Symington, 1981; Hollins & Evered, 1990; Hollins, 1992; Hollins *et al*, 1994; Beaill, 1996, 1998).

### Parent counselling

The first task is to break the news of any suspected disability to parents. The consensus is that it should be told to both parents together, sensitively and honestly, as soon as there is any doubt – even if the doctor is unsure about the answers to their questions. The conveyor of bad news will always be unpopular, but, despite this, he or she should offer further appointments to help the parents to express their feelings and to increase their shared understanding. Such essential counselling may be preferred with a trusted family doctor, an experienced hospital social worker, a genetic counsellor or a member of the child development team (Cunningham & Davis, 1985).

Work with parents at this early stage should reap dividends later, as parents who grieve together are more likely to work well together as parents. Traditionally, mothers become full-time carers of children with disabilities, with fathers having less chance of playing a normal parenting role. There is a tendency for the attachment bond between mother and child to be so distorted that normal sharing in a family triad is not possible.

Unless the father is involved right from the beginning, the mother may find it difficult to let him gradually introduce their child to the outside world. It is not difficult to imagine the consequences of such distorted relationships in later adult life. If separation in infancy is difficult, separation in adulthood will be even harder (Richardson & Ritchie, 1989). 'Letting go' groups for middle-aged or elderly parents, whose disabled sons and daughters are still very dependent on them, are a valued way of introducing change into a family system. However, often it is only after the death of a spouse that the surviving parent will seek help in planning for the future.

In my experience, when parents are brought together, whether in formal or informal settings, they talk endlessly and honestly about experiences that they have in common, finding other parents an invaluable support in their grief and their struggles.

## Case example

Carole, the mother of Robin, a 7-year-old boy with cerebral palsy and uncontrolled epilepsy, said the appointments with the paediatrician offered the only possibility of a cure and she would not waste a moment of that precious time talking of her own suicidal ideation. The paediatrician described this mother as a wonderful, down-to-earth woman who coped marvellously and certainly did not need any involvement with child psychiatry. At her first meeting with me, requested only after a serious overdose, she asked how long her son would live. He had already been in intensive care twice in status epilepticus, and we talked about her somewhat realistic fear of finding him dead in the morning. At our next meeting, she told me that facing up to the severity of his disability had enabled her to have her son christened, and she had made renewed efforts to get her family re-housed to improve the quality of their lives while Robin was still alive to enjoy it.

## Family therapy

Family therapy is a specialist and scarce resource that aims to encourage better coping strategies. It should not be a last resort but should be considered early on if signs of stress in any family member are causing anxiety. Working with family groups when there is an adult member with a disability is also appropriate. For example, it may be useful when issues of dependence and fear about what will happen when parents die have led to more complex patterns of behaviour (Hollins *et al*, 1994; Goldberg *et al*, 1995).

## Case example

Charlie was 27 years old and his weight had dropped to below 6 stone when his parents finally agreed to psychiatric intervention. After several family therapy interviews, all three were able to agree to, and cooperate with, an admission to a unit for people with anorexia nervosa. Confrontation about separation and dependency issues was carefully avoided, but gradually all three began to explore how they could negotiate a permanent separation for Charlie without anyone feeling rejected.

The needs of siblings may also emerge in family therapy. Often parents omit to explain to their other children anything about their sibling's disability, or they fail to update such explanations as each child's understanding develops. The subject of disability may become a taboo at home, with siblings having to face insensitive questioning or comment from children in the playground. Making a family tree at a first family interview can help to elucidate who knows what about loss and illness in different members. Clarifying difficult or taboo areas in a supportive setting such as this can help families to improve communication at home (Wilkins, 1992).

## Case example

In a family with two children, the older of whom had serious communication and behavioural difficulties, it emerged that the 8-year-old daughter had completely misunderstood explanations about her brother's disability. He had been diagnosed as having fragile-X syndrome, and she had had a chromosomal analysis herself. Although her mother had explained to her that her test was fine and that her children would not have the same condition as her brother, two years later her understanding of this was that she herself would gradually lose skills and become disabled like her brother.

## Bereavement counselling

The task here is to help with the work of mourning and restoration (Parkes, 1998; Stroebe & Schut, 1999). On occasion, the counsellor will find that the bereaved person has not been told of his or her loss, and it is still commonplace for people with learning disabilities to be excluded from the funeral. Helping someone to say goodbye might involve the counsellor in revisiting the grave or the home of the person with the bereaved person, and in looking at photographs or other mementos with them. The bereaved person might need permission to express negative feelings about their dead relative, such as feelings about being let down or deserted. The counsellor is in a position to understand the normality of such feelings, whereas a carer might discourage an individual from 'speaking ill of the dead'. A guided mourning approach may be appropriate (Sireling *et al*, 1988).

Bereavement counselling is available to many people through an individual's church, through voluntary organisations such as Cruse Bereavement Care or through specialist health and social service teams. For people with learning disabilities, such counselling may be withheld for a variety of reasons. Counsellors may have little experience of being with people with learning disabilities, and may feel de-skilled when their ordinary communication skills appear inadequate, but specialist learning disability services can support access to mainstream counselling agencies through training and supervision (Read, 1999).

Trying to understand, to explain and to comfort are vital; sometimes, a genuine and sustained attempt to communicate and share will convey enough emotionally. Two books telling the story of the death of a parent in pictures have been published to assist the counsellor and the bereaved person (Hollins & Sireling, 2003*a,b*). An intellectual understanding of the permanence of a loss is less important that an emotional awareness of what has happened. Senses of sight, hearing and touch will reinforce the realisation of loss: the person is not here, the bed is empty, as is the place at the table. At the funeral service, the coffin, some tears and the flowers are seen and perhaps touched and smelt. The funeral music and singing is heard, as are the subdued voices of the mourners.

Looking more closely, the following responses are described by people who have been bereaved: feelings of fear and panic, feelings of disbelief about what has happened, feelings of remorse or feeling out of control, being under- or overactive, losing an appetite for food, being unable to sleep, having a poor memory, hearing the voice of the dead person, wanting to talk to the dead person, forgetting that he or she has died, being cross with other people, crying a lot or being unable to think or work.

For someone with a learning disability, the same reactions may be expressed behaviourally rather than verbally, and may be difficult to interpret accurately. Disturbances of sleep and appetite are relatively easy to notice, but denial of the death or a failure to understand its finality may lead to 'searching behaviour', which is misattributed. Unexplained anger towards objects or people or episodes of self-injury may be harder to understand, and a loss of intellect or other skills, or the loss of bladder control may seem completely unrelated.

Bereavement counselling can be very effective in small groups, where some of the learning emerges through sharing experiences. These might include visits to places that remind the bereaved group members of their deceased relatives and friends or to a cemetery. Each bereaved person could be encouraged to bring a photograph to the session to enable clear communication about the deceased person, and as a measure of the extent to which the person is avoiding reminders of their loss. Hopefully, therapy will continue until the person, either in individual or group sessions, is able to look at the photograph and talk about their deceased relative or friend in a realistic and positive manner.

## Conclusion

In working psychotherapeutically, we must be prepared to tolerate the fact that there is no cure for our patients' organic impairments. The best we can hope for is that secondary and emotional disabilities are diminished, thus contributing immeasurably to someone's quality of life (Hollins, 2000). Even within the counselling or therapeutic relationship, the therapist might have difficulty acknowledging his or her own negative feelings; this skilled supervision is strongly advised, so that issues such as this are properly examined.

A psychodynamic understanding of the impact of a learning disability on the individual, his or her family and other social groups is long overdue. If we do not take into account the unconscious of the individual and the people he or she relates to, we could run the risk of misunderstanding that person's life experiences.

The Institute of Psychotherapy and Disability was formed in 2000 to promote psychotherapy by adequately qualified and experienced disability psychotherapists, committed to treating people with respect (Frankish, 2000; Sinason, 2000).

Throughout the clinical examples given above, it will be apparent that misunderstandings readily occur and that at no point can emotional and intellectual understanding and acceptance be complete. Life for all of us is a dynamic process of achievement, loss and adjustment. Counselling and psychotherapeutic interventions can be carefully targeted to release emotional blocks, to enable systems to interact dynamically and to allow reorganisation to take place.

# References

Beaill, N. (1996) Evaluation of a psychodynamic psychotherapeutic service for adults with intellectual disabilities: rationale, design and preliminary outcome data. *Journal of Applied Research in Intellectual Disabilities*, **9**, 223–228.

—— (1998) Psychoanalytic psychotherapy with men with intellectual disabilities: a preliminary outcome study. *British Journal of Medical Psychology*, **71**, 1–11.

Bicknell, D. J. (1983) Inaugural lecture: The psychopathology of handicap. *British Journal of Medical Psychology*, **56**, 167–178.

Bowlby, J. (1988) *A Secure Base: Parent–Child Attachment and Health Human Development*. New York: Basic Books.

Brafman, A. (2001) *Untying the Knot*. London: Karnac.

Cawley R. H. (1977) The teaching of psychotherapy. *Association of University Teachers of Psychiatry Newsletter*, January, 19–36.

Conboy-Hill, S. (1992) Grief, loss and people with learning disabilities. In *Psychotherapy and Mental Handicap* (eds A. Waitman & S. Conboy-Hill), pp. 150–170. London: Sage.

Cook, D. (1978) *Walter*. London: Penguin.

Cooke, L. B. & Sinason, V. (1998) Abuse of people with learning disabilities and other vulnerable adults. *Advances in Psychiatric Treatment*, **4**, 119–125.

Cunningham, C. & Davis, H. (1985) Early intervention for the child. In *Mental handicap: a Multi-Disciplinary Approach* (eds M. Craft, J. Bicknell, & S. Hollins), pp. 209–228. London: Baillière Tindall.

Frankish, P. (1989) Meeting the emotional needs of handicapped people: a psycho-dynamic approach. *Journal of Mental Deficiency Research*, **33**, 407–414.

Goldberg, D., Magrill, L., Hale, J., *et al* (1995) Protection and loss: working with learning disabled adults and their families. *Journal of Family Therapy*, **17**, 263–280.

Hollins, S. (1992) Group analytic therapy for people with mental handicap. In *Psychotherapy and Mental Handicap* (eds M. Craft, J. Bicknell & S. Hollins), pp. 139–149. London: Sage.

—— (1999) Remorse for being: through the lens of learning disability. In *Remorse and Reparation* (ed. M. Cox), pp. 95–104. London: Jessica Kingsley.

—— (2000) Treating with respect: the growth of therapeutic approaches in the community. *Psychotherapy Review*, **2**, 374–375.

—— & Esterhuyzen, A. (1997) Bereavement and grief in adults with learning disabilities. *British Journal of Psychiatry*, **170**, 497–501.

—— & Evered, C. (1990) Group process and content: the challenge of mental handicap. *Group Analysis*, **23**, 55–67.

— & Grimer, M. (1988) *Going Somewhere: People with Mental Handicaps and their Pastoral Care*. London: SPCK.

— & Sinason, V. (2000) New perspectives: psychotherapy, learning disabilities and trauma. *British Journal of Psychiatry*, **176**, 32–36.

—, — & Thompson, S. (1994) Individual, group and family psychotherapy. In *Mental Health in Mental Retardation: Recent Advances and Practices* (ed. N. Bouras), pp. 233–243. Cambridge: Cambridge University Press.

— & — (2003*a*) *When Mum Died* (3rd edn). London: Gaskell.

— & — (2003*b*) *When Dad Died* (3rd edn). London: Gaskell.

Leudar, I. (1989) Communicative environments for mentally handicapped people. In *Language and Communication in Mentally Handicapped People* (eds M. Beveridge, G. Cont-Ramsden & I. Leudar), pp. 274–300. London: Chapman & Hall.

McConachie, H. & Sinason, V. (1989) The emotional experience of multiple handicap – issues in assessment. *Child Care, Health and Development*, **15**, 75–78.

Morris, D. (1987) *Man Watching*. London: Grafton.

Oswin, M. (1991) *Am I Allowed to Cry? A Study of Bereavement Amongst People who have Learning Difficulties*. London: Souvenir.

Parkes, C. (1998) Coping with loss: bereavement in adult life. *BMJ*, **316**, 856–859.

Parry, G. (2000) *Treatment Choice in Psychological Therapies and Counselling: Evidence Based Clinical Practical Guidelines*. London: Department of Health.

Read, S. (1996) Helping people with learning disabilities to grieve. *British Journal of Nursing*, **5**, 91–95.

— (1999) Creative ways of working when exploring the bereavement counselling process. In *Living with Loss: Helping People with Learning Disabilities Cope with Bereavement and Loss* (ed. N. Blackman), pp. 9–13. Brighton: Pavilion.

Richardson, A. & Ritchie, J. (1989) *Letting Go*. Milton Keynes: Open University Press.

Sinason, V. (1986) Secondary mental handicap and its relationship to trauma. *Psychoanalytic Psychotherapy*, **2**, 31–154.

— (1988) Richard III, Echo & Hephaestus: sexuality and mental/multiple handicap. *Journal of Child Psychotherapy*, **14**, 93–105.

— (1992) *Mental Handicap the Human Condition: New Approaches from The Tavistock*. London: Free Association.

— (2000) Psychotherapeutic work with disabled individuals: the past is alive in the present. *Psychotherapy Review*, **2**, 325–382.

Sireling, L., Cohen, D. & Marks, I. (1988) Guided mourning for morbid grief: a controlled replication. *Behavior Therapy*, **19**, 121–132.

Stroebe, M. & Schut, H. (1999) The dual process model of coping with bereavement: rationale and description. *Death Studies*, **23**, 197–224.

Symington, N. (1981) The psychotherapy of a subnormal patient. *British Journal of Medical Psychology*, **54**, 187–199.

Vanier, J. (1985) *Man and Woman: He Made Them*. London: Longman and Todd.

Wilkins, R. (1992) Psychotherapy with the siblings of mentally handicapped children. In *Psychotherapy and Mental Handicap* (eds A. Waitman & S. Conboy-Hill), pp. 24–45. London: Sage.

# Additional reading

Bichard, S. H., Sinason, V. & Ususkin, J. (1996) Measuring change in mentally retarded clients in long term psychoanalytic psychotherapy. *National Association of Dual Diagnosis Newsletter*, **13**, 6–11.

Hollins, S. & Curran, J. (1996) *Understanding Depression in People with Learning Disabilities*. London: Pavilion Publishing and the Department of Psychiatry of Disability, St George's Hospital Medical School.

—— & Sireling, L. (1999) *Understanding Grief: Working with Grief and People who have Learning Disabilities.* London: Pavilion.

Waitman, A. & Conboy-Hill, S. (eds) (1992) *Psychotherapy and Mental Handicap.* London: Sage.

# CHAPTER 11

# Psychological treatment of common behavioural problems

Andrew Jahoda and Audrey Espie

Historically, psychological interventions for behavioural problems in people with learning disabilities have primarily comprised techniques originating from behavioural analysis, and there is a considerable history of applied and experimental work in the field (for a comprehensive review see Emerson, 1995). The first aim of this chapter is to demonstrate how these procedures have been adopted for two main categories of problem behaviours: aggression and stereotypy. The second aim is to illustrate how methods of working with problem behaviour have moved beyond the behavioural paradigm to encompass other psychological models that are gaining increasing clinical credibility.

Challenging behaviour has been defined by Emerson (1995, 1998) as behaviour presented by people with learning disabilities that poses a serious threat to their own well-being or that of others. This well-being could be defined in terms of physical health, or of exclusion from community facilities and other opportunities of everyday life. Interestingly, he also describes the social nature of challenging behaviour and the notion that it involves breaking cultural norms about acceptable conduct. It is the meaning that is ascribed to the act, as well as its immediate consequences, that determines the social impact of the behaviour. If a person hits out in self-defence or because he or she is in a state of fear or confusion, that person's act of aggression is viewed very differently from that of someone who has become aggressive for no apparent reason. Stereotyped behaviours or stereotypies are behaviours that are also commonly viewed as socially inappropriate. Defining stereotypies is difficult owing to the variety of presentations across a range of populations. However, for the purposes of this chapter, they will be defined as 'frequent, idiosyncratic, repetitive movements and/or vocalisations that can be self-injurious, exhibiting little variation, often constant across settings and having no unequivocal function' (Paul, 1997).

In a study of people with learning disabilities using educational, health and social care resources in two areas of England, Emerson *et al* (2001*a*) found that 10–15% of individuals presented problem behaviours. A label of 'other' was used to describe problem behaviours that did not fit into any specific category, with 9–12% of the population presenting behaviour of this kind. Aggression was the most prevalent category of challenging behaviour (7%) and presented more commonly in people with milder learning disabilities (Emerson *et al*, 2001*a*), followed by destructive behaviour (4–5%) and self-injury (4%). The aggressive individuals had higher levels of self-help and communication skills than those presenting other types of challenging behaviour, such as self-injury. Stereotypy usually falls between the categories of 'other' and 'self-injury', but in specific terms, prevalence rates have varied considerably across institutionalised and community clients. They have ranged from 18% to as high as 67% (Berkson & Davenport, 1962; Forehand & Baumeister, 1976; Rojahn, 1986; Dura *et al*, 1987; Walsh, 1994; Matson & Volkmar, 1997), with higher frequencies in people with more severe learning disability (Matson & Volkmar, 1997; Emerson *et al*, 2001*b*).

As other chapters in this book suggest, there may be other explanations of people's behaviour, originating from neurological problems and mental health difficulties. The dominant psychological model used to work with people presenting challenging behaviour has been behavioural. Consequently, we will begin this chapter with an outline of the behavioural perspective. This will lead on to a description of assessment procedures, highlighting the importance of differential diagnosis and ethical considerations. We will also discuss behavioural treatment approaches and their efficacy. Finally, We will consider alternative approaches to challenging behaviour, with an introduction to the use of anger management.

## Behavioural approaches

A number of assessment manuals have been produced in order to guide the clinical assessment process and the functional analysis of problem behaviour (LaVigna & Donnellan, 1986; Sturmey, 2001). Functional analysis is a means of developing hypotheses about the predisposing and maintaining factors for a person's problem behaviour. It is crucial to the behavioural paradigm that the baseline frequency of the target behaviour is recorded, so that the success of any interventions can be measured against this.

Assessing the contribution of social, psychological and biological factors, both past and present, can lead to a number of hypotheses about how a person's problem behaviour is maintained, usually involving the interaction of several factors. These hypotheses should then inform the development of the interventions that are used. Gardner & Moffat (1990) reviewed the behavioural literature concerning psychological work with people who were frequently aggressive. They set out a framework for the functional analysis of aggression, with the aim of identifying the biological and psychosocial factors involved in the genesis and maintenance of incidents of aggression. There are two distinct types of information to be gathered. First, there are the distal factors – environmental conditions and personal characteristics that may predispose the individual towards being aggressive. For example, living in a barren social environment where there are few positive social interactions, or where individuals themselves lack social skills or problem-solving abilities, may make it more likely that a person will respond aggressively in difficult interpersonal situations. The second stage of the model involves an analysis of proximal factors, such as the topography of the aggressive behaviour and its antecedents and consequences. This would include looking at the triggers of aggression, and the setting conditions or circumstances in which incidents occur. For example, a person might often become abusive when requested to help with household activities by a particular support worker. Moreover, the situation may be more likely to escalate into violence if his or her other flatmates are present and the room is crowded.

The theoretical basis of this work is the operant model of conditioning. This involves identifying the environmental consequences of a particular behaviour, which has the effect of increasing or decreasing the likelihood of the behaviour recurring. If the presentation of a particular behaviour results in the individual obtaining a reinforcing stimulus, then the behaviour is likely to occur again. Similarly, if the presentation of a behaviour results in the removal of a negative stimulus, then that behaviour is also likely to occur again. For example, someone's aggressive behaviour might gain them access to a valued activity or act as an escape route from social situations that they find aversive. Negative consequences can come in the form of punishment or the loss of a positive consequence that was helping to maintain the behaviour.

There are a number of common misunderstandings of the operant model (Clements, 1997b) that can cause confusion among carers and other professionals. One concept that can be difficult to grasp is that operant conditioning concerns the probability or likelihood of behaviour occurring. Moreover, although the stimulus needs to be sufficiently reinforcing to maintain the behaviour, the behaviour and stimulus will not necessarily be paired on every occasion. For example, a person who hits out (behaviour) might sometimes, but not always, be taken out by members of his family for a walk (reinforcing stimulus) to calm down. Indeed, there may be a number of different maintaining factors for a particular behaviour that can vary with context and time (Emerson, 1998). It is also unwise to assume what the individual finds reinforcing or aversive. For example, one person might greatly enjoy a lot of praise and attention, while another finds this aversive.

Reiss & Havercamp (1997) believe that traditional behavioural analysts have failed to take the intrinsic nature of motivation seriously in their examination of problem behaviour. They argue that behavioural analysis has traditionally viewed aberrant behaviour as resulting from either aberrant environments or contingencies and has ignored aberrant motivation. Consequently, they have developed the 'sensitivity theory', in which they argue that people have different levels of motivation to seek particular reinforcers. This means that those who crave attention might seek attention of any kind, even if it is negative. In such a case, simply changing the contingencies may not be enough to reduce the person's continuing wish for attention if the motivation for attention is intrinsic or an end in itself. The logical conclusion of Reiss and Havercamp's position is that assessment and treatment might have to address the individual's motivation alongside environmental factors and contingent stimuli. This theory requires empirical investigation and remains unproven, but it highlights the need to carefully consider what might be reinforcing or aversive stimuli and the intrinsic motivation to engage in certain behaviour. LaVigna & Donnellan (1986) describe a reinforcement inventory to help determine the most effective reinforcement schedules to use in behavioural interventions with people with learning disabilities.

## Assessment procedures

A thorough behavioural analysis is potentially a very large undertaking, and many of the existing guides (e.g. see Sturmey, 2001) are rather unwieldy documents. However, it is important to know both what information is required and how to obtain this. The first stage is to consider how the behavioural problem relates to the person's general physical and mental health or to genetic factors.

### Differential diagnosis

Commencing an assessment of challenging behaviour may involve a number of professionals with complementary skills such as psychiatry, psychology, and speech and language therapy. A differential diagnosis forms part of the assessment of challenging behaviour, and can be fundamental in achieving greater understanding of its function. For example, stereotypies have been observed in populations with mental illness, or may be associated with movement disorders such as tardive dyskinesia and neurological conditions such as Tourette syndrome (Stoessl, 1990; Jankovic, 1992; Fish & Marsden, 1994). Studies have also linked epilepsy with stereotypy (Gedye, 1989, 1991, 1992; Espie & Paul, 1997; Paul, 1997). Epilepsy co-presents in 23% to 50% of people with learning disability (Bicknell, 1985; Coulter, 1993) and seizures are more common in people with more severe physical disabilities. The external manifestation of a seizure may be as subtle as a repetitive eye blink or a brief raising of the arm. This results in confusion for carers, where an external event may be described as a seizure by one carer and labelled as stereotyped behaviour by another. In these cases, assessment should move beyond the initial formulations of professionals within the learning disabilities field, to encompass other specialists such as neurologists. The client may require an electroencephalographic assessment or a thorough examination of motor skills.

The literature in this area also indicates that in cases where the underlying mechanisms are established and understood, such as Parkinson's disease, pharmacological interventions are sometimes considered appropriate. Such clear associations are more elusive in people with learning disabilities and treatment is often pragmatic. Thus, biochemical investigations (Sandman *et al*, 1990; Smith *et al*, 1995) continue to generate hypotheses regarding the role of neurochemical systems, particularly opioid systems, in the development and maintenance of stereotypies – especially in people with autism. Neurochemical theories will not be discussed in detail here (see Jones *et al*, 1995), but pharmacological interventions have been advocated to reduce or eliminate stereotypies. However, efficacy studies (Baumeister, 1991; Campbell *et al*, 1993) suggest that a number of these investigations lack methodological sophistication. There is also concern that prescribing, for example, neuroleptic agents might, at best, reduce stereotypies in those who demonstrated high rates (Aman, 1983; Aman & Singh, 1983; Aman *et al*, 1984, 1989; Aman & Kern, 1989) and, at worst, cause extrapyramidal side-effects resembling the original stereotypies. In addition, these agents may exacerbate seizure frequency in people with a diagnosis of epilepsy and challenging behaviour, and, as Deb & Fraser (1994) point out, they are sometimes prescribed without sufficient monitoring. There is often a need, therefore, to explore non-pharmacological interventions at the outset if assessment indicates no definitive origin. Finally, it is important to note that despite the frequency of motor disorders such as Tourette syndrome, Huntington's disease and dystonic conditions in the general population, they are rarely recognised as a dual diagnosis in people with learning disabilities. This last fact would suggest that a proper assessment protocol incorporating a detailed differential diagnosis is of vital importance.

Other aspects of a person's medical history could also pertain to their problem behaviour. For example, the awareness that someone suffers from chronic earache could help to explain a stereotypy where they frequently slap their ear. A repetitive orofacial movement could be an initial symptom of tardive dyskinesia in someone who has received neuroleptic agents, to reduce stereotypy or aggression, for a considerable number of years. Medical records may indicate accumulative tissue and organ damage caused by self-injurious stereotypies or physical problems, explaining why an individual becomes aggressive if touched by a carer.

## Environmental and personal factors: setting the problem behaviour in context

Developing hypotheses concerning the function of the problem behaviour means gaining insight into the individuals concerned, and their relationships with their social and physical environment. Where possible, this means interviewing the person, and also using other sources of information. Involving the main carers in the assessment process can provide vital information about the individual's history and development, including significant life events and other factors that might help to maintain behaviours. The sudden onset of challenging behaviour could coincide with family bereavement, providing insight into the genesis of problem behaviours. Disruption and distress can be caused by a lack of consistent supportive relationships in a person's life. On the positive side, informants might also indicate where an individual's strengths and interests lie, offering the possibility of increasing their repertoire of skills for engaging with their world, rather than focusing on the elimination of behaviour. There might be vital clues as to the history and nature of the problem behaviour itself, such as whether there had been successful interventions in the past. It might emerge that the challenging behaviour is displayed in one setting and not another. Thus, placing the person and their behaviour into context helps to move beyond a snapshot of pathology and assists the analysis of the function of the behaviour in the individual's wider life.

## Problem behaviour: topography, antecedents and consequences

A clear description of the behaviour (topography) is the starting point for an analysis of the more immediate factors that trigger or maintain episodes of problem behaviour. Although this might sound like a simple process, it can be surprisingly difficult to obtain an agreed account of the problem behaviour. For example, one set of support workers might not regard it as remarkable when someone reaches out and grabs at other people's clothing, while others describe the same actions as a potentially dangerous assault. Typically, family members and support workers are likely to disagree about the nature and extent of problem behaviour. Observing the behaviour first-hand is straightforward where the behaviour is frequent, but may be problematic if it is infrequent. Nevertheless, it is vital to reach an agreed and concrete account of the problem behaviour, and informants must know how to differentiate between different levels of severity and intensity, before being asked to collect data. There are scales designed to elicit the topography of problem behaviour such as the Stereotyped Behaviour Scale (Rojahn *et al*, 2000) and the Non-convulsive Ictal Signs Checklist (Gedye, 1996). Depending upon the degree of sophistication required, these scales can either be completed by a psychologist *in situ* or they may involve interviewing carers. If ethical consent is obtained, a video recording of the behaviour can be made and a behavioural description produced from this.

If the psychologist wants merely to determine how problematic the behaviour is for carers, then analogue ratings provide a straightforward means of collecting subjective information. This involves observers completing analogue charts each time the behaviour is witnessed or each day. These charts could rate on a scale of 0–10 (0 = not a problem, 10 = very severe problem) either the overall difficulty or the severity of each behaviour as it occurs.

To have a clear idea about the antecedents and consequences of a particular problem, it is necessary to determine when an episode of the behaviour starts and finishes. Does the person suddenly hit out or is there an observable build-up in their agitation over a period of some hours? Understanding the typical chronology of an episode of problem behaviour of this nature influences the management or treatment of the behaviour. A slow build-up to aggression might make it possible to introduce distraction or other methods of de-escalation at an early stage, before a serious incident occurs. At this point in the data-gathering exercise, the best tool might be a chart following the classic 'antecedents, behaviour and consequences' format, with the aim of establishing the function of the behaviour. Forms can also request information about the environmental setting, along with information about the affective and physical state of the person displaying the problem behaviour. These incident forms can provide important data for the functional analysis.

There are other methods of obtaining data about the behaviour itself, including simple event recording when the behaviour does not occur at a particularly high rate, through to recording the duration and latency of high-frequency behaviour. Latency is the time between the opportunity to display a particular behaviour and its actual presentation. Small diaries, similar to those often produced for recording seizure events when an individual moves between home and day centre, can provide a carer with a simple, efficient means of recording problem behaviours. Such diaries use a code for each problem behaviour identified in the initial assessment period. These codes, alongside a description of the behaviour, are put at the front of the diary. To record an event, the carer simply enters the date and code and the time and/or duration of each behaviour. This is illustrated in Box 11.1.

---

**Box 11.1** Example of coding and entries in a problem behaviour diary, maintained by a carer

A: While seated in the day centre, John pushes away anyone who approaches
B: John slaps the right-hand side of his face with his palm
C: John slaps the wall with both hands

**Recording**

| Date | Time | Code | Duration |
|---|---|---|---|
| 06/07/03 | 9.03 am | A | 5 s |
| 06/07/03 | 9.08 am | B | 10 s |
| 06/07/03 | 3.30 pm | C | 10 s |

---

Behavioural principles rest on the assumption of scientific objectivity, so it is paradoxical that in everyday clinical practice, data about the person's behaviour are usually collected by informants who are family members or support workers. Far from being objective, these informants usually have an emotional attachment to the person. Involvement in aggressive incidents can make carers fearful or angry with the individual concerned, leading to strong beliefs about the cause of the behaviour. A history of interpersonal conflict will not merely affect how the carers view the person's behaviour and its causes, but also how they view the person as a whole (Wanless, 2000). It is important to bear these factors in mind when interpreting the data from incident sheets completed by support workers or family members. Yet, gaining insight into the beliefs and perceptions of significant others is an important part of the assessment process. The successful treatment of problem behaviours like aggression has to take account of the interpersonal context (Lovett, 1985; Kushlick *et al*, 1997; Clements, 1997*b*).

Iwata *et al* (1994) developed an experimental approach to examining the environmental factors maintaining problem behaviour. This involved systematically exposing the individual with problem behaviours to a series of analogue conditions, with different levels of environmental richness and with varied demands on the person and his or her social attention. This experimental approach has been used as a clinical tool for people with behavioural problems such as self-injury and aggression (Pelios *et al*, 1999). For instance, observations might suggest that a man's aggression increases in particular demanding situations. To test this hypothesis, analogue situations could be set up where active attempts are made to engage the person in structured activity. His aggressiveness might then be compared with situations where materials are made available to him with minimal prompting. While this method holds out great promise, the analogue conditions are presented for time-limited periods. Consequently, clinically significant findings will only be obtained for high-frequency target behaviours.

Finally, the baseline psychological assessment of people with learning disabilities may involve standardised measures such as the Aberrant Behavior Checklist (Aman *et al*, 1985) and the Vineland Adaptive Behavior Scales (Sparrow *et al*, 1984). These tools collect data on adaptive and maladaptive behaviours as well as functional skills, and can be used as repeated measures following an intervention period.

## Ethical issues

Once a comprehensive assessment has been conducted, there are two main areas that require some ethical consideration. First, in light of the fact that the aetiology of stereotyped behaviour, in particular, remains unclear, the psychologist must decide whether or not to intervene. Second, if intervention is deemed necessary, then the nature of that intervention must be considered, as some approaches may be regarded as aversive. This is particularly important in the case of someone with a learning disability, who might be unable to give informed consent to an intervention and, more likely, might not understand the nature of that intervention.

Clinicians must bear in mind the extent to which behaviours are of more concern to the carers than the clients themselves, and also whether the cost of intervening may outweigh the gains. For example, both aversive and non-aversive behavioural interventions continue to be recommended (Mace *et al*, 2001). However, there is longitudinal evidence to indicate that dramatic short-term gains following intensive behavioural interventions are not maintained at 10-year (Jones, 1999) and 7-year follow-up (Emerson *et al*, 2001*b*). Moreover, psychological interventions for problem behaviour need to be viewed in the context of the individual's quality of life. For example, if a severely disabled person's hand-flapping serves the purpose of keeping him/her awake in an unstimulating environment, then the emphasis should be on improving the quality of the environment rather than trying to reduce the person's hand-flapping. The same principle would apply to aggression due to boredom in a particular environment. On the other hand, if, as is commonly believed, there is a progressive relationship between non-injurious stereotypies and self-injurious stereotypies, then the clinician might feel duty-bound to intervene.

## Treatment

Treatment studies using behavioural interventions for stereotypy reported high success rates throughout the 1970s and 1980s (Koegel & Covert, 1972; Epstein *et al*, 1974; Repp *et al*, 1975; Baumeister, 1978; Ollendick & Matson, 1978; Bright *et al*, 1981; LaGrow & Repp, 1984) and these approaches are still advocated today (Lindsay & Walker, 1999). In a review, Allen (2000) also reported the success of behavioural interventions for problems of aggression. Whitaker (1993) carried out an earlier review of intervention studies for aggression, in which he classified behavioural treatments under the categories of 'ecological interventions', 'positive programming' and 'contingency management'. This serves as a good general classification system for behavioural interventions with problem behaviours. Consequently, in this section We will outline the interventions that come under these broad categories, before going on to briefly describe the multiple factors that clinicians often have to tackle in a treatment package.

## Ecological interventions

In some instances, it might be hypothesised that aberrant environments or surroundings that fail to meet the basic need for stimulation or communication are the primary cause of behavioural problems. This leads to interventions that focus on environmental change or enrichment. For example, Fallon & Whitaker (1996) advocated the manipulation of setting events by introducing sessions of physical and cognitive stimulation into the weekly activities of one woman who displayed frequent stereotypies. The aim was to improve the context in which the behaviour occurred, so as to reduce or eliminate it. A functional analysis could hypothesise a link between a man's aggressiveness, his autism and the fact that the rather abstract language used by support workers makes him confused and anxious. In this instance, the emphasis would be on increasing the effectiveness of the support workers' communication, perhaps by the systematic use of non-verbal cues (Clements, 1997a). It is important, however, for those intervening to be realistic when setting goals, as making substantial environmental changes might be beyond the resources of the carers involved.

## Positive programming

There has been an increasing emphasis upon 'positive' treatment strategies, such as functional communication training (Carr & Durand, 1985). Clinicians' preferences for 'positive' approaches are largely due to their values or philosophies, while a pragmatic basis for adopting these 'positive' approaches is their social acceptability (Emerson, 1998). The premise behind functional communication training is that the stereotypy or aggression serves a communicative function. This does not mean that it is an intentional communicative act by the person, but rather that the problem behaviour serves an adaptive purpose in his or her environment. For example, if an aggressive act usually results in an escape from aversive demands, then an intervention could teach the person other ways of communicating a wish to leave a particular setting. Alternatively, the person might be taught how to cope with the stressful situation. Hence, when working with someone who is aggressive or displays stereotypies, the treatment goal is not merely to suppress or eliminate the problem behaviour. Efficacy studies (Thompson *et al*, 1998) recommend that functional communication be combined with other interventions to increase effectiveness. Certainly, Jones *et al* (1995) concluded that a combination of psychological interventions might be most efficacious in the majority of cases. In 21 particularly challenging cases, Hagopian *et al* (1998) reduced problem behaviours by 90% by combining functional communication training with time out.

## Contingency management

Interventions focusing on the consequences of problem behaviour encompass both aversive techniques like time out, and non-aversive techniques such as differential reinforcement or sensory extinction. Time out involves the removal of social reinforcement. Results of such interventions have varied, but the literature indicates that aversive procedures are most efficacious for stereotypies (LaGrow & Repp, 1984; Scotti *et al*, 1991). However, Pelios *et al* (1999) have argued, in a recent review of interventions for self-injury, that rather unsophisticated functional analyses often fail to identify the events that are reinforcing behaviour. Thus, punishment has been used by default. Pelios and colleagues suggest that non-aversive techniques that clearly target maintaining factors could prove just as effective in many such cases. The arguments for and against the use of punishment are well-articulated elsewhere (Emerson, 1995), but this section will briefly describe non-punitive behavioural approaches to aggression.

Two of the main non-aversive techniques are differential reinforcement of other behaviour (DRO) and differential reinforcement of incompatible behaviour (DRI). DRO means delivering reinforcement contingent upon the absence of the problem behaviour for a predetermined period of time. DRI means reinforcing a behaviour that is incompatible with the problem behaviour, for example rewarding a person who engages in hand flapping when they put their hands in their pockets. Emerson (1998) makes reference to the fact that DRO procedures are not particularly effective when adopted for more challenging behaviours. Nevertheless, these strategies have obtained good results with stereotypies (Barton & Broughton, 1980), particularly when momentary DRO procedures are used (Derwas & Jones, 1993; Miller & Jones, 1997). These are less intensive than whole-interval DRO procedures, which reinforce a behaviour when it is displayed for the whole of a predetermined interval. Momentary DRO reinforces a behaviour that is displayed at some point during a predetermined interval.

# Multi-faceted interventions for real-life problems

In most instances, there is likely to be a complex interaction of individual and environmental factors involved in the maintenance of challenging behaviour (Clements, 1997b). Consequently, interventions might have to tackle a number of factors. Even if the intervention focuses on individual change, the environment remains crucial. There would be limited value in teaching new skills if the person were to continue to live in an impoverished environment with few opportunities to lead a more purposeful or socially fulfilling life. Cullen (1993) suggested that the impoverished lives of people with learning disabilities could be one of the major difficulties in maintaining change when working with offenders.

# Shifting to a cognitive–behavioural framework

Behavioural interventions continue to play an important part in treatment plans for people with stereotypies, who often have severe disabilities and communication difficulties. However, there are changing approaches to working with people with mild-to-moderate learning disabilities who are aggressive. Despite the proven effectiveness of behavioural procedures in helping people with learning disabilities to reduce their level of aggressive behaviour, there appear to be significant gaps in the outcome research. In particular, Whitaker (1993) has pointed to the paucity of studies concerning individuals living in community settings or independently. One might speculate on the reason why this continues to be the case. Perhaps there are difficulties maintaining the same level of environmental consistency when people are living in varied community settings. Not only might this lead to difficulty in implementing treatment programmes, but there may also be problems generalising new skills across different contexts. Moreover, Pelios et al's (1999) review indicated that many of the methods described in successful case studies relied upon experimental approaches such as analogue conditions that may have limited utility when working in everyday community settings.

Cullen (1993) proposed a solution to the problem of generalisation when working with people who have milder learning disabilities living in diffuse community settings. He suggested that the emphasis should shift from environmental contingencies to helping people use internal rules to govern their behaviour. One might expect that if individuals learn to use a set of rules to govern their behaviour, then these will prove effective across a variety of contexts. Cullen noted how teaching rule-governed behaviour was successfully used with two men who were frequently aggressive in a work setting (Cole et al, 1985). However, teaching people rules to govern their behaviour assumes that their challenging behaviour stems from an inability to interpret external cues or to generate an appropriate response. This may not be the case. Even where a comprehensive assessment is carried out, there is a danger that the aggression presented by people with learning disabilities will simply be traced back to the fact that they have a learning disability (Murphy, 1993).

By definition, individuals with learning disabilities have deficits in their cognitive functioning and daily living skills, and communication problems are common. It is relatively straightforward to identify such deficits as contributing to aggressiveness, which leads to a circular argument that their aggression is caused by factors relating to their learning disability. Yet, a recent study has shown that aggressive participants with mild learning disabilities were better at perspective-taking than their non-aggressive counterparts, who were matched in terms of cognitive ability (Pert *et al*, 1999). Cognitive–behavioural therapy moves beyond a deficit model (Jahoda *et al*, 2001), and begins to take into account the meaning of inter-personal events for people with learning disabilities.

## Anger management

Benson (1994) and Black *et al* (1988) have both been highly influential in adapting cognitive–behavioural anger management approaches, developed by Novaco (1977), for people with learning disabilities. Anger management places emphasis on the regulation of anger as a key factor in determining how people respond in situations of conflict or potential conflict, with uncontrolled anger making aggressive responses more likely. In turn, anger is mediated by cognitive factors and in particular by how people perceive and appraise interpersonal situations. For example, if people display an attributional bias of hostile intent, then they are more likely to think that others are behaving in a deliberately hostile fashion, causing them to be frequently angry. The interpersonal nature of conflict is also emphasised, as anger is seen as a social emotion (Black *et al*, 1997) and the impact of the person's broader social environment and relationships are taken into account. The goal of the intervention is not to prevent people from becoming angry, but to help reduce the frequency and intensity of their anger, thereby allowing them to cope more constructively with anger-provoking situations.

Just as in behavioural work, a thorough assessment and formulation of the person's anger and aggression is required in order to tailor the intervention to the individual's difficulties (Black *et al*, 1997; Lindsay *et al*, 1998; Taylor *et al*, 2002). The assessment examines the cognitive, behavioural, emotional, somatic and environmental factors underlying the person's anger and aggression. Behavioural and environmental factors are assessed in very much the same way as described in the previous section on behavioural methods, and cognitive and emotional factors are examined in terms of both process and content. Assessment of process considers areas of social-cognitive functioning where the person may have deficits, such as problem-solving ability (Fuchs & Benson, 1995) and emotional recognition (Walz & Benson, 1996). Regarding cognitive content, Black *et al* (1997) have pointed to the importance of adapting the existing cognitive therapy methods for tapping into the cognitive appraisals and beliefs of people with learning disabilities. Black & Novaco's (1993) case study found that their client's responses on a problem-solving assessment revealed a great deal about his cognitive appraisals. Reviewing past incidents might also provide insight into a client's perceptions of interpersonal situations and beliefs about others' actions. Moreover, the cognitive assessment also investigates the role of rumination in maintaining arousal or feelings of anger that can spill over into different situations.

The role of anger in the person's aggression is assessed in several ways. A Provocation Inventory (Novaco, 1983) involves reading the participant a list of provocative situations and asking how angry each situation would make him or her feel. The participant is also asked to keep an anger diary, usually with support from a family member or support worker, in which he or she makes daily recordings of the intensity of his or her anger on a visual analogue scale. A contra-indication to anger management treatment would be the instrumental use of aggression, where the person uses aggression without being angry in order to achieve a particular goal. However, there is debate as to whether one can make a clear distinction between instrumental and reactive aggression (Bushman & Anderson, 2001).

In practice, anger management consists of a package of interventions, with group and individual treatment formats being used. It can be argued that there are advantages in using a group approach to tackle an interpersonal problem like aggression. The three phases of treatment described by Black *et al* (1988) are education, skill acquisition, and practice of new skills.

The educational phase is largely concerned with teaching about the role of anger and both its positive and negative uses. However, Benson (1994) suggested placing anger alongside other emotions like happiness and sadness. Presenting anger as a normal feeling helps to examine how different situations evoke different emotions, introducing the link between a person's perception of events, feelings and behaviour. Moreover, there is the accompanying somatic arousal associated with anger. In order to gain greater self-control in situations of actual and potential conflict, a person has to recognise the early signs of this arousal. Psychologists would describe socialising someone into a particular treatment model in the first stages of an intervention. As part of this process, it may be necessary to teach or negotiate a shared language to allow a person to describe thoughts and feelings more fully during treatment. When working with an individual with learning disabilities, a greater period of time might be required to achieve this goal, and the therapist needs to tailor the approach and materials to the individual concerned.

After the learning phase and the raising of awareness, the individual receives coaching in a range of methods of controlling or modifying their anger. This phase includes relaxation training, in order to help individuals lower their level of arousal in anger-provoking situations. Being calmer makes it less likely that individuals will 'shoot from the hip' or act without thinking, and more likely that they will be able to work out a non-aggressive response. Benson (1994) includes problem-solving training that aims to make people more effective at generating non-aggressive responses. In fact, cognitive work carried out as part of anger management interventions still tends to focus on cognitive processes and skills, thereby continuing to concentrate on the cognitive deficits of people with learning disabilities. Self-instruction and the use of positive self-statements are taught in order to cue individuals' coping strategies in stressful situations. Perhaps the most poorly articulated element of treatment concerns perceptions of interpersonal events or cognitive distortions, when people distort the meaning of events and have a more antagonistic view of the world. Relatively little work has been carried out to tackle cognitive distortions, although it has been recognised that this is an area that requires further development for individuals with learning disabilities (Black *et al*, 1997).

In the final phase of treatment, participants use role-play to practise the new skills they have learned. This might involve a hierarchy of situations, building up from the least to the most stressful. The participants are also encouraged to practise their new skills outside the therapy sessions.

## Evidence for the use of anger management with people with learning disabilities

Whitaker (2001), argued in a recent review that the effectiveness of anger management for people with learning disabilities remains unproven, as there are few controlled studies. One exception was the comparison by Benson *et al* (1986) of the outcomes of a number of treatments based on components of anger management, including relaxation, self-instruction, problem-solving, and a combination of the three. They found that all the groups produced a reduction in the participants' anger and aggression. Unfortunately, no differences were found between the treatment groups, and the lack of a control group made the study inconclusive. Yet a number of case studies and investigations of group interventions point to promising outcomes for cognitive–behavioural interventions (Jahoda *et al*, 2001). Black & Novaco (1993) detailed their work with a man who presented significant problems of aggression. A great change in his behaviour was maintained at follow-up from treatment, which allowed him to make a successful move from long-stay hospital to the community.

There have also been a number of group studies, and Taylor *et al* (2002) recently investigated the efficacy of anger management with a group of offenders with learning disabilities living in a secure hospital. They found a significant reduction in the participants' anger problems. The study by Taylor *et al* also included several improvements to existing anger management protocols, suggested by Black *et al* (1997). First, they included a preparatory phase of treatment, dealing with the crucial issue of motivation to change. If people with learning disabilities have been referred for treatment by someone else and lack insight into their anger problems, or simply do not want to change their behaviour, then they will not be motivated to engage in therapy. Anger management, like other cognitive–behavioural approaches, is built upon a therapeutic alliance between the client and the therapist. Second, Taylor *et al* also followed Black *et al*'s example by emphasising the cognitive component of the anger management work. This meant moving on from a self-instructional approach, which is about learning new skills and ways of thinking in situations of conflict, towards challenging people's assumptions about the world. In particular, they tackled their partici-pants' attributions of hostile intent.

For the intervention to be successful, whether behavioural or cognitive–behavioural, there needs to be an impact upon people's wider lives (Cullen, 1993). Individuals with learning disabilities are often caught in dependent relationships with resulting interpersonal tensions. Thus, even if an intervention proves effective in helping individuals to manage their anger more effectively, thereby reducing their aggression, it is important that others recognise and acknowledge the change. Rose *et al* (2000) took their clients' wider social context seriously in their group intervention, by asking a significant other in each of the clients' lives to attend the group. The group intervention focused on inter-personal skills and problem-solving, with the clients and their workers practising how to deal with situations of conflict. Moreover, the groups also examined ways in which staff could work to reduce conflict and encourage more appropriate responses from their clients. Compared with a waiting-list control group, there were significant reductions in the clients' self-recorded levels of expressed anger and depression. The treatment gains were maintained at follow-up. Although there were no formal recordings of aggressive incidents, the staff reported that there had been reductions in the level of aggression during the treatment phase and that this positive trend had continued after treatment finished.

Rose *et al* (2000) argued that there were considerable advantages to having support workers accompany the clients to the group. The authors felt that there was better generalisation, with workers able to reinforce the strategies and skills the clients were learning in the group, when they were at home or work. In a similar vein, there was better communication between the psychologist leading the group and those providing support in the person's wider life. Rose *et al* believed that this communication helped to ensure that support workers followed through the recommended strategies for the staff team and encouraged the staff to give credit to the clients for the progress they made. Perhaps spending 32 hours in each other's company, in a therapeutic setting, may have increased the mutual understanding and sensitivity of the individuals with learning disabilities and their workers, and helped to build more positive relationships.

## Conclusion

The aim of this chapter has been to introduce the reader to a limited number of psychological approaches to working with common behavioural problems. Although behavioural approaches remain the dominant model in this field, there has been a growing openness to different psychological interventions. In part, this may reflect the fact that the field of learning disability research and treatment is catching up on developments in other clinical domains. It may also reflect the growing sophistication in the field of learning disability in thinking about causal and maintaining factors of behaviour. Traditionally, it has been believed that behavioural difficulties may reflect environmental contingencies at one end of a continuum and intrinsic biological factors at the other. Perhaps recent work has begun to bridge the bio-behavioural gap.

## References

Allen, D. (2000) Recent research on physical aggression in persons with intellectual disability: an overview. *Journal of Intellectual and Developmental Disability*, **25**, 41–57.
Aman, M. G. (1983) Psychoactive drugs in mental retardation. In *Treatment Issues and Innovations in Mental Retardation* (eds J. L. Matson & F. Andrasik). New York: Plenum.
—— & Kern, R. A. (1989) Review of fenfluramine in the treatment of the developmental disabilities. *Journal of the American Academy of Child and Adolescent Psychiatry*, **28**, 549–565.
—— & Singh, N. N. (1983) Pharmacological intervention. In *Handbook of Mental Retardation* (eds J. L. Matson & J. A. Mulick). New York: Pergamon.
——, White, A. J. & Field, C. (1984) Chlorpromazine effects on stereotypic and conditioned behaviour of severely retarded patients – a pilot study. *Journal of Mental Deficiency Research*, **28**, 253–260.

——, Singh, N. N., Stewart, A. W., *et al* (1985) Psychometric characteristics of the Aberrant Behavior Checklist. *American Journal of Mental Deficiency*, **89**, 492–502.

——, Teehan, C. J., White, A. J., *et al* (1989) Haloperidol treatment with chronically medicated residents: dose effects on clinical behaviour and reinforcement contingencies. *American Journal on Mental Retardation*, **93**, 452–460.

Barton, R. E. & Broughton, S. F. (1980) Stereotyped behaviour in profoundly retarded clients: a review. *Behaviour Research of Severe Developmental Disabilities*, **1**, 279–306.

Baumeister, A. A. (1978) Origins and control of stereotyped movements. In *Quality of Life in Severely and Profoundly Retarded People. Research Foundations for Improvement* (ed. C. E. Meyers), pp. 353–384. Washington, DC: American Association on Mental Deficiency.

—— (1991) Expanded theories of stereotypy and self-injurious responding: commentary on 'Emergence and maintenance of stereotypy and self-injury.' *American Journal on Mental Retardation*, **96**, 321–323.

Benson, B. A. (1994) Anger management training: a self-control programme for persons with mental retardation. In *Mental Health in Mental Retardation: Recent Advances and Practices* (ed. N. Bouras), pp. 224–232. Cambridge: Cambridge University Press.

——, Rice, C. J. & Miranti, S. V. (1986) Effects of anger management training with mentally retarded adults in group treatment. *Journal of Consulting and Clinical Psychology*, **54**, 728–729.

Berkson, G. & Davenport, R. K. (1962) Stereotyped movements of mental defectives. I. Initial survey. *American Journal of Mental Deficiency*, **66**, 849–852.

Bicknell, D. J. (1985) Epilepsy and mental handicap. In *Epilepsy and Mental Handicap. Royal Society of Medicine Round Table Series No. 2* (ed. C. Wood), pp. 1–15. London: RSM Press.

Black, L. & Novaco, R. (1993) Treatment of anger with a developmentally handicapped man. In *Casebook of the Brief Psychotherapies* (eds R. A. Wells & V. J. Giannetti), pp. 143–158. London: Plenum.

——, Cullen, C., Dickens, P., *et al* (1988). Anger control. *British Journal of Hospital Medicine*, **22**, 325–329.

——, —— & Novaco, R. W. (1997). Anger assessment for people with mild learning disabilities in secure settings. In *Cognitive Behaviour Therapy for People with Learning Disabilities* (eds B. S. Kroese, D. Dagnan & K. Loumidis), pp. 33–52. London: Routledge.

Bright, T., Bittick, K. & Fleeman, B. (1981) Reduction of self-injurious behaviour using sensory integrative techniques. *American Journal of Occupational Therapy*, **35**, 167–172.

Bushman, B. J. & Anderson, C. A. (2001) Is it time to pull the plug on the hostile versus instrumental aggression dichotomy? *Psychological Review*, **108**, 273–279.

Campbell, M., Anderson, L. T., Small, A. M., *et al* (1993) Naltrexone in autistic children: behavioural symptoms and attentional learning. *Journal of the American Academy of Child and Adolescent Psychiatry*, **32**, 1289–1291.

Carr, E. G. & Durand, V. M. (1985) The social communicative basis of severe behaviour problems. In *Theoretical Issues in Behaviour Therapy* (eds S. Reiss & R. Bootzin), pp. 111–125. New York: Academic Press.

Clements, J. (1997*a*) Sustaining a cognitive psychology for people with learning disabilities. In *Cognitive Behaviour Therapy for People with Learning Disabilities* (eds B. S. Kroese, D. Dagnan & K. Loumidis), pp.162–181. London: Routledge.

—— (1997*b*) Challenging needs and problematic behaviour. In *Adults with Learning Disabilities. A Practical Approach for Health Professionals* (eds J. O'Hara & A. Sperlinger), pp. 82–89. Chichester: John Wiley & Sons.

Cole, C. L., Gardener, W. I. & Karan, O. C. (1985) Self-management training of mentally retarded adults presenting severe conduct difficulties. *Applied Research in Mental Retardation*, **6**, 337–347.

Coulter, D. L. (1993) Epilepsy and mental retardation: an overview. *American Journal on Mental retardation*, **98** (suppl. 1), 1–11.

Cullen, C. (1993). The treatment of people with learning disabilities who offend. In *Clinical Approaches to the Mentally Disordered Offender* (eds K. Howells & C. R. Hollin). Chichester: John Wiley & Sons.

Deb, S. & Fraser, W. (1994) The use of psychotropic medication in people with learning disability: towards rational prescribing. *Human Psychopharmacology*, **9**, 259–272.

Derwas, H. & Jones, R. S. (1993) Reducing stereotyped behaviour using momentary D.R.O.: an experimental analysis. *Behavioural Residential Treatment*, **8**, 45–53.

Dura, J. R., Mulick, J. A. & Rasnake, L. K. (1987) Prevalence of stereotypy among institutionalised non-ambulatory mentally retarded people. *American Journal of Mental Deficiency*, **91**, 548–549.

Emerson, E. (1995) *Challenging Behaviour: Analysis and Intervention in People with Learning Disabilities*. Cambridge: Cambridge University Press.

— (1998) Working with people with challenging behaviour. In *Clinical Psychology and People with Intellectual Disabilities* (eds E. Emerson, C. Hatton, J. Bromley, *et al*), pp. 127–153. Chichester: John Wiley & Sons.

—, Kiernan, C., Alborz, A., *et al* (2001*a*) The prevalence of challenging behaviours: a total population study. *Research in Developmental Disabilities*, **22**, 77–93.

—, —, —, *et al* (2001*b*) Predicting the persistence of severe self-injurious behavior. *Research in Developmental Disabilities*, **22**, 67–75.

Epstein, L. H., Doke, L. A., Sajwaj, T. E., *et al* (1974) Generality and side-effects of over-correction. *Journal of Applied Behavioural Analysis*, **7**, 385–390.

Espie, C. A. & Paul, A. (1997) Epilepsy and learning disabilities. In *The Clinical Psychologist's Handbook of Epilepsy* (eds C. Cull & L. Goldstein), pp. 184–198. London: Routledge.

Fallon, J. & Whitaker, S. (1996) The effect of stimulation on stereotyped behaviour of a woman with a profound learning disability. *Behavioural and Cognitive Psychotherapy*, **24**, 323–329.

Fish, D. R. & Marsden, C. D. (1994) Epilepsy masquerading as a movement disorder. In *Movement Disorders III* (eds C. D. Marsden & S. Fahn), pp. 346–358. Oxford: Butterworth Heinemann.

Forehand, R. & Baumeister, A. A. (1976) Decelerating aberrant behaviour among retarded individuals. In *Progress in Behaviour Modification* (eds M. Hersen, R. M. Eisler & P. M. Miller), pp. 55–96. New York: Academic Press.

Fuchs, C. & Benson, B. A. (1995) Social information processing by aggressive and non-aggressive men with mental retardation. *American Journal on Mental Retardation*, **100**, 244–252.

Gardner, W. I. & Moffat, C. W. (1990) Aggressive behaviour: definition, assessment, treatment. *International Review of Psychiatry*, **2**, 91–100.

Gedye, A. (1989) Extreme self-injury attributed to frontal seizures. *American Journal on Mental Retardation*, **94**, 20–26.

— (1991) Tourette syndrome attributed to frontal lobe dysfunction: numerous etiologies involved. *Journal of Clinical Psychology*, **47**, 233–252.

— (1992) Anatomy of self-injurious stereotypic and aggressive movements – evidence for involuntary explanation. *Journal of Clinical Psychology*, **4**, 766–775.

— (1996) Recognizing involuntary movements with vocalisations and autonomic changes: a non-convulsive ictal signs checklist. *Habilitative Mental Healthcare Newsletter*, **15**, 71–80.

Hagopian, L. P., Fisher, W. W., Sullivan, M. T., *et al* (1998) Effectiveness of functional communication training with and without extinction and punishment: a summary of 21 in-patient cases. *Journal of Applied Behavioral Analysis*, **31**, 211–235.

Iwata, B. A., Dorsey, M. F., Slifer, K. J., *et al* (1994) Toward a functional analysis of self-injury. *Journal of Applied Behavior Analysis*, **27**, 197–209.

Jahoda, A., Trower, P., Pert, C., *et al* (2001) Contingent reinforcement or defending the self? A review of evolving models of aggression in people with mild learning disabilities. *British Journal of Medical Psychology*, **74**, 305–321.

Jankovic, J. (1992) Diagnosis and classification of tics and Tourette syndrome. *Advances in Neurology*, **58**, 7–14.

Jones, R. S. P. (1999) A 10 year follow-up of stereotypic behavior with eight participants. *Behavioral Interventions*, **14**, 45–54.

—, Walsh, P. G. & Sturmey, P. (1995) *Stereotyped Movement Disorders*. Chichester: John Wiley & Sons.

Koegel, R. L. & Covert, A. (1972) The relationship of self-stimulation to learning in autistic children. *Journal of Applied Behavioural Analysis*, **5**, 381–87.

Kushlick, A., Trower, P. & Dagnan, D. (1997) Applying cognitive-behavioural approaches to the carers of people with learning disabilities who display challenging behaviour. In *Cognitive Behaviour Therapy for People with Learning Disabilities* (eds B. S. Kroese, D. Dagnan & K. Loumidis), pp. 55–96. London: Routledge.

LaGrow, S. J. & Repp, A. C. (1984) Stereotypic responding: a review of intervention research. *American Association on Mental Deficiency*, **88**, 595–609.

LaVigna, G. W. & Donnellan, A. M. (1986) *Alternatives to Punishment: Solving Behaviour Problems with Non-Aversive Strategies*. New York: Irvington.

Lindsay, W. R. & Walker, B. (1999) Advances in behavioural methods in intellectual disability. *Current Opinion in Psychiatry*, **12**, 561–565.

—, Overend, H., Allan, R., *et al* (1998) Using specific approaches for individual problems in the management of anger and aggression. *British Journal of Learning Disabilities*, **26**, 44–50.

Lovett, H. (1985) *Cognitive Counselling and Persons with Special Needs: Adopting Behavioural Approaches to the Social Context*. London: Praeger.

Mace, F. C., Blum, N. J., Sierp, B. J., *et al* (2001) Differential response of operant self-injury to pharmacological versus behavioural treatment. *Journal of Developmental and Behavioural Pediatrics*, **22**, 85–91.

Matson, J. L. & Volkmar, F. A. (1997) Autism in children and adults: etiology, assessment and intervention. *Contemporary Psychology*, **42**, 932.

Miller, B. Y. & Jones, R. S. P. (1997) Reducing stereotyped behaviour: a comparison of two methods of programming differential reinforcement. *British Journal of Clinical Psychology*, **36**, 297–302.

Murphy, G. (1993) The treatment of challenging behaviour in people with learning difficulties. In *Violence: Basic and Clinical Science* (eds C. Thompson & P. Cowan). Oxford: Butterworth Heinemann.

Novaco, R. W. (1977) Stress inoculation: a cognitive therapy for anger and in application to a case of depression. *Journal of Consulting and Clinical Psychology*, **45**, 600–608.

— (1983) *Stress Inoculation Therapy for Anger Control. A Manual for Therapists*. Irvine, CA: University of California.

Ollendick, T. H. & Matson, J. L. (1978) Overcorrection: an overview. *Behaviour Therapy*, **9**, 830–842.

Paul, A. (1997) An investigation of epilepsy and stereotyped behaviours in people with learning disabilities using EEG spectral analysis and behavioural methodologies. PhD thesis, University of Strathclyde, UK.

Pelios, L., Morren, J., Tesch, D., *et al* (1999) The impact of functional analysis methodology on treatment choice for self-injurious and aggressive behavior. *Journal of Applied Behavior Analysis*, **32**, 185–195.

Pert, C., Jahoda, A. & Squire, J. (1999) Attribution of intent and role taking: cognitive factors as mediators of aggression with people who have mental retardation. *American Journal on Mental Retardation*, **104**, 399–419.

Reiss, S. & Havercamp, S. M. (1997) Sensitivity theory and mental retardation: why functional analysis is not enough. *American Journal on Mental Retardation*, **6**, 533–566.

Repp, A. C., Deitz, S. M. & Speir, N. C. (1975) Reducing stereotypic responding of retarded persons by the differential reinforcement of other behaviours. *American Journal of Mental Deficiency*, **79**, 279–284.

Rojahn, J. (1986) Self-injurious and stereotypic behaviour of non-institutionalized mentally retarded people: prevalence and classification. *American Journal of Mental Deficiency*, **91**, 268–276.

——, Matlock, S. T. & Tasse, M. J. (2000) The Stereotyped Behaviour Scale: psychometric properties and norms. *Research in Developmental Disabilities*, **21**, 437–454.

Rose, J., West, C. & Clifford, D. (2000) Group interventions for anger in people with intellectual disabilities. *Research in Developmental Disabilities*, **21**, 171–181.

Sandman, C. A., Barron, L. J. & Colman, H. (1990) An orally administered opiate blocker, naltrexone, attenuates self-injurious behaviour. *American Journal on Mental Retardation*, **95**, 93–102.

Scotti, J. R., Evans, I. M., Meyer, L. H., *et al* (1991) A meta-analysis of behavioral research with problem behavior: treatment validity and standards of practice. *American Journal on Mental Retardation*, **93**, 233–256.

Smith, S. G., Gupta, K. K. & Smith, S. H. (1995) Effects of naltrexone on self-injury, stereotypy and social behaviour of adults with developmental disabilities. *Journal of Developmental and Physical Disabilities*, **7**, 137–146.

Sparrow, S. S., Balla, D. A. & Cicchetti, D. V. (1984) *Vineland Adaptive Behavior Scales*. Circle Pines, MN: American Guidance Service.

Stoessl, A. J. (1990) Stereotyped motor phenomena in neurological disease. In *Neurobiology of Stereotyped Behaviour* (eds S. J. Cooper & C. T. Dourish), pp. 260–292. New York: Oxford University Press.

Sturmey, P. (2001) The Functional Analysis Checklist: inter-rater and test–retest reliability. *Journal of Applied Research in Intellectual Disabilities*, **14**, 141–146.

Taylor, J., Novaco, R., Gillmere, B., *et al* (2002) Treatment of anger intensity among offenders with intellectual disability. *Journal of Applied Research in Intellectual Disabilities*, **15**, 151–165.

Thompson, R. H., Fisher, W. W., Piazza, C. C., *et al* (1998) The evaluation and treatment of aggression maintained by attention and automatic reinforcement. *Journal of Applied Behavioral Analysis*, **31**, 103–116.

Walsh, P. G. (1994) A survey of stereotyped behaviours exhibited by adults with learning disabilities living in a residential centre in the west of Ireland. *British Journal of Learning Disabilities*, **22**, 90–93.

Walz, N. C. & Benson, B. A. (1996) Labelling and discrimination of facial expressions by aggressive and non-aggressive men with mental retardation. *American Journal on Mental Retardation*, **101**, 282–291.

Wanless, L. (2000) The Responses of Staff Towards People with Mild to Moderate Intellectual Disabilities Who Engage In Aggressive Behaviour: A Cognitive Emotional Analysis. DPsychol thesis, University of Glasgow, UK.

Whitaker, S. (1993) The reduction of aggression in people with learning difficulties: a review of psychological methods. *British Journal of Clinical Psychology*, **32**, 11–20.

—— (2001) Anger control for people with learning disabilities: a critical review. *Behavioural and Cognitive Psychotherapy*, **29**, 277–293.

# CHAPTER 12

# Psychotropic medication and learning disability

## Zed Ahmed

Psychopharmacology has advanced rapidly in the past two decades. The introduction of serotonin reuptake inhibitor antidepressants and the rebirth of clozapine have meant that the arsenal with which to treat mental illness has increased immensely. As new ligands (compounds that attach to specific receptors) are being developed, our understanding of how drugs work is expanding at a rapid pace. Safety of psychotropic drugs is now of paramount importance and has recently led to the withdrawal of the two most widely used drugs in psychiatry, droperidol and thioridazine, both of which were associated with unacceptable cardiac side-effects. Pharmaceutical companies are starting to pay closer attention to the needs of those with learning disabilities, and have begun to include this population in their drug trials. This is currently evident in the field of epilepsy and it will  hopefully filter down to psychiatry in the near future.

Psychotropic drugs are widely used in individuals with learning disabilities. Surveys show that between 30% and 40% will be on psychotropic medication, and of these about a third will be on anti-epileptics, a third on antipsychotics and the rest on antidepressants, anxiolytics or other psychotropics. Polypharmacy rates vary between 5% and 10%. Looking specifically at antipsychotic medication, there is a 22–45% usage in hospital settings and a 20% usage in the community. Psychotropic medication is used mainly for the treatment of mental illness, epilepsy, sleep problems, hyperactivity and behavioural problems. Between 5% and 35% of antipsychotic medication prescribed is for the control of challenging behaviour.

The basis on which psychotropic medication is used in learning disability is usually inferred from studies carried out on the general psychiatric population. There are very few methodologically sound studies showing evidence that these drugs are effective in those with learning disabilities. People with learning disabilities pose extra challenges when compared with the general psychiatric population. The issue of informed consent is important; this is often lacking, especially in those with an IQ of less than 50. Compliance is better in individuals with learning disabilities because carers are often responsible for administering the drugs. Side-effects are more prominent in individuals with learning disabilities, but communication difficulties hinder their reporting by these individuals. There is therefore a greater onus on the carers to monitor for signs of side-effects, which are often present as changes in behaviour and may be mistaken for worsening of the disorder being treated.

Communication difficulties also lead to problems in diagnosing mental illness and this becomes increasingly problematic as IQ decreases. With limited communication, behavioural changes and biological signs are used to make a diagnosis of mental illness. This greatly reduces the diagnostic validity, such that psychotropic medication is more likely to be used diagnostically, i.e. if someone improves with an antidepressant, then the underlying disorder will be retrospectively diagnosed as depression. Drug dosage used in individuals with learning disabilities is often lower than that used in the general psychiatric population, although the validity of this has not been systematically tested. Lastly, the carers of those with learning disabilities often judge the effectiveness of medication prescribed. Carers' judgement of the efficacy of a drug is influenced by what they expect of it. If their expectation is too high, for example for a drug to totally eradicate a challenging behaviour, a drug may be reported as ineffective if this expectation is not met. Informing carers of what to realistically expect can easily overcome this problem.

This chapter addresses the main categories of psychotropic medication, excluding anti-epileptic drugs. Most of the information presented is from studies of the general psychiatric population. Where specific studies in learning disability are available and relevant, these are mentioned.

# Psychotic disorders

Psychotic disorders are predominantly treated with antipsychotic medication. The most common disorder is schizophrenia. There are various bio-psychosocial theories to explain schizophrenia, but it is believed that the end result is an increase in dopamine transmission in the limbic area of the brain, with a decreased transmission in the prefrontal area. Increase in dopamine in the limbic area leads to the positive symptoms of schizophrenia: delusions, hallucinations, bizarre behaviour and thought disorder. Decreased dopamine in the prefrontal area leads to the negative symptoms: affective flattening, anhedonia, avolition, alogia and asociality.

The dopamine hypothesis of schizophrenia is supported by two observations. First, drugs that lead to an increase in dopamine levels in the brain (such as amphetamines, bromocriptine, cocaine, L-dopa and phencyclidine (PCP)) produce symptoms that are indistinguishable from those in schizophrenia. Second, all antipsychotic drugs are thought to reduce dopamine transmission.

Dopamine is a neurotransmitter that binds to dopamine receptors. Molecular genetics has shown that there are many different types of dopamine receptor, all of which are G-linked protein receptors. Receptors $D_2$ and $D_4$ are thought to be important in the treatment of schizophrenia. Serotonin receptors also play a role in treatment of schizophrenia, as is evident from the use of new atypical antipsychotic drugs that block serotonin receptors 5-HT$_{2A}$ and 5-HT$_6$ as well as the dopamine receptors. There are four main areas of the brain where dopamine transmission is important: the limbic area, prefrontal cortex, basal ganglia and tuberoinfundibular tract. Antipsychotic drugs affect all these areas to varying degrees, which explains their efficacy and their side-effect profile.

Blockade of dopamine in the basal ganglia causes extrapyramidal side-effects; similar blockade at the tuberoinfundibular tract causes hyperprolactinaemia. Antipsychotic drugs do not block just dopamine and serotonin receptors: they also block cholinergic $M_1$, histamine $H_1$ and adrenergic $\alpha_1 + \alpha_2$ receptors. Cholinergic blockade leads to impairment of memory and learning and, in extreme cases, can result in confusion and delirium, especially in the elderly. Peripheral blockade of cholinergic receptors can cause blurred vision, dry mouth, tachycardia, constipation, erectile impotence and urinary retention. These side-effects are compounded if anticholinergic medication is used concurrently to treat extrapyramidal side-effects. Activation of adrenergic $\alpha_1$ receptors leads to smooth-muscle contraction; blockade, on the other hand, leads to muscle relaxation and may cause postural hypotension. Adrenergic $\alpha_2$ receptors regulate the release of noradrenalin and serotonin, and blockade of these receptors leads to an increase in noradrenalin and serotonin levels. Blockade of histamine $H_1$ receptors leads to sedation and an increase in appetite that can result in weight gain.

The side-effects mentioned above are acute, but are usually transient and self-limiting or reversed by other drugs such as anticholinergics. The long-term side-effects, such as tardive dykinesia, tardive akathesia and tardive dystonias, are of greater concern and are more prominent in individuals with learning disabilities. Tardive dyskinesia occurs in 30–45% of those with learning disabilities taking typical antipsychotic drugs. Tardive dyskinesia is defined as involuntary, irregular, choreo-athetoid movements of the head, trunk and limbs. It was first described by Schonecker in 1957 and commonly affects the perioral region, leading to darting, protruding, twisting movements of the tongue. It can be minimal and hardly noticed or severe and incapacitating.

Although antipsychotic drugs can produce tardive dyskinesia, in the early stages they also mask its symptoms such that when they are withdrawn it becomes more evident. Paulson *et al* (1975) reported a 20% prevalence of emergent tardive dyskinesia on stopping antipsychotic medication. Gualtieri *et al* (1986) found a 29% incidence of transient dyskinesia on drug withdrawal. Once tardive dyskinesia develops, it is irreversible in about 50% of cases, even if the antipsychotic drug is stopped. It has serious implications: it is cosmetically disfiguring, causes physical morbidity and, in severe cases, it can affect the muscles of respiration and can be fatal.

Neuroleptic malignant syndrome is another serious consequence of antipsychotic drugs. It is thought to be an idiosyncratic reaction to the drugs, including the atypicals, with an increased prevalence in learning disability. The reported prevalence in those prescribed antipsychotic medication is between 0.02% and 2.44%, and more than 40% of these have a diagnosis of mood disorder (Addonizio *et al*, 1987). Eighty per cent of cases occur within 2 weeks of initiating drug therapy. The cause is thought to be severe antagonism of dopamine receptors in the hypothalamus, leading to impaired heat dissipation with hyperthermia (38.5–40°C) and antagonism of dopamine receptors in the striatum, which leads to muscle rigidity and alteration of calcium mobilisation in muscle cells, causing impaired contractility. Without treatment, neuroleptic malignant syndrome has a mortality rate of up to 20%. It causes muscle breakdown, and the consequent release of myoglobin can lead to renal failure. It is also associated with autonomic instability, altered consciousness and the elevation of creatinine phosphokinase and white cell count. Treatment includes discontinuation of the antipsychotic medication, use of dantrolene as a muscle relaxant, use of the dopamine agonists bromocriptine or amantadine, and basic medical support. Electroconvulsive therapy (ECT) has also been used to treat the syndrome, but its efficacy has not been evaluated.

Greater understanding and legal action in the USA have led to the reappraisal of the use of antipsychotic medication in individuals with learning disabilities, with gradual withdrawal in those without a mental illness or use of the minimum effective dose in those requiring maintenance medication. Because of fears of tardive dyskinesia and other extrapyramidal side-effects, there has been a gradual move away from the use of typical antipsychotics such as haloperidol towards the newer atypicals, of which clozapine is the gold standard and risperidone is the most commonly used. There are no randomised controlled trials looking at the effectiveness of atypical antipsychotics in individuals with learning disabilities, although a number of case report studies have shown their effectiveness. Williams *et al* (2000) showed risperidone and olanzapine to be effective and well tolerated in a case study of 21 individuals with learning disabilities.

## Specific antipsychotics

### Amisulpride

Introduced in 1998, amisulpride is thought specifically to block $D_2$ and $D_3$ receptors in the limbic area of the brain, but not to block any other receptor types. At doses of 50–300 mg it improves negative symptoms of schizophrenia, and at doses above 400 mg it improves positive symptoms. Beyond 800 mg it is associated with extrapyramidal side effects and hyperprolactinaemia. Common side-effects (5–10% of all side-effects reported) include insomnia, anxiety and agitation. Less common effects (0.1–5%) include somnolence and various gastro-intestinal disorders such as constipation, nausea and vomiting.

### Clozapine

First synthesised in 1959, clozapine was labelled atypical because of its ability to block amphetamine-induced locomotor activity without causing catalepsy in rodents and was shown to have the lowest incidence of extrapyramidal side-effects. It was introduced in Europe in 1969. In 1975, six deaths were reported in a geographically restricted region of Finland over a short period of time and it was consequently withdrawn. It was reintroduced in 1989, following a study by Kane et al (1988). This showed, in a double-blind comparison with chlorpromazine in 300 treatment-resistant people with schizophrenia, that clozapine was superior at improving both positive and negative symptoms and that 30% of patients responded at 6 weeks with clozapine, compared with 4% with chlorpromazine.

Subsequent studies have shown that if treatment is continued for 6 months, 60–70% will respond to clozapine. The addition of the $D_2$-specific blocker sulpiride to clozapine may also increase the response rate. Retrospective audit studies of clozapine in individuals with learning disabilities suggest that it is effective for resistant schizophrenia. Antonacci & de Groot (2000) in the USA reported use of clozapine in 33 individuals, of whom 79% responded. The most common side-effect reported was constipation; no one discontinued treatment because of agranulocytosis.

Clozapine is associated with potentially life-threatening agranulocytosis in 0.05–0.5% of those on the drug, with peak incidence within 4–18 weeks of starting treatment. Clozapine reduces the seizure threshold, which is important in those with epilepsy. It causes seizures in a dose-dependent manner, mostly frontal motor seizures and especially myoclonic jerks, which occur in 2% of cases with a dose of less than 600 mg and 6% beyond 600 mg. These require treatment with an anti-epileptic drug; the one most commonly used is sodium valproate. Drugs that affect liver metabolism (such as the selective serotonin reuptake inhibitors (SSRIs)) can increase the plasma level of clozapine by decreasing its metabolism, which might lead to an increased risk of seizures. Weight gain is a major problem, with 30% experiencing an increase in body weight of more than 7%. Reinstein *et al* (1999) have shown that substituting 25% of the clozapine dose with quetiapine (1 mg clozapine = 2 mg quetiapine) can lead to weight loss after 1 month. Owing to its ability to block serotonin receptors, clozapine, as well as the other atypicals, can exacerbate obsessive–compulsive disorder and may necessitate the addition of an SSRI or lithium to boost serotonin levels.

## Olanzapine

Introduced in 1996, olanzapine produces dose-dependent extrapyramidal side-effects, marked increase in appetite, weight gain and somnolence. It is not associated with agranulocytosis or lowering of the seizure threshold.

## Quetiapine

Quetiapine was introduced in 1997. It is structurally related to clozapine, but does not cause agranulocytosis or lower the seizure threshold. It causes fewer extrapyramidal side-effects than risperidone or olanzapine. It has no effect on prolactin levels and is the drug of choice in those with Parkinson's disease. It is associated with headache, agitation, dry mouth, dizziness, weight gain and postural hypotension. Animal studies have linked it to an increased risk of cataracts.

## Risperidone

Risperidone was introduced in 1993. It has a greater tendency to cause extrapyramidal side-effects than the other atypical antipsychotics. It has been shown to improve cognition in schizophrenia compared with typical antipsychotics. It causes moderate weight gain, but this is less than that caused by clozapine or olanzapine. Postural hypotension is common owing to adrenergic $\alpha_1$ blockade; it also causes the greatest rise in prolactin levels of all the atypicals. Risperidone is not associated with an increase in seizure threshold or agranulocytosis.

## Ziprasidone

The latest atypical antipsychotic drug, ziprasidone is useful for treating positive, negative and affective symptoms of schizophrenia. It is available as an intramuscular formulation; it causes little weight gain or elevation of prolactin levels and few extrapyramidal side-effects. The most common side-effects are transient somnolence, nausea and dyspepsia. It very rarely causes postural hypotension. Ziprasidone has been shown to be well-tolerated and effective in Tourette syndrome.

### Zotepine

Zotepine has been used in Japan since 1982 and in Germany since 1990; it was introduced in the UK in 1999. It is associated with improvements in cognitive function. Its major side-effect is weight gain, in 31% of patients, and also somnolence, in 14%. It also causes a significant degree of dry mouth, constipation, akathesia and extrapyramidal side-effects. High doses can lower the seizure threshold.

# Mood disorders

## Depression

Depression is thought to manifest at the neurotransmitter level when there is a decrease in the level of serotonin and/or noradrenalin in the hippocampus and limbic regions of the brain. The precise cause of this decrease is unknown. The effect of serotonin and noradrenalin on the post-synaptic receptors is to trigger the activation of adenylate cyclase and cyclic adenosine monophosphate (cAMP). These are intracellular messengers that in turn lead to production of neurotrophic messengers such as brain-derived neurotrophic factor, neurotrophins 3, 4 and 5, nerve growth factor and neurotrophic factor within the neuron. This cascade of events is thought to be responsible for maintenance of a euthymic mood in response to stresses from the external environment. In animal studies, levels of an endogenous compound 5-HT moduline have been shown to increase when an animal faces stress. It binds to presynaptic $5\text{-HT}_{1B}$ receptors and reduces the release of serotonin, thus inducing a state of depression.

All antidepressants act by effectively increasing brain levels of serotonin and noradrenalin. This increase occurs within hours of taking an antidepressant, although there is a delay of about 2 weeks before the depression begins to lift. This is consistent with the fact that although there is an immediate increase in serotonin and noradrenalin following a dose of antidepressant, the increased production of neurotrophic factors is believed to be delayed by 10–20 days.

Overall, antidepressants will work for 65–75% of people. The symptoms that respond the best are low mood, anhedonia, lethargy, poor appetite, guilt, helplessness, sleep problems and feelings of hopelessness. If psychotic symptoms are present, then the use of an antidepressant or an antipsychotic drug on its own results in a response rate of only 30–40%, whereas combining the two increases the rate to 70–80%. In such cases, it is best to start with the antipsychotic drug: first, improving the psychosis will improve the compliance with the medication; and second, if there are doubts as to whether the diagnosis is a pure psychotic disorder or depression with psychotic symptoms, then the most appropriate drug will have been given first. The dose of antipsychotic required is less in depressive disorders (about 100–300 mg equivalent of chlorpromazine) than in schizophrenia.

Verhoeven *et al* (2001), in an open trial, showed that citalopram was effective (measured by the Clinical Global Impression scale) in 60% of subjects with learning disabilities and depression. In severe and profound learning disability, where behavioural signs are used to make the diagnosis of depression, Langee & Conlon (1992), in a retrospective audit study, showed a 36% response rate with antidepressants. The factors associated with a favourable outcome were higher IQ, presence of psychosis, depressed affect and temper tantrums. Those with hyperactivity and self-injurious behaviour showed only a 20% response rate and 10% of their subjects got worse when treated with antidepressants.

Electroconvulsive therapy has the best response rate for depression, at 80–90%, although it is associated with transient memory problems. It has a mortality rate of 1:10 000, usually a result of a pre-existing cardiac problem. It is most effective in psychotic depression.

## Atypical depression

Atypical depression is usually characterised by: a 50% decrease in mood reactivity; hypersomnia (more than 10 hours sleep at least three times a week); overeating, leading to a weight increase of more than 3 kg in 3 months; leaden paralysis (feeling of heavy limbs for more than 1 hour at least three times per week and continuing for more than 3 months; pathological oversensitivity to interpersonal rejection; and reversal of diurnal variation of mood. Atypical depression responds best to monoamine oxidase inhibitors.

## Treatment-resistant depression

Treatment-resistant depression is defined as one that has not responded to three different antidepressants, one of which is a tricyclic and one an SSRI. There are various strategies for the management of treatment-resistant depression. Lithium augmentation is the most commonly used method, the response rate with which is all or nothing. About 50% respond and the response is usually within 2 weeks. Lithium is used at plasma levels of 0.4–0.6 mmol/l. L-tryptophan, a precursor of serotonin, can be used; it is associated with sedation and nausea. Pindolol, which binds to presynaptic 5-HT$_{1A}$ receptors, leading to an increased release of serotonin, is thought to accelerate and augment the antidepressant effect of an antidepressant. However, the evidence for this is conflicting. Augmentation with tri-iodothyronine has been reported and appears to be effective if there is an underlying history of thyroid disease. The mode of action is unknown.

In those with epilepsy, amoxapine, clomipramine, maprotiline and bupropion are best avoided, as these are most likely to lower the seizure threshold. SSRIs are the drugs of choice, of which citalopram is least associated with a decrease in seizure threshold.

Maintenance treatment is for 4–6 months from the time that the depression resolves, for a person under the age of 50 years and presenting with a first episode. The risk of a further episode of depression after the first episode is 60–80%. If the second episode occurs within 3 years, then the maintenance treatment is for 5 years. If the person is over 50 years of age, or 40 years and with second episode, or there have been 3 or more episodes of depression, then the maintenance is for life.

## Mania

Lithium remains the first-line treatment. Its onset of action is delayed by 5–7 days. Antipsychotic drugs also have an antimanic action and have been shown to act more rapidly than lithium, although lithium has proved to be more effective after 3 weeks. Hypnotics and anxiolytics are used to reduce the overactivity and insomnia of mania. ECT is an effective treatment of mania, with a response rate of 75%, compared with 60% for lithium. For rapid cycling and/or where there is comorbid alcohol or other substance misuse, carbamazepine, sodium valproate and valproate semisodium appear to be more effective than lithium.

# Anxiety disorders

The most studied anxiety disorder is panic attacks. In panic attacks, it is assumed that the post-synaptic $\beta$-adrenergic receptors are hypersensitive and that stimulation of these leads to the central and peripheral manifestations of anxiety. The locus ceruleus is important in regulating the release of noradrenalin, and anything that increases the release of noradrenalin increases anxiety. The release of noradrenalin from the locus ceruleus is controlled by $GABA_A$ receptors and $\alpha_2$-adrenergic receptors. Stimulation of these reduces noradrenalin release. The locus ceruleus is influenced by the Raphe nucleus, which releases serotonin. The effect of this serotonin is to decrease the GABAergic activity at the locus ceruleus, which in turn increases the release of noradrenalin and causes increased anxiety. The Raphe nucleus itself has serotonin autoreceptors $5\text{-HT}_{1A}$ and $5\text{-HT}_{1D}$, stimulation of which reduces its release of serotonin. Consequently, the release of noradrenalin from the locus ceruleus is reduced and causes a reduction in the anxiety level.

Drugs can act on various parts of the above pathway to reduce anxiety. Tricyclic antidepressants, monoamine oxidase inhibitors, SSRIs and beta-blockers all reduce anxiety by reducing the sensitivity of the post-synaptic $\beta$-adrenergic receptors. SSRIs and buspirone also act at the Raphe nucleus by reducing the release of serotonin. Benzodiazepines increase the GABAergic activity at the locus ceruleus.

The treatment of choice for most anxiety disorders is cognitive–behavioural therapy. SSRIs are widely used for various anxiety disorders: panic attacks, generalised anxiety, social phobia, agoraphobia and obsessive–compulsive disorder. They often need to be used in high doses and may take up to 3 months to show a response. In 40% of people with panic attacks, they can cause an activation syndrome with agitation and worsening of the anxiety symptoms. Fluoxetine appears to be the worst culprit, therefore it needs to be started at a low dose and then increased slowly. A benzodiazepine drug may also be prescribed for about 2 weeks to reduce the effect of the activation syndrome. Around 40% of patients relapse when the SSRI is discontinued, so the treatment needs to continue for at least a year. Benzodiazepines act rapidly to reduce anxiety, but are associated with tolerance, dependence (especially in those with a personality disorder with poor impulse control or a history of substance misuse) and a high rate of relapse on discontinuation. Monoamine oxidase inhibitors and buspirone are often used as second-line treatment for anxiety.

## Obsessive–compulsive disorder

Obsessive–compulsive disorder is thought to be due to an imbalance of dopamine and serotonin transmission from the basal ganglia to the frontal cortex through the cingulate gyrus, with a reduction in serotonin and an increase in dopamine transmission. SSRIs are the most effective drug treatment, with a response rate of 30–70%. SSRIs can be augmented with antipsychotic drugs to reduce the dopamine transmission. Atypical antipsychotics with high serotonin antagonism can make the symptoms of obsessive–compulsive disorder worse.

# Dementia

The cognitive defects of dementia of the Alzheimer's type are thought to manifest at the neurotransmitter level, as a consequence of reduced cholinergic transmission. This is supported by the fact that in Alzheimer's, there is cholinergic neuronal damage in the forebrain, mainly in the projections from the nucleus basilis of Meynert that form part of the reticular activating system, affecting both muscarinic and nicotinic receptors, although it is mainly muscrinic $M_2$ receptors that are affected. There is a reduction in the level of the enzyme acetyl transferase, which is responsible for the production of acetylcholine. Also in otherwise healthy subjects, scopolamine, a compound that reduces acetylcholine levels, leads to problems with memory and learning.

There are two approaches aimed at increasing cholinergic transmission. The first is to use xanomeline, which has been shown to be effective at increasing the agonist activity at the post-synaptic muscarinic receptors, although its effect is very short lived. The second is to inhibit the enzyme acetylcholinesterase, responsible for the breakdown of acetylcholine, thus increasing the availability of acetylcholine at the synaptic cleft. This is the approach that is currently used to improve the symptoms of dementia. Tacrine, which has been known for over 50 years, was the first acetylcholinesterase inhibitor to be investigated. It produced modest results, but serious side-effects, such as hepatocelluar injury, led to its removal from the market. In 1997, donepezil was introduced for treatment of mild and moderate dementia of the Alzheimer's type, and showed an improvement rate of about 38%, with minimal side-effects, mostly due to increased cholinergic effects on the gastrointestinal system – transient mild nausea, diarrhoea and insomnia. Two other acetylcholinesterase inhibitors, galantamine and rivastigmine, are also available for the treatment of mild to moderate dementia with efficacy and side-effect profiles similar to those of donepezil.

These anti-dementia drugs may prove to be beneficial in individuals with learning disabilities, especially in Down's syndrome, where the underlying cerebral defects are similar to those in Alzheimer's disease.

## Behavioural disorders

Psychotropic drugs are widely prescribed to control challenging behaviour in people with learning disabilities, and of these the antipsychotics are the most commonly used. In fact, the most common use for antipsychotic drugs in learning disability is for the control of challenging behaviour. Aggressive behaviour, to self, environment or others, is the strongest predictor of the use of psychotropic medication. Individuals with a higher IQ, who are able to move about and target their behaviour at the environment or other people, are more likely to receive psychotropic medication. Other factors such as staff perception of the behaviour, environmental factors, staffing ratio and administrative treatment philosophies also influence the use of psychotropic medication.

It is always difficult in individuals with learning disabilities to judge whether a challenging behaviour is functional or a symptom of an underlying mental illness or personality disorder. This difficulty increases as the IQ decreases, and is most difficult in those without any effective verbal communication. Functional behavioural disorder is best addressed by thorough assessment and modification of the behaviour using psychological, educational and social methods. Those with mental disorder need to be appropriately treated for the disorder, which will lead to an improvement in their behaviour. However, in a significant number of individuals, it cannot be established whether a functional basis or a mental disorder is responsible for a particular challenging behaviour, and in this group, psychotropic medication is most likely to be used on a trial basis. How useful psychotropic drugs are at controlling challenging behaviour remains questionable.

A review of the literature by Brylewski & Duggan (1999), as part of the Cochrane Systematic Review, showed over 500 citations assessing the impact of antipsychotic drugs on challenging behaviour. Of these, only three were methodologically sound, randomised controlled trials, but even these were unable to show whether antipsychotic drugs were beneficial or not in controlling challenging behaviour. Buitelaar *et al* (2001), using a double-blind, randomised, placebo-controlled trial, showed that risperidone significantly reduced levels of aggression in hospitalised adolescents.

Aman *et al* (1984) showed a reduction in stereotypy with chlor-promazine. Gualtieri & Schroeder (1989) treated 15 adults who had severe learning disabilities with fluphenazine in an open double-blind study and found a 30% reduction in self-injurious behaviour over a 6-month period. In another open double-blind study, Singh & Owino (1992) reported an improvement in behaviour in 52 individuals with zuclopenthixol compared with placebo. These findings for the usefulness of zuclopenthixol have also been reported by Izmeth *et al* (1988), but in their study, involving 116 individuals, they used depot zuclopenthixol instead of an oral preparation. Vanden Borre *et al* (1993), in a double-blind placebo controlled cross-over study with risperidone as an add-on therapy, reported risperidone to be better than placebo at controlling behaviour, measured using the Aberrant Behaviour Checklist (ABC) and the Global Clinical Impression scale. Campbell & Spencer (1988) reported that haloperidol significantly reduces stereotypic behaviour in children with autism.

The evidence for use of antipsychotic drugs in managing behavioural problems is strongest for the control of stereotypy. This is further reinforced by animal studies, which show that antipsychotic drugs counteract stimulant drug-induced stereotypy in rats. Other drugs have also been shown to be effective for stereotypy. Lewis *et al* (1995) showed a 60% improvement with clomipramine in a double-blind, placebo-controlled cross-over study. Fluvoxamine has also been shown to reduce challenging behaviour, including stereotypy, with a response rate of 53% in adults with autism.

Apart from antipsychotics, various other drugs have been used to control challenging behaviour. In self-injurious behaviour, it has been hypothesised that there is an increase in endogenous opiate activity that reduces sensitivity to the pain of self-injury and reinforces the behaviour. Naltrexone, an opiate antagonist, has been used to reduce the opiate oversensitivity, with the aim of reducing the self-injurious behaviour. The effectiveness of this approach remains debatable; Sandman & Hetrick (1995) and Sandman *et al* (1997) have published controlled trials to support the use of naltrexone, suggesting a 35–70% reduction in self-injurious behaviour. Willemsen-Swinkels *et al* (1995), in a double-blind, placebo-controlled cross-over trial of 19 subjects, failed to show a reduction in self-injurous behaviour, but reported an adverse increase in stereotyped behaviour with naltrexone.

Beta-blockers, lithium, SSRIs and benzodiazepines have all been used to control aggression, but there are very few controlled trials. Craft *et al* (1987), in a double-blind placebo-controlled trial of 42 subjects treated with lithium, showed a 73% response rate. In a retrospective study, Spreat *et al* (1989) showed a 63% response with a greater than 30% reduction in frequency of aggression with lithium. In uncontrolled open studies, sodium valproate and carbamazepine have also shown some efficacy in the treatment of aggression. There are no controlled studies of SSRIs and aggression. In a retrospective case study, Branford (1994) showed an improvement in perseverative and maladaptive behaviour in 13 out of 37 subjects with paroxetine and fluoxetine.

Caffeine has been implicated in overactivity and sleep disturbances. Caffeinism is thought to occur with consumption of caffeine greater than 600 mg per day (a 250 ml mug of instant coffee has between 85–110 mg of caffeine, tea 55–140 mg and a can of a standard cola drink has 36 mg). It presents with tremor, anxiety, palpitations, restlessness, agitation and poor concentration. In adults with schizophrenia but without learning disability, changing to decaffeinated products makes no difference to levels of anxiety, depression or behavioural disturbance. Searle (1994) noted that there was no improvement in the sleep patterns of 26 people with severe learning disabilities after removal of caffeine from their diet, but there was an increase in general ward disturbance on reintroduction of caffeine.

There has been a gradual trend towards reducing the use of antipsychotic drugs in the treatment of functional challenging behaviour. Most drug-reduction studies have shown that on average about two-thirds of people can successfully stop their antipsychotic medication or have the dose significantly reduced without a deterioration in behaviour. However, about a third experience a marked deterioration of behaviour on reinstatement of the antipsychotic drug. Drug reduction is associated with an emergent dyskinesia, which tends to be temporary in the majority of cases, and weight loss. Carer motivation and levels of experience and training to deal with challenging behaviour are factors that are associated with a successful reduction of antipsychotic medication (Ahmed *et al*, 2000).

# Attention-deficit hyperactivity disorder

Attention-deficit hyperactivity disorder (ADHD) can be classified as inattentive behaviour, impulsive/hyperactive behaviour or a combination of the two. It occurs in 2–5% of children, with a greater prevalence in males. Of those diagnosed in childhood, 10–60% continue to have symptoms in adulthood. Dopamine is thought to play an important role; it causes an inhibitory dopaminergic effect at the striatal/prefrontal level, which normally leads to a decrease in overactivity and impulsivity and an improved attention span. A reduction in this inhibitory dopaminergic effect is thought to be responsible for ADHD. Noradrenergic systems are also important in prefrontal regulation; in particular, $\alpha_{2A}$ noradrenergic agonists have a beneficial effect on cognitive tasks. The aim of treatment is to increase the inhibitory dopaminergic effect using stimulant drugs (methylphenidate, dextroamphetamine or pemoline), or to increase the $\alpha_{2A}$ noradrenergic transmission using clonidine. The response rate in adults is 50%, compared with 70–80% in children. Clonidine is useful if there is a concurrent tic disorder. Handen *et al* (1997) showed that children with learning disabilities and ADHD respond to methylphenidate in a similar fashion to children without learning disabilities.

# Excessive sexual drive

In males, anti-androgen drugs are used to decrease sexual arousal. The most common drug for this application is cyproterone acetate. It works mainly by blocking androgen receptors, but also has progestogenic activity that exerts a negative feedback effect on the hypothalamic receptors, leading to a reduction in gonadotrophin release and therefore to diminished production of testicular androgens. It can cause hepatotoxicity, so liver function needs to be monitored. One in five of those treated develop transient or in some cases permanent gynaecomastia. It is also commonly associated with weight gain and tiredness. It is most effective when the dose is sufficient to reduce the plasma testosterone level to below 250 ng/100 ml.

# References

Addonizio, G., Susman, V. L. and Roth, S. D. (1987) Neuroleptic malignant syndrome: review and analysis of 115 cases. *Biological Psychiatry*, **22**, 1004–1020.

Ahmed, Z., Fraser, W., Kerr, M. P., *et al* (2000) Reducing antipsychotic medication in people with a learning disability. *British Journal of Psychiatry*, **176**, 42–46.

Aman, M. G., White, A. J., & Field C. J. (1984) Chlorpromazine effects on stereotypic and conditioned behaviour of severely retarded patients – a pilot study. *Journal of Mental Deficiency Research*, **28**, 253–260.

Antonacci, D. J. & de Groot, C. M. (2000) Clozapine treatment in a population of adults with mental retardation. *Journal of Clinical Psychiatry*, **61**, 22–25.

Branford, D. (1994) A study of the prescribing for people with learning disabilities living in the community and in National Health Service care. *Journal of Intellectual Disability Research*, **38**, 577–586.

Brylewski, J. & Duggan, L. (1999) Antipsychotic medication for challenging behaviour in people with intellectual disability: a systematic review of randomized controlled trials. *Journal of Intellectual Disability Research*, **43**, 360–371.

Buitelaar, J. K., van der Gaag, R. J., Cohen-Kettenis, P., *et al* (2001) A randomized controlled trial of risperidone in the treatment of aggression in hospitalized adolescents with subaverage cognitive abilities. *Journal of Clinical Psychiatry*, **62**, 239–248.

Campbell, M. & Spencer, E. K. (1988) Psychopharmacology in child and adolescent psychiatry: a review of the past five years. *Journal of the American Academy of Child and Adolescent Psychiatry*, **27**, 269–279.

Craft, M., Ismail, I. A., Krishnamurti, D., *et al* (1987) Lithium in the treatment of aggression in mentally handicapped patients. A double-blind trial. *British Journal of Psychiatry*, **150**, 685–689.

Gualtieri, C. T. & Schroeder, S. R. (1989) Pharmacotherapy for self-injurious behaviour: preliminary tests of the D1 hypothesis. *Psychopharmacology Bulletin*, **25**, 364–371.

—, —, Hicks, R. E., *et al* (1986) Tardive dyskinesia in young mentally retarded individuals. *Archives of General Psychiatry*, **43**, 335–340.

Handen, B. L., Janosky, J. & McAuliffe, S. (1997) Long-term follow-up of children with mental retardation/borderline intellectual functioning and ADHD. *Journal of Abnormal Child Psychology*, **25**, 287–295.

Izmeth, M. G., Kahn, S. Y., Kumarajeewa, D. I., *et al* (1988) Zuclopenthixol decanoate in the management of behavioural disorders in mentally handicapped patients. *Pharmatherapeutica*, **5**, 217–227.

Kane, J., Honigfeld, G., Singer, J., *et al* (1988) Clozapine for the treatment-resistant schizophrenic. A double-blind comparison with chlorpromazine. *Archives of General Psychiatry*, **45**, 789–796.

Langee, H. R. & Conlon, M. (1992) Predictors of response to antidepressant medications. *American Journal on Mental Retardation*, **97**, 65–70.

Lewis, M. H., Bodfish, J. W., Powell, S. B., *et al* (1995) Clomipramine treatment for stereotype and related repetitive movement disorders associated with mental retardation. *American Journal of Mental Retardation*, **100**, 299–312.

Paulson, O. W., Rizvi, C. A. & Carne, G. E. (1975) Tardive dyskinesia as a possible sequelae of long term therapy with phenothiazines. *Clinical Paediatrics*, **14**, 953–955.

Reinstein, M. J., Sirotovskaya, L. A., Jones, L. E., *et al* (1999) Effect of clozapine-quetiapine combination therapy on weight and glycaemic control – preliminary findings. *Clinical Drug Investment*, **18**, 99–104.

Sandman, C. A. & Hetrick, W. P. (1995) *Opiate mechanisms in self injury. Mental Retardation and Developmental Disability Research Review*, **1**, 130–136.

—, —, Taylor, D. V., *et al* (1997) Dissociation of POMC peptides after self-injury predicts responses to centrally acting opiate blockers. *American Journal on Mental Retardation*, **102**, 182–199.

Searle, G. F. (1994) The effect of dietary caffeine manipulation on blood caffeine, sleep and disturbed behaviour. *Journal of Intellectual Disability Research*, **38**, 383–391.

Singh, I. & Owino, W. J. E. (1992) A double-blind comparison of zuclopenthixol tablets with placebo in the treatment of mentally handicapped in-patients with associated behavioural disorders. *Journal of Intellectual Disability Research*, **36**, 541–549.

Spreat, S., Behar, D., Reneski, B., *et al* (1989) Lithium carbonate for aggression in mentally retarded persons. *Comprehensive Psychiatry*, **30**, 505–11.

Vanden Borre, R. Vermote, R. Butiëns, M., *et al* (1993) Risperidone as add-on therapy in behavioural disturbances in mental retardation: a double-blind placebo-controlled cross-over study. *Acta Psychiatrica Scandinavica*, **87**, 167–171.

Verhoeven, W. M., Veendrik-Meekes, M. J., Jacobs, G. A., *et al* (2001) Citalopram in mentally retarded patients with depression: a long-term clinical investigation. *European Psychiatry*, **16**, 104–108.

Willemsen-Swinkels, S. H., Buitejaar, J. K., Nijhof, G. J., *et al* (1995) Failure of naltrexone hydrochloride to reduce self-injurious and autistic behaviour in mentally retarded adults: double-blind placebo-controlled studies. *Archives of General Psychiatry*, **52**, 766–773.

Williams, H., Clarke, R., Bouras, N., *et al* (2000) Use of the atypical antipsychotics olanzapine and risperidone in adults with intellectual disability. *Journal of Intellectual Disability Research*, **44**, 164–169.

# Further reading

Aman, M. G. & Singh, N. N. (1988) Patterns of drug use: methodological considerations, measurement techniques and future trends. In *Psychopharmacology of the Developmental Disabilities* (eds M. G. Aman & N. N. Singh). New York: Springer-Verlag.

Branford, D., Bhaumik, S. & Naik, B. (1998) Selective serotonin re-uptake inhibitors for the treatment of perseverative and maladaptive behaviours of people with intellectual disability. *Journal of Intellectual Disability Research*, **42**, 301–306.

Bzaire, S. (2001) *Psychotropic Drug Directory: The Professionals' Pocket Handbook and Aide Memoire 2001–2002*. London: Quays Books.

Clarke, D. J., Kelley, S., Thinn, K., *et al* (1990) Psychotropic drugs and mental retardation: 1. Disabilities and the prescription of drugs for behaviour and for epilepsy in three residential settings. *Journal of Mental Deficiency Research*, **34**, 385–395.

Collaborative Working Group (1998) Adverse effects of the atypical antipsychotics. *Journal of Clinical Psychiatry*, **12**, 17–22.

Cooper, A. J. (1995) Review of the role of two antilibidinal drugs in the treatment of sex offenders with mental retardation. *Mental Retardation*, **33**, 42–48.

Feldman, H., Gauthier, S., Hecker, J., *et al* (2001) A 24-week, randomized, double-blind study of donepezil in moderate to severe Alzheimer's disease. *Neurology*, **57**, 613–620.

Fraser, W. I., Leudar, I., Gray, J., *et al* (1986) Psychiatric behaviour disorder in mental handicap. *Journal of Mental Deficiency Research*, **30**, 49–59.

Handen, B. L., Janosky, J., McAuliffe, S., *et al* (1994) Prediction of response to methylphenidate among children with ADHD and mental retardation. *Journal of the American Academy of Child Adolescent Psychiatry*, **33**, 1185–1193.

Kalachnik, J. E., Harder, S. R., Kidd-Nielsen, P., *et al* (1984) Persistent tardive dyskinesia in randomly assigned neuroleptic reduction, neuroleptic non-reduction and non-neuroleptic history groups. *Psychopharmacology Bulletin*, **20**, 27–32.

Khan, M. & Farver, D. (2000) Recognition, assessment and management of neuroleptic malignant syndrome. *South Dakota Journal of Medicine*, **53**, 395–400.

Kiernan, C., Reeves, D. & Alborz, A. (1995) The use of anti-psychotic drugs with adults with learning disabilities and challenging behaviour. *Journal of Intellectual Disability Research*, **39**, 263–274.

Lieberman, J. & Safferman, A. (1992) Clinical profile of clozapine: adverse reactions and agranulocytosis. *Psychiatric Quarterly*, **63**, 51–70.

Rao, J. M., Cowie, V. A. & Matthew, B. (1989) Neuroleptic-induced parkinsonian side-effects in the mentally handicapped. *Journal of Mental Deficiency Research*, **33**, 81–86.

Richardson, M. A., Haughiand, G., Pass, R., *et al* (1986). The prevalence of tardive dyskinesia in a mentally retarded population. *Psychopharmacology Bulletin*, **22**, 243–249.

Sallee F. R., Kurlan, R., Goetz, C. G., *et al* (2000) Ziprasidone treatment of children and adolescents with Tourette's syndrome: a pilot study. *Journal of the American Academy of Child Adolescent Psychiatry*, **39**, 292–299.

Shalev, A., Hermesh, H. & Munitz, H. (1989) Mortality from neuroleptic malignant syndrome. *Journal of Clinical Psychiatry*, **50**, 18–25.

Shiloh, R., Nutt, D. & Weizman, A. (2001) *Atlas of Psychiatric Pharmacology*. London: Martin Dunitz.

Tu, J. B. & Smith, J. (1979) Factors associated with psychotropic medication in mental retardation facilities. *Comprehensive Psychiatry*, **20**, 289–295.

# CHAPTER 13

# Epilepsy

## Michael Kerr

Epilepsy has a profound effect on individuals with a learning disability and their families. The depth of this impact on health, quality of life, psychological well-being and life expectancy necessitates assessment and intervention.

Carers of patients with learning disability and epilepsy who have behavioural problems commonly question the impact of the seizures or the anti-epileptic medication. The multi-disciplinary team involved in caring for people with learning disabilities who have epilepsy are uniquely positioned, if appropriately trained, to answer such questions. The issue of epilepsy will touch all involved in the care of people with learning disabilities. With community prevalence estimates of 14–40% (Corbett, 1993) and institutional prevalence of over 40%, people with a learning disability have a greatly increased prevalence of epilepsy compared with the general population, where the prevalence of epilepsy is about 0.7%.

This chapter will address the nature of epilepsy and its treatment in this population, focusing on the role and necessary knowledge base of the psychiatrist and the multi-disciplinary team. This knowledge base is broad but in general it should include the ability, relevant to the professional concerned, to apply the International Guidelines for Epilepsy Management in people with a Learning Disability (IASSID Guidelines Group, 2001). These include:

(1)  An understanding of characteristics of individuals that will affect their epilepsy management – individual assessment.
(2)  The investigation and diagnosis of epilepsy and its differentiation from behavioural disorder.
(3)  Assessing the impact of epilepsy on the individual and on carers.
(4)  An understanding of treatment options.
(5)  The role of the multi-disciplinary team.

# The individual

The starting point in the assessment of an individual with epilepsy and learning disability is an understanding of those characteristics that will influence the diagnostic process and the management plan. Table 13.1 highlights the key areas to be considered and the characteristics of the individual with a learning disability that will impact on the diagnostic process, assessment and the implementation of management plans.

## Investigation and diagnosis of epilepsy and its differentiation from behavioural disorder

Epilepsy is a diagnosis made primarily through good history-taking. Further investigations, such as electroencephalograms (EEGs), might

**Table 13.1** Individual assessment – individual characteristics that impact on seizure diagnosis and management

| Area | Influence on treatment |
| --- | --- |
| Aetiology of the learning disability | May help identify seizure type or syndrome, e.g. in Angelman's syndrome the seizure type is believed to be of a cryptogenic generalised nature (Matsumoto *et al*, 1992); in fragile-X syndrome features similar to benign epilepsy with centrotemporal spikes may be seen (Musumeci *et al*, 1991) |
| Communication difficulties | Key to participation in management choice and understanding of treatment plan |
| Severity of the learning disability | May be an important marker to significant comorbidity |
| Psychiatric and behavioural problems | May influence the diagnostic process with confusion over whether presentation is behaviour or seizure, and through non-participation with investigation; may inhibit interventions for fear of worsening behaviour |
| Physical health | Many individuals with a learning disability have unrecognised physical morbidity (Lennox & Kerr, 1997). This can lead to worsening seizures or misattribution of physical symptoms as medication side-effects |
| Swallowing and feeding difficulties | Swallowing and feeding difficulties are common and are associated with gastro-oesophageal reflux. They are an important consideration when choosing the preparation of anti-epileptic medication |

help to confirm the diagnosis and the type of seizure. Neuroimaging can help with understanding the cause of the epilepsy and therefore guide treatment.

## The history

A good description of the suspected seizure, as experienced by the individual and a witness, is the single most important factor in making the diagnosis. In the UK, epilepsy is not usually diagnosed unless there have been at least two seizures. Furthermore, in the absence of an independent eyewitness account and with little direct history available from the individual, a diagnosis may be difficult to reach. The difficulty of diagnosis by working through a third person when an individual's communication is poor – management by proxy – has important implications, making the process of diagnosis and differential diagnosis particularly difficult.

For a professional to extract an accurate history, he or she must have a comprehensive understanding of seizure types (see Table 13.2). Differentiation from the many medical conditions that can mimic seizures (the most relevant of which are simple faints and cardiac problems) is also important. In addition, confusion as to whether a particular behaviour arises because of epilepsy or is behavioural in nature, is a situation that commonly arises with individuals who have a learning disability. This situation can often be clarified by the use of good communication skills and, where necessary, techniques of behavioural analysis.

## The EEG

Central to the appropriate use of the EEG is an understanding of its limitations. Most commonly, a recording of the electrical activity of the brain for a period of approximately 30 minutes, with the patient at rest, is made. In most cases, some attempt to provoke the signs of epilepsy by asking the individual to over-breathe or by the use of photostimulation is attempted.

The limitations are that, first, one gets only a snapshot in time, and second, a degree of cooperation is needed. More sophisticated EEG techniques are available, but often rely on even better cooperation. These include recordings during sleep (changes are more likely in sleep), over 24 hours (increased time span increases the chance of catching a seizure) and those associated with video recording – 'video-telemetry' – confirm that EEG changes and behaviour occur together.

Despite these limitations, the EEG can have a positive effect on the management of an individual. A positive finding of changes suspicious of epilepsy can help the confidence of the diagnosis through differentiating between partial and generalised seizures and therefore help with treatment choice. Unfortunately, a lack of positive findings can be of little help in resolving issues.

## Neuroimaging

Four forms of neuroimaging may be used in the assessment of an individual with epilepsy. They are: computerised axial tomography (CAT) scans, magnetic resonance imaging (MRI), or (less commonly and in some assessments for neurosurgery) single photon emission tomography (SPET) and photon emission tomography (PET). Like EEGs, brain scanning in epilepsy has its limitations. The most common use is when there is a reason to assess the structure of the brain. This is likely to be indicated when a new patient presents with focal seizures or when an EEG suggests the possibility of focal

**Table 13.2**  Classification and clinical description of seizures (adapted from the Commission on Classification and Terminology of the International League Against Epilepsy (1989) classification of seizures).

| 1. | Partial seizures: seizures originating from one part of the brain |
|---|---|
| A. | Simple partial seizures (consciousness not impaired) – can be simple twitching of muscles, or sensory sensations such as smells or visual hallucinations |
| B. | Complex partial seizures (consciousness impaired) – often complex semi-purposeful behaviour, such as lip-smacking or walking around |
| C. | Partial seizures, secondarily generalised – this is where initial partial features as above progress into generalised seizure; may get initial 'focal' sign like stomach pain or moving head to one side |

| 2. | Generalised seizures: occur all over the brain |
|---|---|
| A. | Absence seizures – sudden brief loss of consciousness; may be atypical and have associated muscle jerks or behaviours |
| B. | Myoclonic seizures – sudden brief jerking of limbs; no associated loss of consciousness |
| C. | Clonic seizures – loss of consciousness, repetitive jerking of heads and limbs, associated frothing at mouth; incontinence of urine is not uncommon |
| D. | Tonic seizures – loss of consciousness with sudden stiffening of muscles |
| E. | Tonic–clonic seizures – sudden loss of consciousness with tonic phase as above followed by clonic phase |
| F. | Atonic seizure – sudden loss of tone to muscles, will fall to ground, often resulting in injury |

**Unclassified seizures – often seizures, like people, do not fit into clear categories; these are often seen in people with learning disabilities**

epilepsy. In some cases, this is used in assessment for epilepsy surgery. Much less commonly, scans (SPET or PET) are used to give insight into the function of the brain or to aid localisation of the focus.

## Assessing the impact of epilepsy on the individual and on carers

It is perhaps easy in the context of a difficult, and often chronic, illness such as epilepsy to lose sight of how the condition is affecting the individual, their family and other carers.

The assessment of this impact is an essential part of the management framework. In addition to that of the family, epilepsy can effect three key aspects of an individual's life: physical health and mortality, emotional health, and social integration.

Physical health is affected through an increase in trauma, hospitalisation and through side-effects of medication. Patients with epilepsy are known to have increased risk of mortality compared with the population in general (Cockerell et al, 1994). Patients with a learning disability are also known to have a lower life expectancy than the general population (Forssman & Akesson, 1970), with an estimated standardised mortality ratio (SMR) of 1.6 (Forgren et al, 1996). A study in London demonstrated that proxy measures of severity of learning disability (institutionalisation, impaired mobility and incontinence) were predictors of early death (Hollins et al, 1998). This higher risk of mortality is increased for those patients with co-existing epilepsy (Forgren et al, 1996).

Emotional health is a more complex problem. Studies have found rates of behaviour disturbance and psychiatric disorder to be significantly higher than normal in people with epilepsy (Lund, 1985) and in people with learning disabilities (Mansell, 1993; Deb, 1997). It is not clear whether individuals with epilepsy and learning disability are at a higher risk of emotional ill-health. Studies in children (Lewis et al, 2000) and adults (Deb, 1997) have been unable to identify a difference in the prevalence of behavioural disorder between the population of people with epilepsy and those without. On an individual basis, it is clear that epilepsy can have a profound impact through ictal and post-ictal mood disturbance.

Epilepsy may also impact on an individual's ability to interact in the community, hampering social integration. This can be through a direct impact on the individual and through the effect of epilepsy on carers. Issues to be alert for with individuals are exclusion from services and restricted community access due to fear of seizures.

# An understanding of treatment options

## Anticonvulsant medication

Anticonvulsant medication is the mainstay of epilepsy management. The use of drugs can be conveniently split into the following parts: the decision to treat; the choice of medication; monitoring and side-effects; treatment in acute situations; and the decision to stop treatment

### The decision to treat

It is common practice in the UK to initiate anticonvulsant medication when an individual has had two or more seizures. In most cases, it is advisable to wait until the diagnosis is as certain as possible and not to treat inappropriately early. For a few individuals, it may be decided that the effects of occasional partial seizures are so slight on the quality of life that there is likely to be little benefit from treatment. The ideal in all cases is to manage epilepsy with just one anticonvulsant, though this will frequently not be possible in this population.

### The choice of medication

The choice of drug should be made following individually based considerations. Readers are referred to the *Clinical Guidelines for the Management of Epilepsy in Adults with an Intellectual Disability* (IASSID Guidelines Group, 2001). First, the seizure type should be assessed, as some drugs (e.g. carbamazepine, phenytoin and vigabatrin) can worsen some types such as absence or myoclonic seizures. Second, potential side-effects should always be fully understood. Each drug has its own range of these and the risks should be considered along with the benefits. Third, monitoring needs, such as the need to measure serum drug levels, should be considered. The drugs, with comment on these considerations, are listed in Table 13.3.

### Monitoring and side-effects

The problems of management by proxy, the complexity of the side-effects of medication and the associated morbidity of people with learning disability stress the importance of a high standard of treatment monitoring in this population. Monitoring will be a shared process, the components of which include the assessment of response to treatment, distinguishing side-effects of treatment and monitoring serum drug levels if necessary.

The initiation of a course of anticonvulsants has certain important implications for the individual concerned. The major one is that the necessary monitoring systems must be set up in advance to accurately assess the impact of the drug. As has been discussed, these outcomes

**Table 13.3** The anticonvulsants

| Drug name | Seizure types | Side-effects | Specific learning disability points |
|---|---|---|---|
| Sodium valproate | All seizures | Stomach irritation, unsteadiness, increased appetite and weight gain | Broad spectrum of action and no need for blood levels an advantage |
| Carbamazepine | All seizures except *absence, myoclonic* | Stomach disturbance, confusion, drowsiness, aggression, visual disturbance and unsteadiness | Will need blood levels |
| Vigabatrin | Partial seizures and secondarily generalised seizures; West syndrome | Drowsiness, fatigue, irritability, depression, confusion, aggression, behavioural problems, psychiatric problems; visual field constriction | Must watch for behavioural side-effects **Only last option because of visual field constriction** |
| Lamotrigine | All seizure types | Headaches, tiredness, rash, nausea, dizziness, drowsiness, insomnia | Studies show better side-effect profile than carbamazepine and phenytoin |
| Gabapentin | Partial seizures | Sleepiness, dizziness, unsteadiness, stomach disturbances and nervousness | Lack of drug interaction and good side-effect profile positive factor |
| Topiramate | Partial and generalised seizures | Unsteadiness, poor concentration, dizziness, depression, double vision, rarely possibility of kidney stones | Can show cognitive slowing, helped by slow titration |
| Phenobarbitone /primidone | All seizure types | Drowsiness, lethargy, mental depression, unsteadiness, unexpected excitement, hyperactivity and confusion | Behavioural disturbance and sedation are significant concerns |
| Phenytoin | All except *absence* and *myoclonic* seizures | Nausea, mental confusion, dizziness, nervousness, drowsiness, sleeplessness, slurred speech and unsteadiness | Blood tests are **absolutely essential** |
| Ethosuximide | Only *absence* seizures | Stomach disturbance, dizziness, headache, depression, and psychiatric illness | Very specific use for absence seizures |
| Clonazepam | All seizure types | Drowsiness, fatigue, poor coordination, increased dribbling, irritability, dependence | Dependence and difficulty of withdrawal significant problem in people with learning disabilities |
| Clobazam | All seizure types | Drowsiness, confusion, aggression, dribbling, unsteadiness, memory problems | Dependence and difficulty of withdrawal significant problem in people with learning disabilities |
| Tiagabine | Partial seizures and secondarily generalised seizures | Tiredness, nervousness, tremor, diarrhoea, confusion, headache | Good profile in partial seizures |
| Oxcarbazepine | Partial and secondarily generalised seizures | Somnolence, rash, hyponatraemia, gastrointestinal disturbance, dizziness, headache | Similar to carbamazepine; better side-effect profile |
| Levetiracetam | Add-on partial seizures and secondarily generalised seizures | Somnolence, asthenia, infection, dizziness, headache | New drug; positive trial results |

may be in a range of modalities, not purely seizure frequency. A basic requirement is that an acceptable outcome should be predicted in advance for an agreed maximum dosage of the drug, and if this is not reached, drug withdrawal should be considered.

The side-effects of medication rightly cause great concern to carers and professionals alike, and the precise impact of the drugs on the individual can be difficult to assess. However, the range of potential side-effects seen with most of the drugs implies that many people with learning disabilities will be experiencing them, even if they are unable to vocalise their experiences. Frequently, an individual may present with behavioural issues that are believed to be the effects of drugs. This is a major issue, as in many cases the individual will have been on the drug concerned for many years and teasing out the effect of the medication may be complex. It is here that the techniques of behavioural analysis may prove useful to differentiate between behaviour caused by seizures, behaviour caused by medication and behaviour independent of seizures and medication.

## Treatment in acute situations

The use of rectal diazepam in a community setting to interrupt the process of status epilepticus is common. Management guidelines for individuals should be established in advance of such a situation. These should cover when to give the drug, stating after what period of time a seizure is said to be prolonged, or a certain number of seizures in a given period of time. They should also cover when to call for help. The Joint Epilepsy Council (http://www.jointepilepsycouncil.org.uk/) supplies an excellent form for the use of rectal diazepam.

## The decision to stop treatment

For some people with a learning disability and epilepsy, in whom the seizures have been well-controlled for some years, the issue of drug withdrawal will be raised. In the population of people with epilepsy as a whole, certain predictors exist that suggest an increased risk of recurrence of seizures. These negative factors include the type of seizure (partial only, tonic–clonic or myoclonic); the seizure-free period (the longer the better, but minimum 2 years); the duration of the epilepsy (the longer the worse); recurrence of seizures on treatment; and having needed more than one drug to gain control.

Despite these factors, which are often negative in people with learning disabilities, drug withdrawal may be possible in some individuals. It must be stressed that the decision to withdraw is a complex one, not without risk and difficult to predict. A recent Cochrane collaboration review on drug withdrawal (Sirven et al, 2001) concluded that there is no evidence to guide the timing of drug withdrawal in adult seizure-free patients.

## *Epilepsy surgery*

In highly selected cases, surgery for epilepsy can offer a real option of significant improvement in seizures. People with learning disabilities should not be excluded from epilepsy surgery programmes by reason of their disability itself. The usual indication for surgery is uncontrolled partial epilepsy, with a clear focus of the seizure confirmed on both EEG and MRI. In addition, there must be no other focus in the brain.

The investigation of this can be prolonged and demand a degree of compliance that some will be unable to tolerate. Also, many individuals with learning disability will have more generalised cerebral damage and therefore be unsuitable for surgery. For some individuals who have repeated atonic seizures resulting in frequent facial or other injury, the surgical operation of corpus callosotomy may offer some amelioration of seizures. This procedure separates the connecting fibres between the two cerebral hemispheres, thus stopping the spread of seizures from one side of the brain to the other and limiting the subsequent atonic attacks.

More recently, vagal nerve stimulation has been introduced as an alternative surgical approach. Licensed for seizures resistant to anti-epileptic drugs, it should be considered as an option only in patients with drug-resistant symptoms following considerable assessment.

## Pathways to care: nurse-led coordination

Two key themes should underpin the delivery of epilepsy care: defined interventions and communication. The clarification of roles is particularly important in community services. Here, all professionals should have a clear understanding of their functions and be able to communicate with others. Within the UK it is through a link with the community learning disability nurse that community epilepsy management should ideally occur.

### *Defined interventions*

The interventions available to learning disability nurses cover a wide range of the needs of people with a learning disability who have epilepsy (see Table 13.4). To date, the efficacy of this range of interventions covering issues of diagnosis, treatment and outcome is not backed up by a strong evidence base, and it is the responsibility of services to closely judge the efficacy of treatment.

### *Communication*

The coordination of the communication systems necessary to manage an individual with learning disability who has epilepsy again will often fall upon the learning disability nurse.

This management of information is of particular importance in people with a learning disability, as the individual history becomes lost so easily and the reporting of the present is so often in the hands of others. One option is to use an already developed information tool – the Epilepsy Profile (available upon request from L. McCarthy, WCLD, Meridian Court, North Rd, Cardiff CF14 3BG). The completion of the profile with accuracy necessitates a skilled professional working with family members, carers and others.

Addressing the present again calls for a highly systematic response. Key features are a reliable system to measure seizure frequency, continued staff training to ensure its accuracy, and ensuring clear communication of medication and medication change – both to carers and to other health professionals. All this leaves the learning disability nurse as the essential link between hospital, home and general practice.

Increasingly, services need to understand the effect of their interventions and communicate this to others. This is the case in the management of epilepsy, but it is undoubtedly complicated by the broad range of social and health outcomes that exist for a person with learning disability and epilepsy.

# Conclusion

Within the UK, the psychiatrist and community learning disability teams have taken on an increasing role in the management of epilepsy.

**Table 13.4** Pathways to care – the role of the community learning disability nurse

| Treatment area | Action |
| --- | --- |
| Diagnosis | Full description of events; collect information from direct carers; use video to train and to record events; advice to parents or carers on seizure types; assessment of behavioural psychological components to seizures; advice on functional analysis of behaviours; help with individuals' communication of his or her experiences; establishment of recording of history |
| Treatment | Explanation of side-effects (for patients and carers); staff training: medication use, first aid, use of rectal diazepam, social and other impact of epilepsy; outcome monitoring; use of disability-sensitive outcome measures such as the Epilepsy Outcome Scale (Espie *et al*, 1998); continued help on seizure recording |
| Community interaction | Support and education to day service; clarification of risk in employment and other settings |
| Family support | Education and advice on epilepsy and its manifestation; advice on safety, risk-taking |

These services are ideally placed to address some of the key health needs in this group and thus achieve health gain. With this mandate comes a responsibility, in terms of training and knowledge. In particular, practitioners should ensure that their knowledge meets the needs as defined at the beginning of the chapter.

# References

Cockerell, O. C., Johnson, A. L., Sander, J. W., *et al* (1994) Mortality from epilepsy: results from a prospective population-based study. *Lancet*, **344**, 918–921.

Commission on Classification and Terminology of the International League Against Epilepsy (1989) Proposal for classification of epilepsies and epileptic syndromes. *Epilepsia*, **26**, 389–399.

Corbett, J. (1993) Epilepsy and mental handicap. In *A Textbook of Epilepsy* (eds J. Laidlaw, A. Richens & D. Chadwick), pp. 631–636. Edinburgh: Churchill Livingstone.

Deb, S. (1997) Mental disorder in adults with mental retardation and epilepsy. *Comprehensive Psychiatry*, **38**, 179–184.

Espie, C. A., Paul, A., Graham, M., *et al* (1998) The Epilepsy Outcome Scale: the development of a measure for use with carers of people with epilepsy plus intellectual disability. *Journal of Intellectual Disability Research*, **42**, 90–96.

Forgren, L., Edvinsson, S., Nystrom, L., *et al* (1996) Influence of epilepsy on mortality in mental retardation: an epidemiological study. *Epilepsia*, **37**, 956–963.

Forssman, H. & Akesson, H. O. (1970) Mortality of the mentally deficient: a study of 12,903 institutionalised subjects. *Journal of Mental Deficiency Research*, **14**, 276–294.

Hollins, S., Attard, M. T., von Fraunhofer, N., *et al* (1998) Mortality in people with learning disability: risk, causes and death certification findings in London. *Developmental Medical Child Neurology*, **40**, 50–56.

IASSID Guidelines Group (2001) Clinical guidelines for the management of epilepsy in adults with an intellectual disability. *Seizure*, **10**, 401–409.

Lennox, N. & Kerr, M. (1997) Primary care and people with an intellectual disability: the evidence base. *Journal of Intellectual Disability Research*, **41**, 365–371.

Lewis, J. N., Tonge, B. J., Mowat, D. R., *et al* (2000) Epilepsy and associated psychopathology in young people with intellectual disability. *Journal of Paediatric Child Health*, **36**, 172–175.

Lund, J. (1985) Epilepsy and psychiatric disorder in the mentally retarded adult. *Acta Psychiatrica Scandinavica*, **72**, 557–562.

Mansell, J. L. (1993) *Services for People with Learning Disabilities and Challenging Behaviour or Mental Health Needs*. London: HMSO.

Matsumoto, A., Kumagai, T., Miura, K., *et al* (1992) Epilepsy in Angleman syndrome associated with chromosome 15q deletion. *Epilepsia*, **33**, 1083–1090.

Musumeci, S. A., Ferri, R., Elia, M., *et al* (1991) Epilepsy and fragile X syndrome: a follow-up study. *American Journal of Medical Genetics*, **38**, 511–513.

Sirven, J., Sperling, M. & Wingerchuck, D. (2001) Early versus late withdrawal of antiepileptic drug for people with epilepsy in remission. *Cochrane Epilepsy Group Newsletter*, **15**, 1–2.

# CHAPTER 14

# Health needs
# and the organisation of health care

Helen Baxter, Christopher Morgan and Michael Kerr

In addition to the physical and psychiatric morbidity shared with the population as a whole, there is evidence that people with learning disabilities have increased health needs (Beange *et al*, 1995). These are due partly to comorbidities associated with specific aetiologies of their learning disability and partly to the deterioration of conditions that may go unreported as a result of problems with communication (Beange *et al*, 1995; Evenhuis, 1997). Conversely, owing to the restricted lifestyle of many individuals with learning disabilities, prevalence rates of common conditions such as cancer and ischaemic heart disease may be lower than in the general population (Carter & Jancar, 1983; Moss & Turner, 1995). These conditions are usually associated with older age groups in the general population and therefore are likely to occur only in individuals with learning disabilities who have survived into old age (Moss *et al*, 1993; Holland, 2000). Furthermore, traditionally subsections of the population with learning disabilities, such as those within institutions, may be protected from certain known risk factors (e.g. smoking) because of their more restrictive environment. However, with the secular trend of increasing life expectancy and the process of deinstitutionalisation, prevalence rates for these conditions are increasing (Carter & Jancar, 1983; Patja, 2001).

In this chapter, we consider the characteristic health needs of people with learning disabilities and how health care systems have been organised to accommodate these needs. Particular emphasis is placed on the changes that have occurred since deinstitutionalisation, as individuals have been moved away from the on-site medical care found in institutions. Mortality rates for this population, barriers to accessing care and potential solutions to these apparent inequalities are discussed.

## Organisation of health care

Many patients with learning disabilities require both health and social care. Following the programme of deinstitutionalisation that occurred in the late 1980s and 1990s, the provision of social care has shifted entirely to local authorities, which supervise a variety of state and charitable bodies. The closure of the old hospitals for the 'mentally handicapped' has meant that health agencies now have a predominantly medical function, providing residential care for only a small minority of patients.

As for the population as a whole, the point of entry into the health care system for patients with learning disabilities is through primary care. Despite conflicting evidence, it appears that patients with learning disabilities have higher general practice consultation rates (Stein & Ball, 1999). This has become an important issue in recent years, following the process of deinstitutionalisation and the relocation of patients into a community setting. The individuals moved out of closed-down institutions tend to have the most-severe learning disabilities and behavioural problems, and it has been shown that patients within staffed community homes have the highest consultation rates (Morgan *et al*, 2000). It seems likely, therefore, that general practice workload for the learning disability population will increase. This is certainly the perception of general practitioners who, although accepting responsibility for the health care of these patients, often feel that they lack the specialist skills to deal with their specific needs.

The relatively small number of patients with whom individual general practitioners will have direct contact further increases this problem (Dovey & Webb, 2000). It has been suggested that regular health screening should be a part of the care offered to people with learning disabilities (Webb & Rogers, 1999). This is contrasted with general practitioners' assertions that they should not be responsible for proactive health promotion and health screening (Bond *et al*, 1997).

As discussed below, patients with learning disabilities present with conditions common in the population as a whole, with a secular trend of increasing prevalence of conditions such as vascular disease and cancers due to increasing life expectancy and changes in lifestyle. In addition, some conditions have increased prevalence among patients with learning disabilities (e.g. sensory problems, dental problems and epilepsy).

## Secondary care

Overall, there is no significant increase in utilisation of non-psychiatric secondary care services by patients with learning disabilities compared with the population as a whole. However, there is wide variation by speciality, with a large excess of admissions within dentistry owing to the need for procedures to be performed under anaesthetic and within medical specialities (especially neurology and general medicine). There is, however, reduced activity within the surgical specialities, owing to reduced fertility rates and possibly to perceived surgical risk or selection bias.

Despite increased health needs, institutionalised patients tend to have no more contact with secondary care than those living in the community and their mean length of stay for medical admissions is significantly reduced. This is evidence that institutions have a non-psychiatric health care function that needs to be considered with their closure (Morgan *et al*, 2000).

# Evidence of health care needs

## *Weight*

Being under- or overweight places the individual at risk of additional morbidities, some of which can be life-threatening. Those underweight are vulnerable to recurrent food aspiration and respiratory infections, whereas the range of health problems associated with obesity includes heart disease, some forms of cancer, hypertension, diabetes and respiratory problems (Burkart *et al*, 1985; Bell & Bhate, 1992; Moss & Turner, 1995; Turner & Moss, 1996). Research has suggested that the weight distribution of the population of people with learning disabilities has a tendency to be clustered at the two ends of the scale (Simila & Niskanen, 1991; Wood, 1994). People with learning disabilities may have more difficulty maintaining a healthy weight because of additional morbidities, physical handicaps, the side-effects of medication, dependence on others to monitor diet, and less access to information on a healthy lifestyle (Springer, 1987; Simila & Niskanen, 1991; Bell & Bhate, 1992; Wood, 1994). As some research has indicated that the polarisation may be increased outside of institutional care, nutritional issues may need particular attention in community settings (Wood, 1994).

### Obesity

The rate of obesity is generally thought to be higher among people with learning disabilities than in the general population. Research in the USA found that in people with learning disabilities, 27.5% of men and 58.5% of women were obese (Rimmer *et al*, 1993), whereas in the American general population estimates of the rates of obesity were 33% for males and 36% for females (Rubin *et al*, 1998). The obesity rates in the English general population have been reported at 19% for males and 21% for females (Office for National Statistics, 2001), compared with rates in a community sample of people with learning disability of 19.1% and 34.6% respectively (Bell & Bhate, 1992). Prevalence rates for obesity, however, need to be treated with caution, owing to problems of definition and methodological issues. Confusion over the differences between the terms 'overweight' and 'obese' have been discussed by

Burkart *et al* (1985), who have highlighted the tendency of many researchers and clinicians to use these terms interchangeably. In addition, the tools used to measure obesity have tended to vary, with some studies relying on the use of height and weight tables and others using measures of tricep skinfold thickness. Caution is also required when using standard measures taken from other populations, as differences may occur in body size and growth rate. This is particularly the case for people with learning disabilities, whose physical make-up may be atypical (Polednak & Auliffe, 1976; Burkart *et al*, 1985; Rimmer *et al*, 1987; Moss & Turner, 1995).

Some characteristics do appear to increase the risk of an individual becoming obese. First, studies have highlighted a greater rate of obesity among females than among males (Fox & Rotatori, 1982; Burkart *et al*, 1985; Emery *et al*, 1985; Simila & Niskanen, 1991; Bell & Bhate, 1992; Rimmer *et al*, 1993). Second, there has been evidence to suggest that obesity may be more of a problem for individuals living in the community than those residing in institutions (Rimmer *et al*, 1993), particularly in family homes (Emery *et al*, 1985; Prasher, 1995; Rubin *et al*, 1998). Finally, some studies have shown that obesity is more common in individuals with mild or moderate learning disabilities than in those with more-severe learning disabilities (Fox & Rotatori, 1982; Rimmer *et al*, 1993), but others have questioned this association (Emery *et al*, 1985; Prasher, 1995). Greater freedom for individuals living in the community without knowledge of healthy living and nutritional issues, combined with a tendency of carers and family members to reward with food treats, may be accelerating the problem.

Research into specific clinical populations of people with learning disabilities is still limited, as many of the syndromes are rare. Clinical populations in which obesity has been observed include Down's, Prader–Willi, Carpenter, Lawrence–Moon–Biedl and Cohen syndromes (Wallen & Roszkowski, 1980). The research evidence has indicated that there is a higher prevalence of obesity in individuals with Down's syndrome (Bell & Bhate, 1992; Prasher, 1995; Rubin *et al*, 1998). However, an earlier decline in weight with age has been identified in those with Down's syndrome than in the general population (Prasher, 1995; Rubin *et al*, 1998). This is believed to be due to the early ageing process that is characteristic of Down's syndrome and it emphasises the need for early weight-reduction strategies for this population, who may become overweight at a younger age than other individuals.

Treatments using behavioural self-control strategies have been found to be successful, particularly when carers are also involved (Jackson & Thorbecke, 1982; Burkart *et al*, 1985). Other authors have argued in favour of increasing levels of physical activity (Robertson *et al*, 2000) or a combination of dietary controls and increased activity levels (Nardella *et al*, 1983). The reliance on others to monitor and inform on diet is likely to be a continuing problem for individuals with learning disabilities and this is highlighted by research by Jackson & Thorbecke (1982), demonstrating the importance of involving the main caregiver in any intervention strategies. However, obesity may not be due solely to the individual's ability to learn about healthy eating and lifestyle. A study in the USA looking at the nutritional knowledge of individuals with learning disabilities found that those who were obese possessed more nutritional knowledge than those who were not obese (Golden & Hatcher, 1997).

### Underweight

Being severely underweight can put an individual at risk for mal-nutrition (Kennedy et al, 1997). Research to date has indicated that low weight in people with learning disabilities is strongly related to difficulties in feeding (Simila & Niskanen, 1991; Wood, 1994). Reliance on being fed by others, a soft diet, food regurgitation and immobility are associated with low weight, therefore it is often those with more-severe disabilities who are more at risk (Springer, 1987; Wood, 1994). A study of underwight patients with learning disabilities revealed a positive association between the severity of feeding difficulties and the degree of undernutrition (Kennedy et al, 1997). This study also found that over 60% of individuals with learning disabilities and neurological handicaps were underweight. Similarly, Springer (1987) found that half of children with nutritional problems were also diagnosed with seizures and cerebral palsy. A study investigating nutritional and feeding problems found that individuals had normal protein levels but that their energy intake (fat and carbohydrates) was reduced and difficult to increase because of swallowing difficulties (Kennedy et al, 1997). As individuals with choreo-athetoid movements need a higher energy intake, they, especially, may require high-carbohydrate drinks to supplement their diet (Kennedy et al, 1997).

## Sensory impairment

There are higher rates of sensory impairment in populations of people with learning disabilities than in the general population. This association has been seen in The Netherlands (van Schrojenstein Lantman-de Valk, 1998), Australia (Beange & Bauman, 1991), Canada (adolescents) (Larson & Lapointe, 1986), the USA (Kappell et al, 1998) and the UK (Cooke, 1989; Aitchison et al, 1990). This problem is exacerbated by the problems of detection, particularly in individuals who have communication difficulties and those who are more severely disabled. Practitioners responsible for an individual's care may have previously relied on carer reports of any difficulties with sight or hearing. However, research findings have suggested that professional testing is needed to accurately assess whether the individual has sensory impairment or not. In a study by Wilson & Haire (1990), it was found that carers failed to predict sensory impairment in half of patients who had difficulties in hearing or vision. This happened even in patients who had been given hearing aids, who did not receive check-ups for any further problems. Similarly, a study in Denmark found that in estimates of visual impairment, the caregivers and clinicians agreed in only a third of cases (Warburg, 1994).

In populations with learning disability, early detection and treatment for sensory impairment has also been advocated to reduce further handicap and increase individuals' acceptance and use of sensory aids. A study of elderly subjects revealed that a quarter had conductive loss of hearing probably caused by unrecognised middle-ear infections, which added to the gradual hearing loss occurring with old age (Evenhuis, 1995a). Special attention should be paid to the elderly, and authors have called for screening for sensory impairment for all those over 50 years of age (van Schrojenstein Lantman-de Valk et al, 1997). Assistive devices such as glasses and hearing aids can help to reduce impairment and have been used successfully by people with learning disabilities (Evenhuis, 1995a,b). Evenhuis (1995a) found that even in the elderly, nearly all were able to use hearing aids after individual habituation training. However, Evenhuis thought that this rate might have been improved had the individuals received the hearing aids earlier in life. In addition, high levels of hearing loss due to impacted earwax have been found in populations with learning disabilities. Crandell & Roeser (1993) found a rate of occurrence of impacted earwax in individuals with learning disabilties seven times higher than would be expected in the general population. Similarly, in a study of elderly subjects in The Netherlands, earwax had to be removed in the majority of cases before assessment could take place – for some individuals, this happened annually (Evenhuis, 1995a).

People with mild learning disabilities can be screened for hearing loss by the general practitioner using a screening audiometer or whispered speech (Evenhuis, 1995a). Even when people have moderate or severe learning disabilities, they can still be screened for hearing loss using subjective tests with conditioning responses (Evenhuis et al, 1992). In addition, auditory brain-stem response audiometry has been used successfully in difficult-to-test adults with learning disabilities (Evenhuis et al, 1992). Syndromes known to have particular associations with hearing impairment include Down's (Brookes et al, 1972; Keiser et al, 1981), fragile-X and Noonen syndromes. For individuals with fragile-X or Noonen syndrome, these hearing difficulties are usually due to the high prevalence of otitis media (chronic inflammation of the middle ear associated with perforations of the eardrum) (Hangerman et al, 1987; Udwin & Dennis, 1995).

Aitchison *et al* (1990) discovered that over half of adults with learning disabilities in an institution in the UK had one or more eye abnormalities, and Sacks *et al* (1991) detected eye abnormalities other than refractive errors or strabismus in a third of individuals in a work activity centre in the USA. In a Danish population with learning disabilities, one-fifth were found to have a moderate visual impairment (half of which could be cured by glasses), compared with 1.5% of people in the general population (Warburg, 1994). As with hearing difficulties, visual problems are difficult for carers to detect. McCulloch *et al* (1996) identified 86% internal ocular disorders that staff were unaware of prior to a clinical examination. It has been stated that a reduction of excess impairment should be possible by an active diagnostic process at a young age, as such impairment is often caused by congenital or childhood conditions (Hestnes *et al*, 1991; Evenhuis, 1995*b*).

People with severe or profound learning disabilities are more likely to be affected by visual impairments and therefore need appropriate screening (van Schrojenstein Lantman-de Valk *et al*, 1997). Findings in Hong Kong and the UK have suggested a high prevalence of visual impairment in severe learning disability (McCulloch *et al*, 1996; Kwok *et al*, 1997). Research has suggested that visual impairment in this population is largely due to optic nerve or cortical dysfunction, which may have an association with the presence of epilepsy and/or cerebral palsy (Warburg, 1994; McCulloch *et al*, 1996).

There is a particularly high prevalence of visual problems among individuals with Down's syndrome. Out of 30 individuals with Down's syndrome, Hestnes *et al* (1991) found only one person without eye problems. Van Schrojenstein Lantman-De Valk *et al* (1994) discovered that elderly people with Down's syndrome showed a six to seven times higher prevalence of visual impairment than elderly people without learning disabilities. Woodhouse *et al* (1997), in a study of children with Down's syndrome, suggested that poor visual acuity in this population may be due to physiological changes in the visual cortex at a young age. Hestnes *et al* (1991) found a significantly higher rate of keratoconus (cone-shaped cornea) in patients with Down's syndrome than in patients without Down's syndrome. Individuals with Prader–Willi or Noonan syndromes are also prone to ophthalmic problems (Udwin & Dennis, 1995).

## Mental health

Puri *et al* (1996), in a study of adults with learning disabilities, found that those with psychotic disorders other than schizophrenia and mood disorder died significantly younger than those without. At 27.1% (Lund, 1985) and 47.9% (Cooper, 1997), the rates of psychiatric illness in individuals with learning disabilities are higher than those found in the general population. However, prevalence of mental illness within the the population with learning disabilities often varies depending on whether or not the estimate includes behavioural disorder. The relationship between behavioural problems and mental illness can cause confusion, as they are sometimes strongly linked. Abnormal behaviours have been found to mask the symptoms of underlying dementia in the elderly and have also been shown to be associated with the prevalence of psychiatric symptoms, particularly depression (Aylward *et al*, 1997; Moss *et al*, 2000). However, if behavioural disorder is omitted from prevalence estimates, then rates of psychiatric illness in populations of people with learning disabilities can drop considerably (Prosser, 1999; see also Chapter 8, this volume).

## Epilepsy

Epilepsy is a common comorbidity for patients with learning disabilities. Estimates of the prevalence of epilepsy in learning disability range from 14% to 44% (compared with 0.5–1% in the general population), with the relative prevalence greatest in the younger age groups (Bowley & Kerr, 2000). There is a strong association between prevalence of epilepsy and severity of learning disability (Richardson *et al*, 1981), with the highest prevalence figures reported among institutionalised patients (Mariani *et al*, 1993). Epilepsy among this population is also more complex than within the population as a whole, with more intractable cases. With the process of deinstitutionalisation, therefore, primary care services must be prepared for this common comorbidity among those with learning disabilities.

## Dental disease

Studies have shown that people with learning disabilities have high levels of poor oral hygiene, gum disease and calculus (Shaw *et al*, 1989; Kendall, 1992). Research looking at the manual dexterity of individuals with learning disabilities has found no relationship with oral health, suggesting that it is not physical ability that is influencing the low levels of oral health found in this population. Indeed, prevalence of tooth decay and loss of teeth has not been found to be particularly high when related to the UK general population (Kendall, 1992). Although previous studies have suggested that individuals with learning disabilities receive less restorative care than others, more recent work has indicated a positive trend that is more in line with the general population (Kendall, 1992).

Some forms of medication have been found to cause periodontal problems for the individual. Phenytoin, an anti-epileptic drug, has shown an association with gingivitis (Majola *et al*, 2000). Also, in some clinical populations, dental abnormalities have been associated with specific conditions such as Angelman's syndrome, where prognathism and deformation of primary dentition is common, and fragile-X syndrome, in which a high, arched palate and dental overcrowding are observed (Udwin & Dennis, 1995). These abnormalities and predispositions could put individuals at risk for dental problems, and therefore additional attention may be necessary.

## Incontinence

In a study population of 202 adults with learning disabilities in Sydney, Australia, 13% reported a problem with faecal or urinary incontinence. Beange *et al* (1995) and Cooper (1998) found rates of incontinence at 17.4% for those aged 20–64 years and 49.3% for those aged 65 and above. Incontinence can be a major difficulty for the individual and the carers, and it becomes an increasing problem with age. Sensory impairment and mobility problems that increase with old age are likely to worsen the situation. Incontinence can occur as challenging behaviour in response to trauma, as a learnt behaviour or a means of communication (Stanley, 1996). In some individuals, incontinence will be a result of their disability. However, the sudden presence of incontinence in an individual could be due to infection or an indication of other morbidities (Lennox & Beange, 1999).

## Respiratory disease

Around half of the deaths of people with learning disabilities are caused by respiratory disease (the rate in the general population is about 8%; Carter & Jancar, 1983). Mortality rates in learning disability of 50.3% (Carter & Jancar, 1983), 42.8% (Puri *et al*, 1996) and 58%, rising to 75% for individuals with severe learning disabilities (Chaney *et al*, 1979) have been recorded. Chaney *et al* noted that the majority of those with severe learning disabilities died from infectious respiratory disease, whereas among the more able death was likely to be due to non-infectious respiratory disease. Those who are immobile and who have additional physical disabilities are thought to be at greater risk for respiratory disease (Chaney *et al*, 1979). In addition, those with food-aspiration problems and those who are underweight are also more susceptible to respiratory disease (Kennedy *et al*, 1997). Recurring colds and chest infections are a particular problem for individuals with Down's syndrome (Adlin, 1993). However, research has suggested that it is the more able with Down's syndrome who are more likely to die from respiratory infection (Chaney *et al*, 1979). This finding is the reverse of the pattern found in the rest of the population of people with learning disabilities.

## Heart disease and abnormalities

People with learning disabilities (not including Down's syndrome) are generally believed to have fewer risk factors for heart disease due to lifestyle, for example they have less access to alcohol and cigarettes (Adlin, 1993; Moss & Turner, 1995). However, as stated above, they are at a high risk for obesity, which is strongly related to heart disease. Thus, as rates of obesity rise within the population, so does the risk for heart problems. Carter & Jancar (1983) noted that deaths from myocardial infarction rose to 8% in the period 1976–1980, from less than 1% in 1930–1950. Logically, as people with learning disabilities are given more freedom and choice in the move into the community, the risk for heart disease is likely to increase to rates more similar to those for the general population. In addition, the absence of education on healthy lifestyle issues means that they may not be able to make informed choices about their health. A study by Rimmer *et al* (1993) found that of 324 adults with learning disabilities, 23% were considered to be at borderline high risk and 17% at high risk of cardiovascular disease.

As would be expected from the normal ageing process, cardiovascular disorders are found at higher rates in older people with learning disabilities (van Schrojenstein Lantman-de Valk *et al*, 1997; Cooper, 1998). This may be due to the 'healthy ageing' of people with learning disabilities: those with severe disabilities die younger, so that patterns of illness in older people with learning disabilities are comparable with those in older people in the general population (Moss *et al*, 1993; Holland, 2000). People with Down's syndrome are at particular risk from heart problems, owing to both their vulnerability to heart defects from birth and to their susceptibility to premature ageing. Adlin (1993) reported rates of 30–50% for mitral valve prolapse, 5–10% for aortic regurgitation and 40% for congenital heart disease in people with Down's syndrome. Other syndromes that are known to have an association with heart defects are Noonen syndrome (pulmonary stenosis, atrial septal defect, hypertrophic cardiomyopathy), Prader–Willi syndrome (rhabdomyomata of the heart and arrhythmias) and fragile-X syndrome (mitral valve prolapse) (Udwin & Dennis, 1995).

## Cancer

Cancer, although a major health issue in the general population, has not been of such significant concern for those with learning disabilities. This could well be due to the differences in life expectancy, particularly among those with severe disabilities. In a study by Carter & Jancar (1983), cancer accounted for only about 15% of deaths in institutionalised populations, although rates were found to rise as longevity increased, from 10% in 1967 to 15% in 1980 and 17.5% in 1976–1985. The types of cancer found in people with learning disabilities are also notable: cancers of the gastrointestinal tract are more common, but breast and prostate cancers are much less common (Cooke, 1997). In more recent years, increased independence, especially among those with milder learning disabilities, might be affecting these differences as individuals begin to adopt a lifestyle that places them at greater risk (Moss & Turner, 1995). Greater freedom and choice may lead to higher levels of smoking, use of alcohol and obesity, all of which can increase the risks of having cancer.

# Mortality

Studies of mortality within populations with learning disabilities will tend to overestimate mortality rates, as these populations will be skewed towards profound and severe cases. Certain conditions such as Down's syndrome (Van Allen *et al*, 1999) and cerebral palsy (Strauss & Shavelle, 1998) will predict higher mortality rates, as will severity of learning disability in general (Hayden, 1998). The impact of the severity of disability on mortality risk is greatest in the younger age groups, indicating a survivor effect.

In terms of underlying cause of death, patients with learning disabilities mirror the population as a whole. The secular trend of increasing life expectancy for those with learning disabilities ensures that this tendency increases as patients reach ages where cardiovascular disease and cancers are common and adopt lifestyles in the community that provide associated risk factors.

The most common cause of death among people with learning disabilities is cardiovascular disease (Patja, 2001). Respiratory diseases appear in excess among younger age groups and those with more severe learning disabilities. Deaths from cancers, accidents and suicides are reduced compared with the general population, although mortality from cancer is increasing with increased longevity (Patja *et al*, 2001).

Severity of the learning disability remains the strongest predictor of premature mortality. Death in childhood for those with cerebral palsy is predicted by severity: those with severe spastic quadriplegia and learning disability are more likely to die in childhood than are those with moderate and mild disability. Relative mortality for those with Down's syndrome is comparable with the population as a whole in younger age groups, but from age 35 onwards there is an increase predominantly due to the development of Alzheimer's disease.

# Barriers to health care

Although people with learning disabilities often require more attention to their health, in practice they have been found to receive the same level of care as the general population (Whitfield *et al*, 1996). Studies have identified many untreated common conditions among patients with learning disabilities (Howells, 1986; Wilson & Haire, 1990; Beange & Bauman, 1991; Webb & Rogers, 1999) and low levels of health promotion and preventative care (Wilson & Haire, 1990; Beange *et al*, 1995; Kerr *et al*, 1996; Whitfield *et al*, 1996). It is believed that this may be due to several barriers identified by research, which will need to be overcome if people with learning disabilities are to have access to the health services appropriate to their needs. Mobility problems (Minihan *et al*, 1993), difficult behaviour (Lennox & Kerr, 1997) and communication issues (Wilson & Haire, 1990; Lennox *et al*, 1997) have all been highlighted as barriers to health care, as have general practioners' lack of specialist knowledge (Lennox *et al*, 1997; Aspray *et al*, 1999) and the additional time and resources required by many patients with learning disabilities (Kerr *et al*, 1996; Chambers *et al*, 1998).

As these barriers exist both within the health services and as a result of the learning disabilities, tackling them is complex. Steps have been made in research, looking at health promotion (Jones & Kerr, 1997), health-screening (Martin *et al*, 1997; Webb & Rogers, 1999), education of general practitioners (Kendrick *et al*, 1995) and carer knowledge of the health issues for people with learning disabilities (Matthews & Hegarty, 1997).

## Conclusions

As a subset, people with learning disabilities share many common health needs with the general population. However, for a variety of reasons their care has to be specifically tailored to meet these needs.

The process of deinstitutionalisation provides new challenges. People with learning disabilities who are discharged from institutions are likely to have greater physical and psychiatric morbidity and yet they are moving into a care setting that in itself leads to increased primary and secondary care consultation. This places an increased burden on general practitioners that requires liaison with specialist community learning disability teams. In addition, there is a strong case for routine screening for conditions such as sensory problems. Many general practitioners believe this area to be beyond their role, and the conflict needs to be resolved.

The positive secular changes in longevity for this population will also provide new challenges. The prevalence of cancer and cardiovascular disease will increase and this will be accelerated by exposure to risk factors such as smoking and to factors related to obesity. It is important that this changing profile of morbidity is recognised and that those with learning disabilities are not excluded from public health campaigns directed at the population as a whole.

# References

Adlin, M. (1993) Health care issues. In *Older Adults with Learning Disabilities* (eds E. Sutton, A. F. Factor, B. A. Hawkins, *et al*), pp. 49–90. Baltimore, MD: Paul H. Brookes.

Aitchison, C., Easty, D. L. & Jancar, J. (1990) Eye abnormalities in the mentally handicapped. *Journal of Mental Deficiency Research*, **34**, 41–48.

Aspray, T. J., Francis, R. M., Tyler, S., *et al* (1999) Patients with learning disability in the community: have special needs that should be planned for. *BMJ*, **318**, 476–477.

Aylward, E. H., Burt, D. B., Thorpe, L. U., *et al* (1997) Diagnosis of dementia in individuals with learning disability. *Journal of Learning Disability Research*, **41**, 152–164.

Beange, H. & Bauman, A. (1991) Health care for the developmentally disabled. Is it really necessary? In *Key Issues in Mental Retardation Research* (ed. W. Fraser), pp. 155–162. London: Routledge.

—, McElduff, A. & Baker, W. (1995) Medical disorders of adults with mental retardation: a population study. *American Journal on Mental Retardation*, **99**, 595–604.

Bell, A. J. & Bhate, M. S. (1992) Prevalence of overweight and obesity in Down's syndrome and other mentally handicapped adults living in the community. *Journal of Learning Disability Research*, **36**, 359–364.

Bond, L., Kerr, M., Dunstan, F., *et al* (1997) Attitudes of general practitioners towards health care for people with learning disability and the factors underlying these attitudes. *Journal of Learning Disability Research*, **41**, 391–400.

Bowley, C. & Kerr, M. (2000) Epilepsy and intellectual disability. *Journal of Intellectual Disability Research*, **44**, 529–543.

Brookes, D. N., Wooley, H., Kanjilal, G. C., *et al* (1972) Hearing loss and middle ear disorders in patients with Down's syndrome. *Journal of Mental Deficiency Research*, **16**, 21–29.

Burkart, J. E., Fox, R. A. & Rotatori, A. F. (1985) Obesity of mentally retarded individuals: prevalence, characteristics and intervention. *American Journal of Mental Deficiency*, **90**, 303–312.

Carter, G. & Jancar, J. (1983) Mortality in the mentally handicapped. A 50 year survey at the Stoke Park group of hospitals (1930–1980). *Journal of Mental Deficiency Research*, **27**,143–156.

Chambers, R., Milsom, G., Evans, N., *et al* (1998) The primary care workload and prescribing costs associated with patients with learning disability discharged from long-stay care to the community. *British Journal of Learning Disabilities*, **26**, 9–12.

Chaney, R. H., Eyman, R. K. & Miller, C. R. (1979) Comparison of respiratory mortality in the profoundly mentally retarded and in the less retarded. *Journal of Mental Deficiency Research*, **23**, 1–7.

Cooke, L. B. (1989) Hearing loss in aging mentally handicapped persons. *Australian and New Zealand Journal of Developmental Disabilities*, **15**, 321–328.

— (1997) Cancer and learning disability. *Journal of Learning Disability Research*, **41**, 312–316.

Cooper, S. (1997) Epidemiology of psychiatric disorders in elderly compared with younger adults with learning disabilities. *British Journal of Psychiatry*, **170**, 375–380.

— (1998) Clinical study of the effects of age on the physical health of adults with mental retardation. *American Journal on Mental Retardation*, **102**, 582–589.

Crandell, C. C. & Roeser, R. J. (1993) Incidence of excessive/impacted cerumen in individuals with mental retardation. A longitudinal investigation. *American Journal on Mental Retardation*, **97**, 568–574.

Dovey, S, & Webb, O. J. (2000) General practitioners' perceptions of their role in care for people with learning disability. *Journal of Learning Disability Research*, **44**, 553–561.

Emery, C. L., Watson, J. L., Watson, P. J., *et al* (1985) Variables related to body-weight status of mentally retarded adults. *American Journal of Mental Deficiency*, **90**, 34–39.

Evenhuis, H. M. (1995*a*) Medical aspects of ageing in a population with learning disability. II: Hearing impairment. *Journal of Learning Disabiltiy Research*, **39**, 27–33.

—— (1995*b*) Medical aspects of ageing in a population with learning disability. I: Visual impairment. *Journal of Learning Disability Research*, **39**, 19–25.

—— (1997) Medical aspects of ageing in a population with intellectual disability. Mobility, internal conditions and cancer. *Journal of Intellectual Disability Research*, **41**, 8–18.

——, Van Zanten, G. A., Brocaar, M. P., *et al* (1992) Hearing loss in middle-age persons with Down syndrome. *American Journal on Mental Retardation*, **97**, 47–56.

Fox, R. & Rotatori, A. F. (1982) Prevalence of obesity among mentally retarded adults. *American Journal of Mental Deficiency*, **87**, 228–230.

Golden, E. & Hatcher, J. (1997) Nutritional knowledge and obesity of adults in community residences. *Mental Retardation*, **35**, 177–184.

Hangerman, R., Altshul-Stark, D., McBogg, P., *et al* (1987) Recurrent otitis media in boys with fragile-X syndrome. *American Journal of Diseases of Children*, **141**, 184–187.

Hayden, M. F. (1998) Mortality among people with mental retardation living in the United States. Research review and policy application. *Mental Retardation*, **36**, 345–359.

Hestnes, A., Sand, T. & Fostad, K. (1991) Ocular findings in Down's syndrome. *Journal of Mental Deficiency Research*, **35**, 194–203.

Holland, A. J. (2000) Ageing and learning disability. *British Journal of Psychiatry*, **176**, 26–31.

Howells, G. (1986) Are the medical needs of mentally handicapped adults being met? *Journal of the Royal College of General Practitioners*, **36**, 449–453.

Jackson, H. J. & Thorbecke, P. J. (1982) Treating obesity of mentally retarded adolescents and adults. An exploratory program. *American Journal of Mental Deficiency*, **87**, 302–308.

Jones, R. G. & Kerr, M. P. (1997) A randomised control trial of an opportunistic health screening tool in primary care for people with learning disability. *Journal of Learning Disability Research*, **41**, 409–415.

Kappell, D., Nightingale, B., Rodriguez, A., *et al* (1998) Prevalence of chronic medical conditions in adults with mental retardation. Comparison with the general population. *Mental Retardation*, **36**, 269–279.

Keiser, H., Montague, J., Wold, D., *et al* (1981) Hearing loss of Down's syndrome adults. *American Journal of Mental Deficiency*, **85**, 467–472.

Kendall, N. P. (1992) Oral health of a group of non-institutionalised mentally handicapped adults in the UK. *Community Dental Oral Epidemiology*, **19**, 357–359.

Kendrick, T., Burns, T. & Freeling, P. (1995) Randomised controlled trial of teaching general practitioners to carry out structured assessments of their long term mentally ill patients. *BMJ*, **311**, 93–98.

Kennedy, M., McCombie, L., Dawes, P., *et al* (1997) Nutritional support for patients with learning disabilility and nutrition/dysphagia disorders in community care. *Journal of Learning Disability Research*, **41**, 430–436.

Kerr, M., Richards, D. & Glover, G. (1996) Primary care for people with an intellectual disability – a group practice survey. *Journal of Applied Research in Intellectual Disabilities*, **9**, 347–352.

Kwok, S. K., Ho, P. C. P., Chan, A. K., *et al* (1997) Occular defects in children and adolescents with severe mental deficiency. *Journal of Intellectual Disability Research*, **40**, 330–335.

Larson, C. P. & Lapointe, Y. (1986) The health status of mild to moderate learning handicapped adolescents. *Journal of Mental Deficiency Research*, **30**, 121–128.

Lennox, N. G. & Kerr, M. P. (1997) Primary health care and people with an intellectual disability: the evidence base. *Journal of Intellectual Disability Research*, **41**, 365–372.

Lennox, N. G., Diggens, J. N. & Ugoni, A. M. (1997) The general practice care of people with intellectual disability: barriers and solutions. *Journal of Intellectual Disability Research*, **41**, 380–390.

Lennox, N. G. & Beange, H. (1999) Adult healthcare. In *Management Guidelines for People with Developmental and Learning Disabilities* (eds N. Lennox & J. Diggens), Melbourne: Theraputic Guidelines.

Lund, J. (1985) The prevalence of psychiatric morbidity in mentally retarded adults. *Acta Psychiatrica Scandinavica*, **72**, 563–570.

Majola, M. P., McFadyen, M. L., Connolly, C., *et al* (2000) Factors influencing phenytoin-induced gingival enlargement. *Journal of Clinical Periodontology*, **27**, 506–512.

Mariani, E., Ferini-Strambi, L., Sala, M., *et al* (1993) Epilepsy in institutionalised patients with encephalopathy: clinical aspects and nosological considerations. *American Journal of Mental Retardation*, **98**, 27–33.

Martin, D. M., Roy, A. & Wells, M. B. (1997) Health gain through health checks: improving access to primary health care for people with learning disability. *Journal of Learning Disability Research*, **41**, 401–408.

Matthews, D. & Hegarty, J. (1997) The OK health check: a health assessment checklist for people with learning disabilities. *British Journal of Learning Disabilities*, **25**, 138–143.

McCulloch, D. L., Sludden, P. A., McKeown, K., *et al* (1996) Vision care requirement among intellectually disabled adults: a residence-based pilot study. *Journal of Learning Disability Research*, **40**, 140–150.

Minihan, P. M., Dean, D. H. & Lyons, C. M. (1993) Managing the care of patients with mental retardation: a survey of physicians. *Mental Retardation*, **31**, 239–246.

Morgan, C. Ll., Ahmed, Z. & Kerr, M. P. (2000) Health care provision for people with a learning disability. A record linkage study of the epidemiology and factors contributing to hospital care uptake. *British Journal of Psychiatry*, **176**, 37–41.

Moss, S. & Turner, S. (1995) *The Health of People with Learning Disability*. Manchester: Hester Adrian Research Centre.

—, Goldberg, D., Patel, P., *et al* (1993) Physical morbidity in older people with moderate, severe and profound mental handicap, and its relation to psychiatric morbidity. *Social Psychiatry and Psychiatric Epidemiology*, **28**, 32–39.

—, Emerson, E., Kiernan, C., *et al* (2000) Psychiatric symptoms in adults with learning disability and challenging behaviour. *British Journal of Psychiatry*, **177**, 452–456.

Nardella, M. T., Sulzbacher, S. I. & Worthington-Roberts, B. S. (1983) Activity levels of persons with Prader–Willi syndrome. *American Journal of Mental Deficiency*, **87**, 498–505.

Office for National Statistics (2001) *Social Trends*. London: Stationery Office.

Patja, K. (2001) Cause specific mortality of people with learning disability in a population-based, 35 year follow up study. *Journal of Learning Disability Research*, **45**, 30–40.

—, Iivanainen, M., Raitasuo, S., *et al* (2001) Suicide mortality in mental retardation: a 35 year follow-up study. *Acta Psychiatrica Scandanavica*, **103**, 307–311.

Polednak, A. P. & Auliffe, J. (1976) Obesity in an institutionalised adult mentally retarded population. *Journal of Mental Deficiency Research*, **20**, 9–15.

Prasher, V. (1995) Overweight and obesity amongst Down's syndrome adults. *Journal of Learning Disability Research*, **39**, 437–441.

Prosser, H. (1999) An invisible morbidity. *The Psychologist*, **12**, 234–237.

Puri, B. K., Lekh, S. K., Langa, A., *et al* (1996) Mortality in a hospitalized mentally handicapped population: a 10-year survey. *Journal of Learning Disability Research*, **39**, 442–446.

Richardson, S. A., Koller, H., Katz, M., et al (1981) A functional classification of seizures and its distribution in mentally retarded population. *American Journal of Mental Deficiency*, **85**, 457–466.

Rimmer, J. H., Kelly, L. E. & Fujiura, G. (1987) Accuracy of anthropometric equations for estimating body composition of mentally retarded adults. *American Journal of Mental Deficiency*, **91**, 626–632.

——, Braddock, D., Fujiura, G., et al (1993) Prevalence of obesity in adults with mental retardation: implications for health promotion and disease prevention. *Mental Retardation*, **31**, 105–110.

Robertson, J., Emerson, E., Gregory, N., et al (2000) Lifestyle related factors for poor health in residential settings for people with learning disabilities. *Research in Developmental Disabilities*, **21**, 469–486.

Rubin, S. S., Rimmer, J. H., Chicoine, B., et al (1998) Overweight prevalence in persons with Down syndrome. *Mental Retardation*, **36**, 175–181.

Sacks, J. G., Goren, M. B., Burke, M. J., et al (1991) Ophthalmologic screening of adults with mental retardation. *American Journal on Mental Retardation*, **95**, 571–574.

Shaw, L., Shaw, M. J. & Foster, T. D. (1989) Correlation of manual dexterity and comprehension with oral hygiene and peridontal status in mentally handicapped adults. *Community Dental Oral Epidemiology*, **17**, 187–189.

Simila, S. & Niskanen, P. (1991) Underweight and overweight cases among the mentally retarded. *Journal of Mental Deficiency Research*, **35**, 160–164.

Springer, N. S. (1987) From institutional to foster care: impact on nutritional status. *American Journal of Mental Deficiency*, **91**, 321–327.

Stanley, R. (1996) Treatment of continence in people with learning disabilities: 2. *British Journal of Nursing*, **5**, 492–498.

Stein, K. & Ball, D. (1999) Contact between people with learning disability and general practitioners: a cross-sectional case note survey. *Journal of Public Health Medicine*, **21**, 192–198.

Strauss, D. & Shavelle, R. (1998) Life expectancy of adults with cerebral palsy. *Developmental Medicine of Child Neurology*, **40**, 369–375.

Turner, S. & Moss, S. (1996) The health needs of adults with learning disabilities and the Health of the Nation strategy. *Journal of Learning Disability Research*, **40**, 438–450.

Udwin, O. & Dennis, D. (1995) Psychological and behavioural phenotypes in genetically determined syndromes. A review of research findings. In *Behavioural Phenotypes* (eds G. O'Brien & W. Yule), pp. 90–208. London: Mac Keith Press.

Van Allen, M. I., Fung, J. & Jurenka, S. B. (1999) Health concerns and guidelines for adults with Down syndrome. *American Journal of Medical Genetics*, **89**, 100–110.

van Schrojenstein Lantman-de Valk, H. M. J. (1998) *Health Problems in People with Learning Disabilities*. Maastricht: UnigraphicMaastricht.

—— & Haveman, M. J., Maaskant, M. A., et al (1994) The need for assessment of sensory functioning in aging people with mental handicap. *Journal of Learning Disability Research*, **38**, 289–298.

——, Maaskant, M. A., Haveman, M. J., et al (1997) Prevalance and incidence of health problems in people with intellectual disability. *Journal of Intellectual Disability Research*, **41**, 42–51.

Wallen, A. & Roszkowski, M. (1980) Patterns of weight disorders in institutionalised menatally retarded adults. *Nutritional Reports International*, **21**, 469–477.

Warburg, M. (1994) Visual impairment among people with developmental delay. *Journal of Learning Disability Research*, **38**, 423–432.

Webb, O. J. & Rogers, L. (1999) Health screening for people with learning disability: the New Zealand experience. *Journal of Learning Disability Research*, **43**, 497–503.

Whitfield, M., Langan, J. & Russel, O. (1996) Assessing general practitioners'care of adult patients with learning disability: case control study. *Quality in Health Care*, **5**, 31–55.

Wilson, D. N. & Haire, A. (1990) Health care screening for people with mental handicap living in the community. *British Medical Journal*, **301**, 1379–1381.

Wood, T. (1994) Weight status of a group of adults with learning disabilities. *British Journal of Learning Disabilities*, **22**, 97–99.

Woodhouse, J. M., Pakeman, V. H. & Saunders, K. J. (1997) Visual acuity and accommodation in infants and young children with Down's syndrome. *Journal of Learning Disability Research*, **40**, 49–55.

# CHAPTER 15

# Health morbidity in adults with Down's syndrome

## Vee Prasher

Research and clinical experience suggest that people with Down's syndrome are living longer than previously and that some individuals are now surviving into their sixth or seventh decade of life (Baird & Sadovnick, 1989). The population of people with Down's syndrome, and in particular those over 50 years of age, will continue to increase during the next few decades (Stratford & Steele, 1985; Steffelaar & Evenhuis, 1989). As people with Down's syndrome reach middle age, they have an increased risk of health (both physical and psychiatric) morbidity (Jacobson & Janicki, 1985; Prasher, 1994, 1995a). Therefore, all professionals, but particularly psychiatrists, involved in the care of a person with Down's syndrome must be aware of the clinically significant physical and psychiatric issues. The following discussion does not focus on the phenotypic characteristics of Down's syndrome, as these are often an inherent part of the syndrome and not a 'health problem' as such. I review only those physical and psychological problems with significant clinical implications for adults with Down's syndrome, and of which psychiatrists working in the field of learning disabilities should have some knowledge.

## Physical health

It might be argued that, in today's modern National Health Service, physical disorders in adults with Down's syndrome should be managed by the primary health services (principally by the general practitioner), with support from the specialist medical and surgical services. However, the quality of primary health services for people with learning disabilities vary markedly from one health region to another. As many physical problems in adults with Down's syndrome affect or are affected by the psychological state of the individual, a psychiatrist may need to become involved in the management of a physical problem that may appear initially to be outside their remit.

## Cardiological aspects

A century has elapsed since congenital heart malformations in infants with Down's syndrome were first described. Since then, an association between cardiac pathology and Down's syndrome has been established (Goldhaber *et al*, 1986). Such cardiac abnormalities may be the main cause of death in both children and adults. Although cardiac abnormalities are usually diagnosed and managed in childhood, children with Down's syndrome may survive into adulthood, where the presence of such pathology might give cause for concern or might present for the first time.

Mitral valve prolapse, aortic regurgitation, tricuspid valve prolapse and pulmonary valve fenestrations are the most common abnormalities to be found (Goldhaber *et al*, 1986). Up to 50% of adults with Down's syndrome have pathology affecting at least one heart valve, although it may be asymptomatic. Detection of valvular pathology is important to prevent subsequent heart failure and complications during surgical or dental procedures, where prophylactic antibiotic cover is required to prevent the occurrence of bacterial endocarditis.

Prasher (1994) reported the mean resting heart rate for adults with Down's syndrome (aged 16 years and over) to be 65 beats/minute (72 beats/minute for the non-learning disability population), and a mean systolic blood pressure of 115 mmHg (120 mmHg for the non-learning disability population), with a mean diastolic blood pressure of 75 mmHg (80 mmHg for the non-learning disability population). Richards & Enver (1979) investigated the effects of ageing on blood pressure in Down's syndrome, and found that both the systolic and the diastolic blood pressures increased with age, but less steeply than for the non-learning disability population. For all ages, blood pressure readings for the Down's syndrome group were significantly below those for the non-learning disability population and below those for the non-Down's syndrome population with other learning disabilities.

It has previously been reported that the prevalence of atherosclerotic coronary artery disease in adults with Down's syndrome is low (Murdoch *et al*, 1977a). Adults with Down's syndrome are therefore described as an 'atheroma-free model'. The precise underlying reasons for this low prevalence still remain to be determined, but probably include the lower resting blood pressure and heart rate, possible triplication of protective genes (cystathionine B-synthase) and the reduced effect of environmental factors (such as the low prevalence of smoking).

Regular screening for cardiovascular disorders, in particular heart murmurs, hypertension and heart failure, is recommended. Screening should be undertaken by the general practitioner or by the responsible psychiatrist if psychotropic medication is being initiated that may affect the cardiovascular system. Subsequent management of any detected disorder should follow established guidelines.

## Ophthalmological conditions

Ocular abnormalities are very common in people with Down's syndrome and virtually all structures of the eye have been reported to have some associated abnormality (Caputo *et al*, 1989; Catalano, 1990). Strabismus (30–69%), cataracts (11–50%), nystagmus (6–29%), blepharitis (4–67%), keratoconus (3–30%) and all forms of refractive error (astigmatism, hypermetropia and myopia) occur more commonly in individuals with Down's syndrome than in other age-matched individuals.

Keratoconus (conical cornea) may be unilateral or bilateral and can lead to reduced visual acuity. Acute keratoconus (hydrops) can occur. Cataracts are often bilateral, incidence increases with age and, without surgical intervention, they can lead to blindness. The esotropic form of strabismus (inward deviation of the eyes) is more common than exotropia (outward deviation of the eyes). Nystagmus is more likely to occur in individuals who also have strabismus, and fine rapid horizontal nystagmus is more common than pendular nystagmus. Unless the nystagmus is associated with underlying pathology (e.g. a space-occupying lesion), there is usually no need for further medical intervention.

Deterioration in vision or the presence of ocular disorders can lead to deterioration in behaviour or a decline in intellectual and social functioning. A psychiatric disorder (e.g. dementia) may be misdiagnosed. Regular screening and the regular assessment of vision and associated eye pathology should be undertaken in all adults with Down's syndrome. Such testing should take place every 1–2 years. Significant clinical pathology should be further investigated by an ophthalmologist. The majority of disorders can benefit from correction of any associated refractive error with suitable glasses, but occasionally surgical intervention may be necessary.

## Audiological problems

Several studies have reported a high prevalence of both conductive and sensorineural hearing loss in adults with Down's syndrome (Mazzoni *et al*, 1994; Yeates, 1995). Evenhuis *et al* (1992) assessed hearing function in 35 institutionalised people with Down's syndrome over 35 years of age, and found a hearing loss of 20 dB and over in 56 of 59 ears tested. Thirty-two per cent had unexplained high levels of loss (>50 dB).

It has been demonstrated that individuals with impaired hearing have impaired social functioning (Wright *et al*, 1991; Lonigan *et al*, 1992) and that hearing loss may be a factor in the decline of cognitive functioning (Saxon & Witriol, 1976; Libb *et al*, 1985). Exclusion of hearing deterioration should therefore be made before diagnosing a psychological disorder such as depression or dementia.

With the appropriate assessment, hearing loss in most adults with Down's syndrome should be detected (although cooperation with testing can be extremely difficult). Otoscopy, tympanometry and audiometry are the principal techniques used, with modification for individuals with increasing severity of learning disability. Treatment should involve reducing the background noise (e.g. keeping the volume of the television or radio low), prescription of a well-fitting hearing aid and the use of other non-verbal forms of communication (e.g. pictures). Successful management is often dependent on the degree of carer involvement and community support provided.

## Thyroid dysfunction

The most important endocrine disorder in people with Down's syndrome is thyroid dysfunction. Other endocrine abnormalities include an under-developed pituitary gland (Benda, 1949), an abnormal response to growth hormone (Wisniewski et al, 1989) and abnormal levels of gonadotrophin hormones (Pueschel, 1988).

Over the past 40 years, many reports have highlighted an association between Down's syndrome and thyroid dysfunction, showing altered plasma levels of thyroxine, tri-iodothyronine and thyroid-stimulating hormone (Prasher, 1999a). The lifetime prevalence of thyroid dysfunction in Down's syndrome is about 25%. There is an increase in the prevalence of acquired thyroid dysfunction with increasing age, with hypothyroidism being more common than hyperthyroidism. An association between thyroid dysfunction and autoimmune thyroiditis has been reported (Vladutin et al, 1984).

The clinical presentation of thyroid dysfunction in people with Down's syndrome remains an area of controversy. In the past, similarities between Down's syndrome and hypothyroidism led to a misdiagnosis of the syndrome and to inappropriate treatment with thyroid extract (Benda, 1949). The recognition of thyroid disease (especially hypothyroidism) can be very difficult in individuals with Down's syndrome (Mani, 1988). A healthy adult with Down's syndrome is short in stature, has dry skin and thinning hair, may be overweight, has a slow heart rate and may not be very active. These features are frequently found in hypothyroidism and make the diagnosis difficult. A high index of suspicion for thyroid dysfunction is therefore required. However, other findings that may suggest the presence of a thyroid disorder include: an abnormal electrocardiogram with abnormalities consistent with hypothyroidism (Murdoch et al, 1977b), detection of a goitre (Hollingsworth et al, 1974) and the presence of alopecia areata (Du Vivier & Munro, 1975).

Adults with Down's syndrome do need regular monitoring of their thyroid status, but evidence is lacking regarding how frequently thyroid function tests should be undertaken. If previous tests were normal, every 2–3 years is reasonable for individuals with a past history of thyroid disease. For individuals presently on thyroxine replacement treatment tests every 1–2 years should be done. The treatment of hypothyroidism (with thyroid hormone replacement) and the treatment of hyperthyroidism (with anti-thyroid drugs, surgery and radioiodine) should not be too dissimilar to that for typical adults.

## Musculoskeletal aspects of health

A number of different musculoskeletal abnormalities have been reported in individuals with Down's syndrome. Two of the most clinically significant involve the cervical spine: atlanto-occipital instability and atlanto-axial instability. Cervical spine instability is one of the most potentially serious orthopaedic conditions encountered in Down's syndrome. From a review of the literature (Pueschel *et al*, 1992; Machlachlan *et al*, 1993), the prevalence of atlanto-axial instability in adults with Down's syndrome can range from 7% to 40%, depending on the age of the population studied, the method of assessment and the criteria used to detect the instability.

The rate of clinical neurological complications secondary to atlanto-axial instability remains uncertain. Pueschel & Scola (1987) examined 404 persons with Down's syndrome and found that 59 (14%) displayed atlanto-axial instability. Fifty-three (13%) had asymptomatic instability and six (1.4%) had symptoms requiring surgical intervention. The most common neurological symptoms included brisk deep tendon reflexes, extensor plantar responses, ankle clonus, paralysis of the limbs, muscle weakness, gait abnormalities and difficulty walking. Local neck pain, neck mobility and head tilt may also be observed. A history of neck trauma can be elicited in some cases, and surgical intervention can benefit some individuals (Taggard *et al*, 2000). Acute conditions are more likely to respond to medical intervention than is chronic symptomatology.

Restrictions to participation in sporting activities for people with Down's syndrome have been previously recommended. These restrictions have included training for competition gymnastics, diving, diving start in swimming, butterfly stroke in swimming, high jump, pentathlon, soccer, alpine skiing and even warm-up exercises that place pressure on the head and neck. However, these restrictions remain controversial. At present in the UK, most clinicians would argue that these recommendations are too restrictive. Qualified caution is still, however, required. Findings from research suggest that routine screening for atlanto-axial instability by cervical X-ray examination is not of any significant clinical value. However, any adult with Down's syndrome presenting with central neurological symptomatology should be assessed for cervical spine pathology.

## Obesity

In 1984, Knight & Eldridge reported that within the general adult population (aged 16–64 years), 34% of males and 24% of females were overweight and 6% of males and 8% of females were obese. For people with learning disabilities as a whole, about 16% of males and 21% of females have been reported to be overweight, with 16% of males and 25% of females obese (Fox & Rotatori, 1982; Bell & Bhate, 1992). Prasher (1995b) found that only 11% of adults with Down's syndrome had a 'desirable weight' (a body mass index, calculated as weight in kg/ (height in m)$^2$, of 21–24). Twenty-seven per cent were 'overweight' (body mass index 25–29) and 47% could be described as being 'obese' (body mass index >29).

Being overweight or obese is therefore a health issue, not only for the general population, but in particular for adults with Down's syndrome (Rubin et al, 1998). This may reflect poor diet control, low levels of physical activity, a lower basal metabolic rate or associated medical problems (e.g. thyroid dysfunction). It remains important, however, that a good body weight is maintained, ideally from childhood. The basic principles of managing obesity in the general population also apply to adults with Down's syndrome. Appropriate support from a dietician and the close involvement of carers can have a significant impact on outcome.

## Epilepsy

Until recently, research studies had differed on whether any association exists between epilepsy and Down's syndrome (Kirman, 1951; Johannsen et al, 1996). During the past two decades, such an association has been established, in particular between seizures and dementia of the Alzheimer's type in older adults with Down's syndrome (Evenhuis, 1990; Prasher & Corbett, 1993). Prasher (1995c) found a point prevalence rate for epilepsy of 15.9%. This was probably an underestimate, as subjects with partial complex seizures were excluded from the study. A bimodal distribution of seizure onset was found, with early-onset seizures in childhood and late-onset seizures in middle age. This latter peak was thought to be due most probably to the presence of underlying changes of Alzheimer's disease. Tonic-clonic seizures only were the most common form of seizure disorder.

The classification, assessment and management of seizures in adults with Down's syndrome is generally the same as in the general population (Betts, 1998). Anti-epileptic drugs should be started at a low dose and gradually increased. Psychiatrists must be aware of the presence of comorbid problems (e.g. bradycardia, increased renal anomalies) that may influence the type of drugs used. Non-drug treatment, such as counselling and social support, psychological treatments and alternative therapies, may be considered as a complement or alternative to anticonvulsant therapy.

## Other physical health issues

Respiratory problems, especially recurrent respiratory infections and obstructive sleep apnoea, are recognised conditions associated with Down's syndrome. Gastrointestinal and genito-urinary problems (e.g. duodenal stenosis, Hirschsprung's disease, hydronephrosis, obstructive uropathy and renal agenesis, distal hypospadias, cryptochidism) can persist from birth or childhood into adulthood, but most should have been managed at an earlier age. Dermatological problems (xerosis, atopic dermatitis, tinea pedis, alopecia areata) are also common in adults with Down's syndrome. Some are easily managed (e.g. tinea pedis), whereas others are less easy to treat (e.g. alopecia areata).

Adults with Down's syndrome are susceptible to many physical illnesses, affecting virtually all organs and bodily systems. Regular screening and appropriate management are essential to maintaining a good quality of life. Psychiatrists caring for people with learning disabilities must be fully aware of many of the physical conditions associated with Down's syndrome. The provision of high-quality psychiatric care cannot occur in isolation of physical health care.

# Mental health

Recently, there has been considerable interest in the presentation of psychiatric disorders in people with learning disabilities. The accurate diagnosis of mental illness in learning disability is imperative, as later management will in large part be determined by this. However, the accurate diagnosis of mental disorders is highly problematic because of underlying cognitive impairment, impairment of communication, compounding medical conditions (e.g. sensory loss), poor test compliance and lack of standardisation of measuring instruments for people with learning disabilities. To impose the diagnostic psychopathology found in the general population on people with learning disabilities may be inappropriate. Do psychiatric disorders present in learning disability as they do in the general population? Should we try to fit abnormal behaviour occurring in people with learning disabilities into diagnostic criteria (ICD–10, DSM–IV) developed for people without learning disabilities?

A limited number of studies have investigated the prevalence rates of the differing forms of mental disorder in adults with Down's syndrome (Myers & Pueschel, 1991; Collacott, 1992; Prasher, 1995a). Myers & Pueschel (1991) investigated 497 people with Down's syndrome for psychiatric morbidity, of whom 164 were over 20 years of age (adults). Of the adults, 1.3% had an attention-deficit disorder or a hyperactivity disorder, 1.3% a conduct or oppositional disorder, 1.2% aggressive behaviour, 4.1% compulsive behaviour, 1.3% eating problems, 5.5% self-injurious behaviour, 1.3% showed affective syndromes and 6.1% were found to have dementia. Prasher (1995*a*) studied the prevalence of psychiatric morbidity in 201 adults with Down's syndrome according to ICD–10 diagnostic criteria (World Health Organization, 1993). Twenty-nine per cent of the sample was diagnosed as having a current mental disorder. Dementia of the Alzheimer's type was present in 13.5%, a depressive episode in 5.0%, obsessive–compulsive disorder in 4.5%, conduct disorder in 4.0% and anxiety-related disorders in 2%.

Research findings appear to show that the spectrum of psychiatric disorders seen in the non-learning disability population also occurs in adults with Down's syndrome. Although the overall prevalence rate for the presence of a mental disorder is higher in the Down's syndrome population, a different epidemiological profile of mental disorders is seen. Dementia of the Alzheimer's type is markedly more common in adults with Down's syndrome. Whether depression, pervasive developmental disorders and obsessive–compulsive disorders are also more common, or are overrepresented because of misdiagnosis, remains to be further researched. Alcohol-related disorders and drug misuse can occur, but are significantly less common.

## *Dementia of the Alzheimer's type*

Alzheimer's disease is the principle illness associated with Down's syndrome (Berg *et al*, 1993; Hutchinson, 1999). The hallmark of Alzheimer's is the presence of extracellular amyloid plaques and intra-neuronal neurofibrillary tangles. The former are minute areas of degeneration, consisting of granular deposits of aluminium and silicate, remnants of neuronal processes, and the latter are paired helical filaments. The amyloid plaques are usually spherical in shape, measuring 5–150 μm in diameter. Neurofibrillary tangles are filaments, 14–18 nm in diameter, coiled anti-clockwise around each other with a periodic of 70–90 nm. Parallel bundles are cross-linked by thin filaments at regular intervals (for a detailed review see Berg *et al*, 1993).

Identification of clinical dementia, particularly early in Down's syndrome, has proven to be extremely difficult because of problems in detecting cognitive and non-cognitive psychopathology (Janicki *et al*, 1996; Aylward *et al*, 1997; Dalton *et al*, 1999). For example, it is not easy to detect mild memory disturbance in people with pre-existing severe cognitive impairment. However, it is now established that the prevalence of dementia of the Alzheimer's type increases markedly with age: at

30–39 years of age it is 2–3%, 40–49 years (9–10%), 50–59 years (36–40%), 60–69 years (55%) (Prasher, 1995d; Holland et al, 1998). Such rates suggest that dementia of the Alzheimer's type can occur in individuals with Down's syndrome in their early 30s and that by the age of 55, of those still alive, more will have dementia than not (further information available from the author upon request). Prasher & Krishnan (1993), in a literature review of 98 published case reports of people with Down's syndrome and a high diagnostic probability of dementia, found the mean age at onset of dementia was 51.7 years (range 31–68 years). The mean age at onset for males was 53.6 years (range 31–68 years) and for females 49.8 years (range 36–66 years); there was a statistically significant difference between genders, with females showing an earlier age of onset than males. The mean duration of dementia for the sample as a whole was 6 years. No statistically significant difference in the duration of dementia between the genders was found.

Dalton & Crapper-McLachlan (1986) reviewed 35 case reports of people with Down's syndrome for whom a clinical description had been given in relation to the development of Alzheimer's disease. The most frequently occurring symptom/sign was the presence of epilepsy (88% of subjects), followed by focal neurological signs (46%) and personality change (46% of cases). Other symptoms and signs were (in order of frequency) incontinence, apathy, inactivity, loss of conversation, electro-encephalogram changes, loss of self-help skills, tremor, myoclonus, visual or auditory effects, walking impairment, stubbornness, unco-operative behaviour, depression, memory loss, flexed posture, increased muscle tone, disorientation and hallucinations or delusions.

Lai & Williams (1989) studied 96 individuals with Down's syndrome over 35 years of age. Three phases of clinical deterioration were recognised. In the initial phase, memory impairment, temporal disorientation and reduced verbal output were evident in the higher-functioning individuals. For those with more-severe learning disability, the first indications of dementia were apathy, inattention and reduced social interactions. In the second phase, loss of self-help skills such as dressing, toileting and use of food utensils were seen. The gait was often slowed and shuffling. In the final phase, the patients were non-ambulatory and bedridden, often assuming flexed postures. Sphincter incontinence was present and pathological reflexes such as sucking, palmar grasp and glabellar reflexes were prevalent. Seizures occurred in 41 (84%) of the 49 patients with dementia, but were present in all 23 who died. Four had a pre-existing seizure disorder, 23 had the onset within 2 years of mental decline, and in 14 seizures developed more than 3 years after the dementia began.

Most of the seizures were of a generalised and tonic-clonic type, but several had partial complex seizures; all were easily controlled with anticonvulsants. Seven patients also developed myoclonus. Ten patients

(20%) in the group with dementia had the flexed posture, bradykinesia, masked faces and cogwheel rigidity of Parkinsonism. Four had a coarse resting tremor. The picture, therefore, of dementia of the Alzheimer's type in this Down's syndrome population is generally similar to that seen in the general population. Detection of early symptoms, for example decline in short-term memory, is more difficult, and emphasis on non-cognitive features (e.g. personality change) may be required. The age at onset is significantly younger in the Down's syndrome population, but the characteristic course and outcome appear to be the same irrespective of the underlying level of intellectual function.

A number of different methods of diagnosing or screening for dementia in adults with Down's syndrome have been proposed (Table 15.1) and a neuropsychological test battery for the diagnosis of dementia in individuals with learning disabilities has been developed (Burt & Aylward, 2000). Many of these tests require further evaluation, but it is unlikely that one specific test will be able to detect dementia in a population with such a wide range of abilities, communication skills, confounding health disorders and varying degrees of test compliance. Information from tests should be taken together with the findings from a detailed clinical assessment in diagnosing dementia of the Alzheimer's type according to recognised ICD–10 diagnostic criteria (World Health Organization, 1992).

Several genetic markers for Alzheimer's disease in the general population have been determined. Mutations in the amyloid precursor protein gene (Goate *et al*, 1991) and presenilin genes (van Broeckhoven, 1995) have been linked to the development of Alzheimer's in particular families. The presence of an apolipoprotein ε4 allele is a high-risk factor for the onset of dementia, whereas presence of an ε2 allele is a

**Table 15.1** Procedures used to detect dementia in adults with Down's syndrome

| Measure | Reference |
| --- | --- |
| *Neuropsychological tests* | |
| Dementia questionnaire for persons with Mental Retardation (pmre) | Evenhuis (1992) |
| Dementia Scale for Down's Syndrome | Gedye (1995) |
| Adaptive Behaviour Scale | Prasher *et al* (1994) |
| *Neurophysiological tests* | |
| Electroencephalography | Visser *et al* (1996) |
| Evoked potentials | Blackwood *et al* (1988) |
| *Neuroimaging assessments* | |
| Computed tomography | Schapiro *et al* (1992) |
| Single photon emission computed tomography | Deb *et al* (1992) |
| Positron emission tomography | Azari *et al* (1994) |
| Magnetic resonance imaging | Aylward *et al* (1999) |

protective factor (Corder *et al*, 1993). In adults with Down's syndrome it has been hypothesised that triplication of the amyloid precusor protein gene (found on chromosome 21) is the main reason for development of Alzheimer's disease. A case report of a 78-year-old adult with partial trisomy 21 strongly supports this hypothesis (Prasher *et al*, 1998*a*). In people with Down's syndrome, as in the general population, the apo-lipoprotein ε4 allele increases the risk for dementia of the Alzheimer's type (Deb *et al*, 2000). The effect in Down's syndrome is, however, less than that in the general population, probably because it is overwhelmed by the effects of the triplication of the amyloid precursor protein gene.

During the past decade, a number of acetylcholinesterase (AChE) inhibitors have been developed to improve brain cholinergic function in patients with Alzheimer's disease (Burns *et al*, 1999). Donepezil, rivastigmine and galantamine have now been approved by the National Institute for Clinical Excellence (2001) for widespread but monitored clinical use in the UK. A few case studies of the effects of donepezil in adults with Down's syndrome with and without dementia of the Alzheimer's type have been reported (Kishnani *et al*, 1997; Hemingway-Eltomey & Lerner, 1999).

Prasher *et al* (2002) completed a 24-week double-blind placebo-controlled trial of donepezil in adults with Down's syndrome and dementia of the Alzheimer's type. They found that donepezil (5 or 10 mg) administered once a day was generally well tolerated and safe. There appeared to be some efficacy in the treatment of symptoms of mild to moderate dementia in this population, although the sample size of the study was too small to be statistically significant. The authors concluded that further research was required to evaluate fully whether AChE inhibitors are an efficacious treatment for dementia of the Alzheimer's type in Down's syndrome. However, from the available information there is now cautious optimism regarding the treatment of dementia in people with Down's syndrome.

## Age-associated functional decline

Age-associated functional decline is objectively identified decline in cognitive and/or adaptive behaviour consequent to the ageing process that is thought to be within normal limits given the person's age. The decline seen is therefore not attributable to a specific mental or physical disorder. There are problems in the field of learning disability in defining the expected decline with increasing age in a population that previously would rarely have survived beyond middle age. Individuals with age-associated functional decline may show early signs of impairment of memory, attention or concentration. A minor degree of deterioration may be seen in overall intellectual functioning. Associated with or in the absence of intellectual decline, there may be a decline in day-to-day functioning (independence, level of self-care skills, mobility, speed of activity).

To date, most research into age-associated functional decline has focused on the investigation of changes in 'adaptive behaviour' (Prasher *et al*, 1998*b*), which is defined as 'the effectiveness or degree with which the individual meets the standards of personal independence and social responsibility expected of his/her age or cultural group' (Grossman, 1977). Zigman *et al* (1987) were able to show that, for individuals with Down's syndrome at all levels of disability, adaptive competence declined with increasing age to a greater extent than for controls with learning disabilities other than Down's syndrome. The decline seen is usually due to an underlying illness (in particular, dementia of the Alzheimer's type), but a decline is also seen in healthy older people with Down's syndrome (Prasher *et al*, 1998*b*). Although research has now begun to investigate age-associated functional decline in Down's syndrome (Prasher *et al*, 1998*b*; Devenny *et al*, 2000), further studies are required to investigate its specifics. Which particular areas of cognitive functioning are affected? How best can we discriminate age-associated functional decline from early dementia of the Alzheimer's type?

## Affective disorders

There have been few epidemiological studies reporting the prevalence of depression in adults with Down's syndrome (Collacott & Cooper, 1992; Prasher, 1995*a*). Myers & Pueschel (1991), in their study of 164 adults with Down's syndrome, identified 10 (6.1%) cases of depression, 1 of bipolar affective disorder and 1 of organic affective disorder. Collacott (1992) found the lifetime prevalence of depression in adults with Down's syndrome to be 11.3% and that of bipolar affective disorder to be 0.5%. A study of 201 adults with Down's syndrome (Prasher, 1995*a*) found a point prevalence rate for a depressive episode of 5.0%. The aetiology of affective disorders in people with learning disabilities remains multi-factorial and includes the underlying genetic make-up, presence of secondary organic brain pathology (e.g. epilepsy), the occurrence of coexisting physical or psychiatric illness (e.g. dementia) and the experience of 'life events' (Prasher, 1999*b*).

The spectrum of clinical symptomatology of affective disorders seen in the general population can also occur in adults with Down's syndrome. However, in diagnosing a depressive episode in the latter group, more significance is often given to behavioural features (increased aggression, being withdrawn, decline in social skills) and to changes in biological features (disturbed sleep, weight loss) than to cognitive features (e.g. memory decline, deterioration in attention and concentration). Thoughts of self-harm and suicidal behaviour are uncommon, but do occur (Hurley, 1998).

It used to be thought that Down's syndrome precludes the development of mania (Sovner *et al*, 1985). However, several case reports of mania in Down's syndrome have now been described (Haeger, 1990; Cooper & Collacott, 1993). Cooper & Collacott (1993) reviewed the published cases of mania in people with Down's syndrome and concluded that the mean age of first-episode onset was 33.7 years. No case in a female was described, no family history of affective disorder was found and symptoms similar to those in the general population were evident.

The approach to the management of depression and mania in adults with Down's syndrome is similar to that for the general population. With appropriate caution and monitoring, antidepressants, electroconvulsive therapy, psychotherapy and behavioural therapy can be used to treat a depressive episode. Neuroleptics and mood stabilisers are used to treat mania. Carers and non-health professionals must be involved in the management of treatment, often playing a significant role. Limited research data are available regarding the prognosis for adults with Down's syndrome and affective disorders, but available evidence suggests that some individuals do suffer ongoing impairments (Collacott & Cooper, 1992; Prasher & Hall, 1996).

Whether affective disorders are more common in people with Down's syndrome than in the general population, or in people with learning disabilities of other aetiologies, still remains to be resolved. A large epidemiological study using standardised criteria for an affective disorder is required. The short-term response to long-term treatment and prognosis is still unknown and further research is needed.

## *Obsessive–compulsive disorder*

The prevalence of obsessive–compulsive disorder (OCD) is reported to be 1.6% to 2.5% in the general population. Rituals and other repetitive behaviours in people with learning disabilities may be difficult to distinguish from compulsive behaviour and this must be borne in mind before a diagnosis of OCD is made. Obsessional repetitive thoughts can occur in people with Down's syndrome, but may be difficult to diagnose because of impaired language function. Obsessive–compulsive acts are probably more likely to be detected. Myers & Pueschel (1991) found a rate of 1.7% in individuals with Down's syndome, a rate similar to that in the general population. Prasher & Day (1995) found a point prevalence rate of 4.5% for OCD in adults with Down's syndrome. O'Dwyer *et al* (1992) reported two cases of OCD in individuals with Down's syndrome. The first was a 19-year-old male with acute onset of checking and ordering of items and the second was a 37-year-old female presenting with a 9-year history of washing and ordering.

## Autism (pervasive developmental disorders)

Over the past two decades there has been growing interest in a possible association between autism (pervasive developmental disorders) and Down's syndrome. Lund (1988) found 5 of 44 persons with Down's syndrome (11.4%) to have infantile autism, as compared with 19 (6.9%) of 258 controls with other learning disabilities. Several case reports of pervasive developmental disorders in adults with Down's syndrome have been reported (Ghaziuddin *et al*, 1992; Kent *et al*, 1998). The definition of 'autism' and the exclusion of other disorders that could account for the behaviour (e.g. behavioural phenotype, depression, OCD) are important factors that influence prevalence rates. At present there is evidence in the literature suggesting an association, but further, methodologically improved, epidemiological studies are still required.

## Other psychiatric disorders

Although several studies have investigated the prevalence of schizophrenia in people with learning disabilities (Wright, 1982; Turner, 1989), few cases of schizophrenia in individuals with Down's syndrome have been reported (Eaton & Menolascino, 1982; Duggirala *et al*, 1995). These reports failed to give details of phenomenology or to fully investigate an organic-induced psychosis. To date, therefore, there is no strong evidence to suggest that people with Down's syndrome are particularly susceptible to, or are protected from, developing schizophrenia.

Studies within the learning disability population as a whole have reported increased rates of anxiety disorders (Malpass *et al*, 1960; Knights, 1963). For adults, Lund (1988) found neurotic traits in 25 of 44 (57%) subjects with Down's syndrome, but diagnosis using diagnostic criteria revealed none with a neurosis. It would appear that people with Down's syndrome may suffer less from phobic/anxiety disorders than do people without learning disabilities, but, as with many other psychiatric illnesses, no firm conclusions can be made at present. Other psychiatric disorders reported in adults with Down's syndrome are anorexia nervosa (Cottrell & Crisp, 1984; Morgan, 1989), Tourette syndrome (Barabas *et al*, 1986), paraphilias (Myers & Pueschel, 1991) and multiple personality disorder (Fotheringham & Thompson, 1994).

Studies investigating psychiatric morbidity in adults with Down's syndrome have often suffered from numerous methodological flaws. These include: retrospective case-note studies; small sample sizes; isolated case reports; the definition of learning disability or the level of disability not given; assessment measures not standardised for people with learning disabilities; and other possible causes of the symptomatology not given. Many studies have been of institutionalised populations, which are liable to selection bias. The overall prevalence rate of psychiatric disorders in adults with Down's syndrome appears to be higher than that in the general population. Dementia of the Alzheimer's type and, possibly, depression are common disorders in people with Down's syndrome, but an increase in prevalence rates of other psychiatric disorders has not been confirmed. Overall, behavioural and conduct disorders may be underdiagnosed in people with Down's syndrome. The 'Prince Charming' label often given to people with Down's syndrome may prove to be detrimental, as underlying behavioural and personality problems may be being missed.

## Conclusions

Adults with Down's syndrome have a high prevalence of physical and mental disorders. The medically significant physical disorders that psychiatrists should be aware of include: cardiac problems, ophthalmic and audiological pathology, thyroid dysfunction, atlanto-axial instability, obesity and epilepsy. Psychological disorders that are particularly associated with adults with Down's syndrome are: dementia of the Alzheimer's type, age-associated functional decline, affective disorders, obsessive–compulsive disorder, and autism (pervasive developmental disorders).

Individuals with Down's syndrome may not be able to communicate any distress they experience associated with a given illness. Ill health may be masked and this can result in missed or misdiagnosed psychiatric and physical morbidity. Complications can follow, which may ultimately prove to be fatal. To ensure that appropriate health care is provided to adults with Down's syndrome, health services must be aware of the diagnosis, treatment and management of the medical and psychiatric disorders that occur in this population. An active screening programme implemented by both primary and secondary health services is required. This programme should be ongoing and at the very least should monitor sensory function, thyroid status, mental state, prescribed medication and the level of adaptive behaviour. The improved life expectancy of people with Down's syndrome makes them more susceptible than ever to physical, psychological and social morbidity. The development of a good-quality, comprehensive health service is essential to ensure a high quality of life for adults with Down's syndrome. Psychiatrists in the field of learning disability arguably play a central role, and therefore their knowledge of the many health issues affecting this vulnerable population must be of a high standard.

## References

Aylward, E. H., Burt, D. B., Thorpe, L. U., et al (1997) Diagnosis of dementia in individuals with intellectual disability. *Journal of Intellectual Disability Research*, **41**, 152–164.

—, Li, Q., Honeycutt, N. A., *et al* (1999) MRI volumes of the hippocampus and amygdala in adults with Down's syndrome with and without dementia. *American Journal of Psychiatry*, **154**, 564–568.

Azari, N. P., Pettigrew, K. D., Pietrini Horwitz, B., *et al* (1994) Detection of an Alzheimer disease pattern of cerebral metabolism in Down's syndrome. *Dementia*, **5**, 69–78.

Baird, P. A. & Sadovnick, A. D. (1989) Life tables for Down's syndrome. *Human Genetics*, **82**, 291–292.

Barabas, G., Wardell, B., Sapiro, M., *et al* (1986) Coincident Down's and Tourette syndrome. Three case reports. *Journal of Child Neurology*, **1**, 358–360.

Bell, A. J. & Bhate, M. S. (1992) Prevalence of overweight and obesity in Down's syndrome and other mentally handicapped adults living in the community. *Journal of Intellectual Disability Research*, **36**, 359–364.

Benda, C. E. (1949) *Mongolism and Cretinism* (2nd edn). New York: Grune & Stratton.

Berg, J. M., Karlinsky, H. & Holland, A. J. (1993) *Alzheimer Disease, Down's Syndrome and their Relationship*. Oxford: Oxford University Press.

Betts. T. (1998) *Epilepsy Psychiatry and Learning Difficulty*. London: Martin Dunitz.

Blackwood, D. H. R., St Clair, D. M., Muir, W. J., *et al* (1988) The development of Alzheimer's disease in Down's syndrome assessed by auditory event-related potentials. *Journal of Mental Deficiency Research*, **32**, 439–453.

Burns, A., Rossor, M., Hecker, J., *et al* (1999) The effects of donepezil in Alzheimer's disease: results from a multinational trial. *Dementia and Geriatric Cognitive Disorders*, **10**, 237–244.

Burt, D. B. & Aylward, E. H (2000) Test battery for the diagnosis of dementia in individuals with intellectual disability. *Journal of Intellectual Disability Research*, **44**, 175–180.

Caputo, A. R., Wagner, R. S., Reynolds, D. R., *et al* (1989) Down's syndrome. Clinical review of ocular features. *Clinical Pediatrics*, **28**, 355–358.

Catalano, R. A. (1990) Down's syndrome. *Survey of Ophthalmology*, **34**, 383–398.

Collacott, R. A. (1992) The effect of age and residential placement on adaptive behaviour of adults with Down's syndrome. *British Journal of Psychiatry*, **161**, 675–679.

— & Cooper, S.-A. (1992) Adaptive behaviour after depressive illness in Down's syndrome. *Journal of Nervous and Mental Disease*, **180**, 468–470.

Cooper, S.-A. & Collacott, R. A. (1993) Mania and Down's syndrome. *British Journal of Psychiatry*, **162**, 739–743.

Corder, E. H., Saunders, A. M., Strittmatter, W. J., *et al* (1993) Gene dose of apolipoprotein E type 4 allele and the risk of Alzheimer's disease in late onset families. *Science*, **261**, 921–923.

Cottrell, D. J. & Crisp, A. H. (1984) Anorexia nervosa in Down's syndrome – a case report. *British Journal of Psychiatry*, **145**, 195–196.

Dalton, A. J. & Crapper-McLachlan, D. R. (1986) Clinical expression of Alzheimer's disease in Down's syndrome. *Psychiatric Perspectives on Mental Retardation*, **9**, 659–670.

—, Mehta, P. D., Fedor, B. L., *et al* (1999) Cognitive changes in memory precede those in praxis in aging persons with Down's syndrome. *Journal of Intellectual and Developmental Disability*, **24**, 169–187.

Deb, S., de Silva, P. N., Gemmell, H. G., *et al* (1992) Alzheimer's disease in adults with Down's syndrome: the relationship between regional cerebral blood flow equivalents and dementia. *Acta Psychiatrica Scandinavica*, **86**, 340–345.

—, Braganza J., Norton, N., *et al* (2000) APOE ε4 influences the manifestation of Alzheimer's disease in adults with Down's syndrome. *British Journal of Psychiatry*, **176**, 468–472.

Devenny, D. A., Krinsky-McHale, S. J., Sersen, G., *et al* (2000) Sequence of cognitive decline in dementia in adults with Down's syndrome. *Journal of Intellectual Disability Research*, **44**, 654–665.

Duggirala, C., Cooper, S.-A. & Collacott, R. A. (1995) Schizophrenia and Down's syndrome. *Irish Journal of Psychological Medicine*, **12**, 30–33.

Du Vivier, A. & Munro, D. D. (1975) Alopecia areata, autoimmunity and Down's syndrome. *BMJ*, **1**, 191–192.

Eaton, L. F. & Menolascino, F. J. (1982) Psychiatric disorders in the mentally retarded: types, problems, and challenges. *American Journal of Psychiatry*, **139**, 1297–1303.

Evenhuis, H. M. (1990) The natural history of dementia in Down's syndrome. *Archives of Neurology*, **48**, 318–320.

—— (1992) Evaluation of a screening instrument for dementia in ageing mentally retarded persons. *Journal of Intellectual Disability Research*, **36**, 337–347.

——, van Zanten, G. A., Brocaar, M. P., *et al* (1992) Hearing loss in middle-age persons with Down's syndrome. *American Journal on Mental Retardation*, **97**, 47–56.

Fotheringham, J. B. & Thompson, F. (1994) Case report of a person with Down's syndrome and multiple personality disorder. *Canadian Journal of Psychiatry*, **39**, 116–119.

Fox, R. & Rotatori, A. F. (1982) Prevalence of obesity among mentally retarded adults. *American Journal of Mental Deficiency*, **87**, 228–230.

Gedye, A. (1995) *Dementia Scale for Down's Syndrome: Manual.* Vancouver: Gedye Research and Consulting.

Ghaziuddin, M., Tsai, L. Y. & Ghaziuddin, N. (1992) Autism in Down's syndrome: presentation and diagnosis. *Journal of Intellectual Disability Research*, **36**, 449–456.

Goate, A. M., Chartier-Harlene, C. M. & Mullan, M. (1991) Segregation of a missense mutation in the amyloid precursor protein gene with familial Alzheimer's disease. *Nature*, **353**, 844–846.

Goldhaber, S. Z., Rubin, I. L., Brown, W., *et al* (1986) Valvular heart disease (aortic regurgitation and mitral valve prolapse) among institutionalised adults with Down's syndrome. *American Journal of Cardiology*, **57**, 278–281.

Grossman, H. J. (ed.) (1977) *Manual on Terminology and Classification in Mental Retardation.* Washington, DC: American Association on Mental Deficiency.

Haeger, B. (1990) Mania in Down's syndrome (letter). *British Journal of Psychiatry*, **157**, 153.

Hemingway-Eltomey, J. M. & Lerner, A. J. (1999) Adverse effects of donepezil in treating Alzheimer's disease associated with Down's syndrome (letter). *American Journal of Psychiatry*, **156**, 1470.

Holland, A. J., Hon, J., Huppert, F. A., *et al* (1998) Population-based study of the prevalence and presentation of dementia in adults with Down's syndrome. *British Journal of Psychiatry*, **172**, 493–498.

Hollingsworth, D. R., Mckean, H. E. & Roeckel, I. (1974) Goitre, immunological observations, and thyroid function tests in Down's syndrome. *American Journal of Diseases of Children*, **127**, 524–527.

Hurley, A. D. (1998) Two cases of suicide attempt by patients with Down's syndrome. *Psychiatric Services*, **49**, 1618–1619.

Hutchinson, N. J. (1999) Association between Down's syndrome and Alzheimer's disease: review of the literature. *Journal of Learning Disabilities for Nursing, Health and Social Care*, **3**, 194–203.

Jacobson, J. W. & Janicki, M. P. (1985) Functional and health status characteristics of persons with severe handicaps in New York State. *Journal of the Association for Persons with Severe Handicaps*, **10**, 51–60.

Janicki, M. P., Heller, T., Seltzer, G. B., *et al* (1996) Practice guidelines for the clinical assessment and care management of Alzheimer's disease and other dementias among adults with intellectual disability. *Journal of Intellectual Disability Research*, **40**, 374–382.

Johannsen, P., Christensen, J. E. J., Goldstein, H., *et al* (1996) Epilepsy in Down's syndrome – prevalence in three age-groups. *Seizure*, **5**, 121–125.

Kent, L., Perry, D. & Evans, J. (1998) Autism in Down's syndrome: three case reports. *Autism*, **2**, 259–267.

Kirman, B. H. (1951) Epilepsy in mongolism. *Archives of Disease in Childhood*, **26**, 501–503.

Kishnani, P. S., Sullivan, J. A., Walter, B. K., *et al* (1997) Cholinergic therapy for Down's syndrome. *Lancet*, **353**, 1064–1066.

Knight, I. & Eldridge, J. (1984) *The Heights and Weights of Adults in Great Britain*. London: HMSO.

Knights, R. M. (1963) Test anxiety and defensiveness in institutionalized and noninstitutionalized normal and retarded children. *Child Development*, **34**, 1019–1026.

Lai, F. & Williams, R. S. (1989) A prospective study of Alzheimer disease in Down's syndrome. *Archives of Neurology*, **46**, 849–853.

Libb, J. W., Dahle, A. J., Smith, K., *et al* (1985) Hearing disorders and cognitive function of individuals with Down's syndrome. *American Journal of Mental Deficiency*, **90**, 353–56.

Lonigan, C. J., Fischel, J. E., Whitehurst, G. J., *et al* (1992) The role of otitis media in the development of expressive language disorder. *Developmental Psychology*, **28**, 430–440.

Lund, J. (1988) Psychiatric aspects of Down's syndrome. *Acta Psychiatrica Scandinavica*, **78**, 369–374.

Machlachlan, R. A., Filder, K. A, Yeh, H., *et al* (1993) Cervical spine abnormalities in institutionalised adults with Down's syndrome. *Journal of Intellectual Disability Research*, **37**, 277–285.

Malpass, L. F., Mark, S. & Palermo, D. S. (1960) Responses of retarded children to the Children's Manifest Anxiety Scale. *Journal of Educational Psychology*, **51**, 305–308.

Mani, C. (1988) Hypothyroidism in Down's syndrome. *British Journal of Psychiatry*, **153**, 102–104.

Mazzoni, D. S., Ackley, R. S. & Nash, D. J. (1994) Abnormal pinna type and hearing loss correlations in Down's syndrome. *Journal of Intellectual Disability Research*, **38**, 549–560.

Morgan, J. R. (1989) A case of Down's syndrome, insulinoma, and anorexia. *Journal of Mental Deficiency Research*, **33**, 185–187.

Murdoch, J. C., Rodger, J. C., Rao, S. S., *et al* (1977a) Down's syndrome: an atheroma-free model? *BMJ*, **2**, 226–228.

—, Ratcliffe, W. A., Mclarty, D. G., *et al* (1977b) Thyroid function in adults with Down's syndrome. *Journal of Clinical Endocrinology*, **44**, 453–458.

Myers, B. A. & Pueschel, S. M. (1991) Psychiatric disorders in a population with Down's syndrome. *Journal of Nervous and Mental Disease*, **179**, 609–613.

National Institute for Clinical Excellence (2001) *Guidance on the Issue of Donepezil, Rivastigmine and Galantamine for the Treatment of Alzheimer's Disease*. London: NICE.

O'Dwyer, J., Holmes, J. & Collacott, R. A. (1992) Two cases of obsessive–compulsive disorder in individuals with Down's syndrome. *Journal of Nervous and Mental Disease*, **180**, 603–604.

Prasher, V. P. (1994) Screening of physical morbidity in adults with Down's syndrome. *Down's Syndrome Research and Practice*, **2**, 59–66.

— (1995a) Prevalence of psychiatric disorders in adults with Down's syndrome. *European Journal of Psychiatry*, **9**, 77–82.

— (1995b) Overweight and obesity amongst Down's syndrome adults. *Journal of Intellectual Disability Research*, **39**, 437–441.

— (1995c) Epilepsy and associated effects on adaptive behaviour in adults with Down's syndrome. *Seizure*, **4**, 53–56.

— (1995d) Age-specific prevalence, thyroid dysfunction and depressive symptomatology in adults with Down's syndrome and dementia. *International Journal of Geriatric Psychiatry*, **10**, 25–31.

—— (1999a) Down's syndrome and thyroid disorders: A review. *Down's Syndrome Research and Practice*, **6**, 25–42.

—— (1999b) Presentation and management of depression in people with learning disability. *Advances in Psychiatric Treatment*, **5**, 447–454.

—— & Corbett, J. A. (1993) Onset of seizures as a poor indicator of longevity in people with Down's syndrome and dementia. *International Journal of Geriatric Psychiatry*, **8**, 923–927.

—— & Day, S. (1995) Brief report: obsessive–compulsive disorder in adults with Down's syndrome. *Journal of Autism and Developmental Disabilities*, **25**, 453–458.

—— & Hall, W. (1996) Short-term prognosis of depression in adults with Down's syndrome. Association with thyroid status and effects on adaptive behaviour. *Journal of Intellectual Disability Research*, **40**, 32–38.

—— & Krishnan, V. H. R. (1993) Age of onset and duration of dementia in people with Down's syndrome. A study of 98 reported cases. *International Journal of Geriatric Psychiatry*, **8**, 915–922.

——, Krishan, V. H. R., Clarke, D. J., *et al* (1994) The assessment of dementia in people with Down's syndrome. Changes in adaptive behaviour. *Journal of Developmental Disabilities*, **90**, 120–130.

——, Farrer M. J., Kessling, A. M., *et al* (1998a) Molecular mapping of Alzheimer-type dementia in Down's syndrome. *Annals of Neurology*, **43**, 380–383.

——, Chung, M. C. & Haque, M. S. (1998b) Longitudinal changes in adaptive behaviour and Down's syndrome. Interim findings from a longitudinal study. *American Journal on Mental Retardation*, **103**, 40–46.

——, Huxley, A., Haque, M. S., *et al* (2002) A 24-week, double-blind, placebo-controlled trial of donepezil in patients with Down's syndrome and Alzheimer's disease – Pilot study. *International Journal of Geriatric Psychiatry*, **17**, 270–278.

Pueschel, S. M. (1988) The biology of the maturing person with Down's syndrome. In *The Young Person with Down's syndrome: Transition from Adolescence to Adulthood* (ed. S. M. Pueschel), pp. 23–34. Baltimore, MD: Paul H. Brookes.

—— & Scola, F. H. (1987) Atlantoaxial instability in individuals with Down's syndrome: epidemiologic, radiographic and clinical studies. *Pediatrics*, **80**, 555–560.

——, Scola, F. H. & Pezzullo, J. C. (1992) A longitudinal study of atlanto-dens relationships in asymptomatic individuals with Down's syndrome. *Pediatrics*, **89**, 1194–1198.

Richards, B. W. & Enver, F. (1979) Blood pressure in Down's syndrome. *Journal of Mental Deficiency Research*, **23**, 123–135.

Rubin, S. S., Rimmer, J. H., Chicoine, B., *et al* (1998) Overweight prevalence in persons with Down's syndrome. *Mental Retardation*, **36**, 175–181.

Saxon, S. A. & Witriol, E. (1976) Down's syndrome and intellectual development. *Journal of Pediatric Psychology*, **1**, 45–57.

Schapiro, M. B., Haxby, J. V. & Grady, C. L. (1992) Nature of mental retardation and dementia in Down's syndrome. Study with PET, CT, and neuropsychology. *Neurobiology of Aging*, **13**, 723–734.

Sovner, R., Hurley, A. D. & LaBrie, R. (1985) Is mania incompatible with Down's syndrome. *British Journal of Psychiatry*, **146**, 319–320.

Steffelaar, J. W. & Evenhuis, H. M (1989) Life expectancy, Down's syndrome, and dementia. *Lancet*, **1**, 492–493.

Stratford, B. & Steele, J. (1985) Incidence and prevalence of Down's syndrome: a discussion and report. *Journal of Mental Deficiency Research*, **29**, 95–107.

Taggard, D. A., Menezes, A. H. & Ryken, T. C. (2000) Treatment of Down's syndrome-associated craniovertebral junction abnormalities. *Journal of Neurosurgery*, **93** (suppl. 2), 205–213.

Turner, T. H. (1989) Schizophrenia and mental handicap: an historical review, with implications for future research. *Psychological Medicine*, **19**, 301–314.

**285**

van Broeckhoven, C. (1995) Presenilins in Alzheimer's disease. *Nature Genetics*, **11**, 230–232.

Visser, F. E., Kuilman, M., Oosting, J., *et al* (1996) Use of electroencephalography to detect Alzheimer's disease in Down's syndrome. *Acta Neurologica Scandinavica*, **94**, 97–103

Vladutin, A. O., Chung, T. C., Victor, A., *et al* (1984) Down's syndrome and hypothyroidism. A role for thyroid autoimmunity? *Lancet, i*, 1416.

Wisniewski, K. E., Torrado, C. & Castello, S. (1989) Treatment in growth hormone deficient Down's syndrome children with recombinant human growth hormone. *Down's Syndrome Papers and Abstracts for Professionals*, **12**, 1–2.

World Health Organization (1992) *The ICD–10 Classification of Mental and Behavioural Disorders. Clinical Descriptions and Diagnostic Guidelines*. Geneva: WHO.

—— (1993) *The ICD–10 Classification of Mental and Behavioural Disorders. Diagnostic Criteria for Research*. Geneva: WHO.

Wright, E. C. (1982) The presentation of mental illness in mentally retarded adults. *British Journal of Psychiatry*, **141**, 496–502.

Wright, P. F., Thompson, J. & Bess, F. H. (1991) Hearing, speech and language sequelae of otitis media with effusion. *Pediatric Annals*, **20**, 617–621.

Yeates, S. (1995) The incidence and importance of hearing loss in people with severe learning disability. The evolution of a service. *British Journal of Learning Disabilities*, **23**, 79–84.

Zigman, W. B., Schupf, N., Lubin, R. A., *et al* (1987) Premature regression of adults with Down's syndrome. *American Journal of Mental Deficiency*, **92**, 161–168.

# CHAPTER 16

# Forensic psychiatry and learning disability

## Susan Johnston

People with intellectual impairment are considered potentially vulnerable and are therefore subject to protection in law in a wide variety of fields in our society. The direction of strategy for service development and support systems is towards social inclusion as a right. Within this social context, the situation of the offender with a learning disability poses philosophical, ethical and pragmatic dilemmas for agencies and services. People should receive care in the most local, accessible and unrestrictive setting that is feasibly commensurate with their identified risk. Personal autonomy and self-determination must be balanced against the risks posed to individuals and society by their behaviour.

Children commit many potentially dangerous acts without the intent to harm, but recklessly and naïvely, as part of the developmental process and the learning of appropriate impulse control and social rules. Aberrant behaviours in children are seen within an experiential and developmental context and attributed accordingly. Only when such behaviours persist beyond the normally associated age framework do they attract additional attention and intervention above the normal parenting or learning mechanisms. For adults with learning disabilities, it may be difficult to distinguish behaviours that are developmentally congruent from those acts perpetrated with malicious or reckless intent. In the context of pre-existing behavioural disorder, particular difficulties may arise in determining the boundary between severe challenging behaviour and criminal behaviour.

The appropriate developmental, constitutional and dynamic factors related to the assessment of an individual who has perpetrated a chargeable offence must be assessed sensitively, with knowledge and critique of the relationship of these factors to the offence. Consideration of the vulnerability of the individual in progressing through the criminal justice system should support appropriate social learning, while not jeopardising the legal process or disadvantaging the individual from the protections afforded by investigation of alleged offences.

The criminal justice system will determine whether an offence has been committed and whether it is in the public interest for prosecution to be pursued. The investigation of an alleged crime may also act to clarify the circumstances of allegations and refute false allegations against gullible suspects.

Anecdotally, particular offence profiles have been associated with people with learning disabilities, as indeed people with learning disabilities have been thought to be overrepresented in offender populations. The indiscriminate application of the inevitable deterioration paradigm presented a bleak prospect for the management of such individuals. Although extensive research remains lacking, there is a growing body of knowledge examining the pathways into the criminal justice system, discriminating offence and offender characteristics and successful means of intervention (Johnston & Halstead, 2000). Increasingly, attention is also given to the needs of people coming into contact with the criminal justice system as witnesses, to advance their social rights to justice.

This chapter briefly introduces and highlights some key themes in the consideration of the assessment and management of the offender with a learning disability. It considers the role that psychiatrists might play within the criminal justice system in relation to offenders and witnesses. Finally, it addresses some of the dilemmas in the provision of services for such individuals.

## Historical, social and legal perspectives

As early as the 17th century, it is recorded that special provision was made for the royal pardoning of offences committed by those with intellectual disabilities. During the past century, the legislative framework for the detention of people with intellectual disability began to be shaped towards the one we have today in the present mental health legislation, last enacted in 1983 (1984 in Scotland and Northern Ireland).

In the early 1900s, a Royal Commission Review of the services available for those with an intellectual disability resulted in the Mental Deficiency Act 1913. This made provision for those identified to be removed from situations of extreme vulnerability, abuse and exploitation or inappropriate incarceration in prisons, poor houses and local asylums and placed in institutions designed for their 'care, control or training'. With hindsight, it is seen that this social agenda became corrupted by the new science of genetics and the popularist rise of the eugenics movement. The criteria for detention were undoubtedly broader than modern concepts: they were not restricted to those with demonstrable intellectual disability *per se*, but paradoxically recognised the complex social deficits associated in many individuals. Tredgold (1915) observed:

'It is often assumed that by the 'normally' developed mind is meant that which has attained a certain standard of school knowledge, and that inability to reach this standard is the criterion of mental deficiency. This is not so. It is true that many defectives, as defined by Act of Parliament, are also lacking in scholastic attainment, but this is not invariable; and on the other hand, there are many individuals of very poor scholastic ability who are by no means legal defectives. The definitions given in the Mental Deficiency Act of 1913 make it quite clear that the standard of normality is that of the capacity for independent adaptation to ordinary social requirements, and that mental defect is a state in which the individual is without this capacity save without some degree of care, supervision, and control. In other words, the criterion is not primarily of educational but social disability.'

At this time, if charged with an offence, the only diversion from a required custodial sentence was by use of the Lunacy or Mental Deficiency Acts, the latter being applicable if conduct disorder was demonstrable as arising within the developmental period of less than 18 years of age.

The over-inclusive criteria of the Mental Deficiency Act 1913 were reviewed in a further Royal Commission Review, led by Lord Percy (Department of Health, 1957):

'This has led to the supposition that mental defectives must be a more homogenous category than they really are.

'We have no doubt, however that those who interpret the present Mental Deficiency Acts as including, among the feeble-minded and moral defectives, patients whose intelligence is within the normal range but whose moral development is incomplete or abnormal in other respects, are correctly interpreting the intention behind the present Acts. It may well be that the law and terminology should be changed, but if we say that the term "mental defective" should in future be restricted to persons of low intelligence we still have to decide how to deal with the far more difficult problems which arise in regard to the feeble minded and moral defectives of higher intelligence who are also covered by the present Mental Deficiency Acts.

'Although most of those who are at present described as feeble-minded are subnormal or at least below average in intelligence, what distinguishes them and moral defectives and psychopaths most clearly from normal people is their general social behaviour.'

The resultant Mental Health Act 1959 (1960 for Scotland and Northern Ireland) introduced the recognition of the concept of psychopathy (not Scotland), which included individuals with intellectual deficiency. The new act clearly differentiated those individuals from the more vulnerable who were displaying acts as a consequence of their arrested or incomplete development of mind, considered as mental subnormality or severe subnormality, dependent on the severity of 'subnormality'.

Mental health reform in 1983 (1984 in Scotland and Northern Ireland) produced another change in terminology, with 'mental impairment' and 'severe mental impairment' replacing 'subnormality'. The Mental Health Act 1983 (1984 for Scotland and Northern Ireland) introduced the requirement for seriously aggressive or irresponsible behaviour in addition to the intellectual and social dysfunction associated with arrested or incomplete development of mind. This aimed to restrict the potential for the long-term detention of individuals who lacked adequate skills to live independently, but whose behaviour was otherwise unproblematic.

The revisions of Mental Health legislation in 1959 and 1983 considered the requirements for persons in contact with the criminal justice system, identifying specific detention sections to mirror civil detention requirements for assessment or treatment with an acknowledgement of the stage reached in the criminal process from remand to post-conviction.

Further mental health legislation is pending, following the Richardson Review of the Mental Health Act 1999, which will again consider the needs of those involved with the criminal justice system.

## Challenging behaviour or offence?

Service provision and legislation alike may fail to distinguish between offenders with learning disability and those with similar needs. As a practitioner, one can recognise the individual who has no knowledge of the unlawful nature of the act, whose action had no malicious intent, but resulted in damage, distress or injury, who is nevertheless arrested and charged for an offence. Without contact with the criminal justice system, this would be regarded under the rubric of challenging behaviour. In contrast, there are individuals whose repeated antisocial acts, despite all interventions and precautions, are never prosecuted (Kiernan & Dixon, 1991). As is evident from the legislative reviews, the population of those with learning disabilities who have been convicted of offences is a widely heterogeneous group.

The size of the problem remains uncertain. Definitional discrepancies, the reluctance of those with mild learning disabilities to see themselves so described, and changes to services for education and support have made the population hard to identify at a macro-level. There are the vulnerable individuals, the gullible, the easily led, those in the wrong place at the wrong time, those who have let events overtake them. In contrast, there are individuals who place themselves in risky situations, create and take risks, are repeated offenders with poor scholastic ability, communication and adaptive living skills, factors that might constitute an 'intellectually impaired criminal' profile.

Population studies have indicated that the prevalence of offending in the population with learning disabilities is low, perhaps around 1%, but that the group with borderline ability are slightly overrepresented in offender populations. Although the incidence of property offences is low, there is a broad offence profile, and Lund (1990) has suggested an increase in crimes of violence and arson. Although the rate of female offending is less than that for men, Hodgins (1992) found that, in population cohort studies, women with learning disabilities were more likely than either their counterparts without learning disabilities or men to develop violent tendencies. Lund (1990) also suggested, supported by the work of Gudjonsson *et al* (1993) and Lyall *et al* (1995*a*), that those with learning disabilities are overrepresented in police custody, being more easily detected and arrested.

Clinical studies of imprisoned offender populations similarly appear to give conflicting results. In the USA, MacEachron (1979) reviewed studies of prisoners, finding prevalence rates of learning disability of between 2.6% and 39.6%. Variation in assessment modalities, definitions and the differential application of legal processes were cited for the differences. In the prison population of New South Wales, in Australia, Hayes (1991) assessed 12–13% as having learning disabilities. In the UK, surveys of convicted prisoners do not show overrepresentation of those with learning disabilities (Craft & Craft, 1984; Murphy *et al*, 1995). A survey of the prison population of England and Wales (Singleton *et al*, 1998) shows interesting trends. However, some mechanism appears to be reducing the conviction rate of men more than women when relative populations of remand and sentenced prisoners are compared (Fig. 16.1). The data indicates that over 10% of both males and females on remand have a Quick Test score of less than

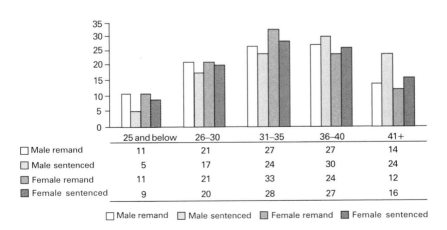

| | 25 and below | 26–30 | 31–35 | 36–40 | 41+ |
|---|---|---|---|---|---|
| ☐ Male remand | 11 | 21 | 27 | 27 | 14 |
| ☐ Male sentenced | 5 | 17 | 24 | 30 | 24 |
| ▨ Female remand | 11 | 21 | 33 | 24 | 12 |
| ▧ Female sentenced | 9 | 20 | 28 | 27 | 16 |

☐ Male remand  ☐ Male sentenced  ▨ Female remand  ▧ Female sentenced

**Fig. 16.1** Computerised Quick Test scores of prisoners (from Singleton *et al*, 1998, with permission).

**291**

25. Despite the limitations of the Quick Test, this prevalence of prisoners with learning disability is greatly in excess of the earlier studies of Brooke *et al* (1996), although similar to that of Faulk (1976).

The widely held view that the presence of a learning disability in itself predisposes to criminal behaviour cannot be substantiated on the available published evidence. Hayes (1991) writes that 'there seems no clear evidence for either over-representation or under-representation of intellectual disability clients in the sex offender population'. However, if factors associated with resisting temptation, difficulties in negotiating the criminal justice system, modifying behaviour in light of experience and receiving appropriate service support are seen with increased frequency in individuals with learning disabilities, the diagnosis may act as a proxy risk factor for these underlying deficits.

## The criminal justice process

The criminal justice process has many steps, summarised in Fig. 16.2. At all of these steps, there is provision for diversion from the system for those with learning disabilities, as discretionary powers and defined in statute. The decisions may be appropriate, justified and valid, but may be subject to positive and negative confounding variables of judgement (Conley *et al*, 1992; Lyall *et al*, 1995*b*; Mikkelsen & Stelk, 1999) as well as to the vagaries of local resources and service allocation. Statute identifies particular dispensations to ensure that the defendant with a disability has a fair trial and that justice may be done (Police and Criminal Evidence Act (PACE) 1984; Criminal Procedure (Insanity and Unfitness to Plead) Act 1991; Youth Justice and Criminal Evidence Act 1999). The clinician working with an offender or witness with a learning disability should be familiar with this process and contribute by interacting with the system and fellow professionals in the most appropriate way.

It is the responsibility of the police to investigate, arrest and compile the evidence for the Crown Prosecution Service, and to consider whether

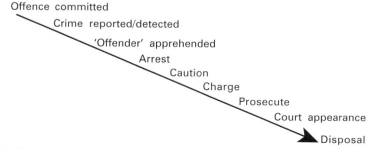

**Fig. 16.2** The criminal process.

a prosecution is progressed. At the time of arrest and before questioning, the police are required to inform the suspect of his or her rights, given in the 'caution' and 'notice to detained persons'. The Police and Criminal Evidence Act (PACE) 1984 requires the identification of those with disabilities so that they may have the services of an 'appropriate adult'. The recognition of those with learning disabilities in the custody suite of a busy police station is difficult, however. Police officers have limited training to help them recognise the features of the variety of forms of mental disorder (Lyall *et al*, 1995*b*). The suspect may wish to mask a disability, but careful observation of behaviour, literacy skills, history of special educational needs and residential or day care provision should assist the identification process.

The vulnerabilities experienced by perpetrators on the commission of an act may well affect them throughout their progress through the criminal justice system and contribute to the increased likelihood of their being processed rather than diverted from the system. They may actively seek to evade detection for fear of losing face, thereby alienating themselves from assistance and support. Individuals who have poorly developed socialisation skills may also react in the pressure of custody and interview by expressing aberrant behaviour as a consequence of their lack of adequate coping mechanisms and internal controls of anger. The inability to foresee the intermediate consequences of their actions, in combination with maladaptive social learning, predisposes such individuals to display impulsive acts, dissociate or act unreasonably. Limited communication skills or specific language deficits, if masked, will mislead interviewers and may impair the veracity of testimony. The desire to please (acquiescence) and ability to be led (suggestibility) in an interview may discredit otherwise factually accurate statements. The failure to appreciate the significance and possible consequences of an admission of guilt may contribute to false confessions in an attempt to end a stressful situation (Gudjonsson *et al*, 1993; Clare & Gudjonsson, 1995; Pearse *et al*, 1998; Everington & Fulero, 1999). The following legislation makes specific provision for the interviewing, processing and disposing of both suspects and witnesses in contact with the criminal justice system.

## Police and Criminal Evidence Act 1984 (PACE)

Having identified a mentally disordered offender, the police are obliged to offer an 'appropriate adult'. Within the PACE provision, the role of the 'appropriate adult' is to advise the suspect and provide active observation of the interview. They may facilitate communication by advising the interviewing officers or legal representation of the most appropriate means of interviewing the suspect, but must not answer on the suspect's behalf. Although the 'appropriate adult' can be a relative or guardian, it is most commonly requested that he or she be a professional person who has had some training in the role and has a knowledge of the suspect or the suspect's disability. It cannot be a police officer, cadet or special officer. The requirement for the presence of an appropriate adult may be overridden only by a senior officer, at least a superintendent – if delay in progressing with the interview is considered to contribute to immediate harm or serious loss or damage. The interview must cease when the immediate risk has been averted.

## Mental Health Act 1983

As stated above, the provision of mental deficiency and mental health legislation has been the means to ensure that appropriate therapeutic settings were made available for those whose capacity to make judgements was impaired. Early legislation required that a person either signed into hospital as a voluntary patient or, if lacking capacity, was 'signed in' as a formally detained patient. The orders were subject to periodic review, but additional appeal mechanisms against detention by application to a Mental Health Review Tribunal were instituted with the Mental Health Act 1983.

Part II of the Act describes the situations under which patients may be compulsorily detained in a hospital or registered mental nursing home for assessment, treatment or, in the case of guardianship, for residence and treatment. Part III of the Act describes the equivalent provisions for those who are involved with the criminal justice system. For the purposes of assessment, Section 35 relates to the remand to hospital for the preparation of a report of the mental condition of the accused, on the evidence that the accused is suspected of having a mental illness, severe mental impairment, mental impairment or psychopathic disorder. It is valid for 28 days and is renewable on two further occasions up to a maximum of 12 weeks. The order must be supported by the written or oral evidence of one registered medical practitioner and enacted within 7 days. Section 36 refers to the remand of an accused person to hospital for treatment of mental illness or severe mental impairment only. It is similarly valid for 28 days and subject to renewal for up to 12 weeks. Section 38 confers powers on the Crown Court to make an interim hospital order, during which the treatability of a presumed condition can be assessed prior to a possible final hospital treatment order disposal. It is granted for 12 weeks and is renewable to a maximum of 12 months. Section 37 confers power on the Crown Court to dispose of a convicted person to hospital for treatment of mental illness, severe mental impairment, mental impairment or psychopathic disorder. For all categories, the disorder must be of a nature or degree that makes it appropriate for hospital admission. If it is thought that the subject has mental impairment and/or psychopathic disorder, an additional requirement is that such treatment is likely to alleviate or prevent a deterioration of the condition. In circumstances where it appears to the Court that it is necessary to protect the public from serious harm, Section 41 may be applied to restrict discharge from hospital. For prisoners in custody, Section 48 allows for remanded prisoners to be transferred to hospital for urgent treatment of mental illness or severe mental impairment. Section 47 allows for the transfer of sentenced prisoners to hospital for treatment of mental illness, severe mental impairment, mental impairment or psychopathic disorder subject to the treatment requirements of Section 37. Additional restrictions (Section 49) may also be applied. With the exception of Section 35, all recommendations must have the written evidence of at least two registered medical practitioners, one of whom may be required to give oral evidence in Court.

Clinical practice and opinion varies as to the appropriateness of a primacy or inclusive model for the use of mental health detention criteria where people with learning disabilities are concerned. Common to the categories of severe mental impairment, mental impairment and psychopathic disorder are abnormally aggressive or seriously irresponsible conduct. The impairment categories require the presence of arrested or incomplete development of mind, which includes (severe) impairment of intelligence and social functioning, whereas psychopathic disorder (whether or not including significant impairment of intelligence) is a persistent disorder of mind. The presence of mental illness superimposed would always warrant detention under that category, irrespective of the degree of impairment, to mitigate against unnecessarily prolonged detention on recovery from the mental illness. For individuals with intellectual impairment whose personality disorders predominate, the duality of classification, although seemingly unnecessary on legal grounds, may highlight the complex synergistic relationship of the conditions, which confers both vulnerability within penal settings and disruption within ordinary care settings.

## Criminal Procedure (Insanity) Act 1964 and Criminal Procedure (Insanity & Unfitness to Plead) Act 1991

The provisions of the Criminal Procedures (Insanity) Act 1964 were intended to provide the means by which those with such disability at the time of trial as to jeopardise their defence could be detained in hospital until they regained 'fitness'. In practice, this led to the indeterminate detention of individuals with learning disabilities under conditions of high security, without the benefit of trial, and unable to regain 'fitness'. Consequently, the criteria for 'fitness' were applied liberally to avoid such courses of action and were considered on a balance of probability rather than categorical framework.

The Act was revised and enacted in 1992, with more flexible considerations of the disposal options after a finding of 'unfitness'. In practice the Crown, defence or court can raise the question of 'fitness to plead'. Although a jury makes the finding of fitness, only two appropriately qualified medical practitioners, at least one of whom must 'have special experience in the field of mental disorder', can assess and report to the court. Traditionally considered on balance, 'fitness' is in fact categorical (each factor considered on balance).

A defendant must be capable of understanding proceedings so that he (or she) can:

- put forward any proper defence he might have; **and**
- challenge a juror to whom he might have cause to object; **and**
- give instructions to his lawyers (this means he must be capable of telling his lawyers what his case is and whether he agrees or disagrees with what the witnesses have to say); **and**
- follow the evidence

Fitness to plead should be assessed as near to each appearance in court as is practical, given the variable quality of 'fitness' in some people. Fitness to plead may be adversely affected by mental illness and states of excessive arousal. The evidence supporting fitness to plead is gained from direct patient interview, depositions and full interview transcripts. On the finding of unfitness, the deciding jury is dismissed and a new jury sworn to hear a 'trial of the facts'. Should the defendant be found to have perpetrated the act with which he or she is charged, a full range of disposals is available for the Court to consider. Dependent on the facts of the case, the defendant may receive absolute discharge, supervision orders akin to probation orders or hospital treatment orders at the most appropriate level of security, with or without restriction.

## Youth Justice & Criminal Evidence Act: Part 2 Criminal Evidence 1999

This new legislation is designed to afford additional protection to youths and vulnerable adult witnesses, to maximise the usefulness of their testimony and, if victims, to advance their potential for justice. Founded on the practices developed for child witnesses, it applies to youths under 17 years of age and to those with mental or physical disorders or disabilities that the court considers likely to affect the quality of their evidence, rendering them 'unable to give their best ... because of their fear and distress ... of testifying'.

For each case, the court must consider the circumstances, the relationships between witness and defendant and the defendant's conduct towards the witness. Additional specific measures decided on the individual merit of each witness may include:

- screens in court
- no wigs or gowns
- live TV-link evidence
- clearing the court of press and public
- video interview as evidence-in-chief
- pre-recorded videotaped cross-examination
- communication through an intermediary
- use of communication aids
- restriction of direct examination of the witness by the defendant.

Professionals are increasingly asked to assess and support witnesses with learning disabilities, and the Youth Justice Act and a review by Kebbell & Hatton (1999) provide useful guidelines for this.

## Reporting to the criminal justice system

The most commonly considered means of engaging with the criminal justice system as a psychiatrist is by the preparation of a 'court report'. However, given the nature of the criminal justice process and the available avenues for diversion, it is important that engagement is both timely and structured. It may be appropriate, as the medical practitioner responsible for the specialist aspect of care of designated out-patients and in-patients, to submit a witness statement at the stage of the police case preparation for consideration by the Crown Prosecution Service. Depending on the features of the case, the statement may support progress through the justice system or suggest early diversion and appropriate service interventions to inform further decision-making. The decision to proceed remains that of the Crown Prosecution Service.

The prosecution or defence may request reports for court in criminal cases. In either case, the brief for the report should clearly state the stage of the case and required considerations. A typical full report should consider the following:

- personal and medical or psychiatric background
- circumstances of the index offence (including client's account)
- mental state evaluation
- summary and opinion of:
  - diagnosis and formulation
  - fitness to plead
  - mental disorder
  - treatability
  - risk of reoffending
  - risk assessment/dangerousness
- recommendations for disposal.

---

**Box 16.1**   Custodial or non-custodial disposals, depending on fitness/unfitness to plead

*Fit to plead*
Fine
Community service
Probation with or without conditions of residence and/or treatment
Custodial sentence
Hospital order with or without a restriction order

*Unfit to plead*
Hospital disposal with or without restriction (specified by Secretary of State)
Guardianship order
Supervision and treatment order
- defendant must be able to cooperate with social worker or probation officer
- defendant must be able to cooperate with medical treatment
- order should be for a period of not more than 2 years
Absolute discharge

---

The report should be based on a full appraisal of the available information, which would normally require access to depositions, including interview tapes and witness statements, previous reports, probation pre-sentence reports and at least one client interview. It must be written in clear, unambiguous language and adequately explain any technical or psychiatric terminology. If there is no medical recommendation appropriate for the particular case, this must be clearly stated. Recommendations for disposal 'respectfully' given for the court's consideration must be realistic, commensurate with the likely sentencing options in the event of conviction and supported by the agencies empowered to deliver them.

The court can decide custodial or non-custodial disposals, determined on the case characteristics shown in Box 16.1.

# Offence assessment and management

Beyond an assessment of the severity of the offence and the likelihood of recurrence as determined by risk assessment, the full assessment of an offender with a learning disability considers the psychiatric, psychological and social factors that have contributed to the offence, the characteristics of the offence and the likely intervention that is required.

The practice of offender assessment broadly follows that of a psychiatric assessment, with consideration of personal, developmental and family background, social and educational attainment, and inter-personal relationships, noting deficiencies and needs. Consideration of

**Table 16.1** Effects on sexual matters of misconceptions about people with developmental delay (from Fedoroff & Fedoroff, 2001, with permission)

| Misconception | Effect |
|---|---|
| They do not like or need sex | Sexual issues are ignored |
| They cannot control their sex drives | Sexuality is suppressed; sexual information is withheld |
| They cannot take responsibility for their sexual activities | Sex is forbidden, maladaptive or criminal sex is tolerated |
| Their parents or guardians need to be kept informed of all sexual issues | Sex is not discussed or condoned |
| They are emotionally handicapped | Relationships are suspect |
| They make things up | Sexual concerns are ignored |

the account of the offence should include both corroborated and perpetrator accounts of the index offence, with consideration of any associated positive or negative setting factors, and the offender's attitude to any victim(s) and to the offence itself. Mental state examination should not only reflect current functioning, but also refer to the mental state at the time of the offence, providing, if possible, adequate evidential support.

Studies of hospitalised offenders with learning disabilities (Day, 1988; Kearns & O'Connor, 1988) have described clinical features of selected in-patient offender populations, citing high rates of comorbidity with mental illness, personality disorders, and social and educational

**Table 16.2** Potential effects of comorbid conditions on sexual behaviours (from Fedoroff & Fedoroff, 2001, with permission)

| Condition | Features | Effect |
|---|---|---|
| Autism | Social isolation | Asocial behaviour |
| Asperger syndrome | Misperceived social cues | Misdiagnosed paraphilic disorders |
| Attention-deficit disorders | Impulsivity | Judgement errors |
| Mood disorders | Altered drive | Desire disorders |
| Dementia | Impaired cognition (adult onset) | Communication and judgement errors |
| Psychotic disorders | Delusions | Sexual dysfunction secondary to medication |
| Anxiety disorders | Fear; ritualistic behaviour | Courtship errors |
| Epilepsy(s) | Seizures | Stigmatisation; desire disorders; ?paraphilia |
| Endocrine disorders | Hormone abnormalities | Fertility problems; sexual dysfunction |
| Sleep disorders | Altered level of consciousness | Sleep sex syndromes; irritability |
| Substance misuse | Addictive behaviour | Sexual dysfunction |

**Table 16.3** Potential institutional effects on sexual behaviours (after Fedoroff & Fedoroff, 2001)

| Feature | Effect |
|---|---|
| Group housing | Lack of privacy |
| Segregation by gender | Increased same-gender experience |
| Dependence on caregivers | Increased risk of sexual abuse |
| Regulations | Lack of individualisation; sexual rebellion |
| Pervasive institutional responsibility | Decreased freedom |
| Isolation | Decreased socialisation |
| Institutional ethos | Decreased control, responsibility |

deficiencies. Studies of sex offenders with learning disabilities allowed Fedoroff & Fedoroff (2001) to describe putative links between aspects of specific features seen in people with learning disabilities, the attitudes of their carers and settings in which they are cared for that may contribute to their potential for offending. Although described for sexual offending potential, the principles could be pertinent to other offence profiles (Tables 16.1–16.3). Denial of emotional expression of basic human feelings, lack of appropriate educational intervention, organic deficits and restricted living experiences all contribute to imbalanced emotional expression and dysfunctional situational understanding. Other factors, including poor socialisation, impaired impulse control, undue personal sensitivity, poor concentration and hyperactivity, may all be more frequent in persons with learning disabilities and may contribute to greater rates of recidivism. Circumscribed preoccupations, as seen in autistic-spectrum disorders, may be significant in some fire-setting behaviours. Under these circumstances, aberrant and offending behaviour may develop.

To date, there is little evidence suggesting differential offence characteristics between those with and without learning disabilities. Murrey *et al* (1992) compared the features of sex offenders who had mental impairment, psychopathic disorder or mental illness, finding few criminological discriminating factors, although Blanchard *et al* (1999) found that offenders with learning disabilities were more likely to offend against younger children and male children. (Lindsay *et al* (1999) give an extensive review of the available literature on the assessment and management of sexual offenders with learning disabilities.) The research in relation to anger, aggression and violence in learning disability is complex, with considerable overlap between concepts and interventions for forensic and for challenging behaviour (Edmondson & Conger, 1996).

This broad conceptual framework for understanding the factors underpinning offending in those with learning disabilities reinforces the need for multidimensional management of these individuals.

# Risk assessment

The vast majority of offenders with learning disabilities are dealt with by local courts and, if convicted, receive non-custodial sentences. The prevalence of mental disorder is high in the offender population with learning disabilities. Multiple and complex problems are common, and alcohol and substance misuse are increasingly significant factors. Services must balance the undoubted needs for therapeutic intervention and offence-focused work with a reappraisal of adaptive and communicative skills, and provide rehabilitative education and life-skills training.

There is always a delicate balance to be reached between appropriate guidance in decision-making for those with very limited ability and the necessary restrictions placed on those with the capacity to decide and who choose to act aberrantly. This dilemma is particularly acute when working with offenders with learning disabilities and a dissocial or borderline personality disorder. Without structure, they may default and transgress – they often resist the structures around them and test out new staff or situations, but coping without the boundaries placed around them by relationships with staff, procedures or physical precautions is too stressful. It requires a skilled team to phase their level of intervention without it becoming oppressive and to devise a plan for the gradual transfer of responsibility back to individuals of those aspects of their lives that they can manage. The therapeutic pathway for the reduction of violent behaviour may be conceived as the progress from the requirement for static physical control, to dynamic physical and situational control with or without pharmacological control, reliant on procedural control until the person can, through therapy, exercise internalised personal control. All of these interventions require skilled teams of staff from many professions working together to a multidimensional model.

Clinicians refer to services and organisations develop units. How do we blend the tensions of scarce resources and expertise with economies of scale and retain the practices of individual services delivered as locally as possible, for what is a minority population? The majority of offenders with learning disabilities are supported by community teams in their home area, but alternatives are required for those for whom this is either not desirable or not possible.

Most local services have access to a small number of open and minimally secure beds, for those whose disorder is of a nature and degree that requires assessment or treatment in hospital. The experience of service users requires us to acknowledge their difficulties and to provide them with the appropriate degree of service to aid their preferred, if acceptable, lifestyle in the least restrictive setting possible. It does not mean that they must fend for themselves if they lack skills or are left to reoffend if we can provide a management plan to educate and support them. Unlike general forensic services, which have a more comprehensive range of low- and medium-secure beds, below the level of high-security hospitals (three for England and Wales and one for Scotland and Northern Ireland), learning disability services have developed in a more piecemeal fashion. In the independent sector there is a flourishing provision of beds offering a medium-secure setting of varying intensity and duration, but the NHS has only a small number of medium secure beds, unevenly distributed across health regions. All 80 of the high-security NHS beds for people with learning disabilities are now shared between just two sites: Rampton Hospital for England and Wales and the State Hospital Carstairs for Scotland and Northern Ireland. It is also important that commissioners and providers of services appreciate the duration and intensity of work required to provide sufficient support to reduce the likelihood that apparently able individuals will reoffend. Victims of assault or property crimes are also entitled to the recognition of the wrong done against them and protection from further victimisation.

How do we reconcile the principles of normalisation with diversion schemes? Are the latter not a form of positive discrimination? Of course, if either option is applied without individual discretion, there will be problems. Glaser & Deane (1999) reported on the effects of subjecting offenders with learning disabilities in Australia to the normal rules of society and on the resultant requirement for special support services.

There are occasions when individuals with capacity must be allowed to appreciate the impact of their behaviour and the social sanctions applied to other members of society: they should be given the opportunity to understand that actions have consequences. How do we balance the tension between the care and support we are trained to give with the boundary-setting and need to apply potentially oppressive restrictions for some individuals? Our clients and patients may be offenders, but a significant majority have been subjected to abuse, at times extreme, and are therefore themselves victims – perhaps with features of post-traumatic stress disorder – rejected by society, family and themselves.

Finally, there are individuals who, despite having adequate intellectual ability and development to live independently, cannot do so, because of their emotional vulnerability, personality disorder or impulsivity: how do we provide an acceptable quality of life for what might be the rest of their days?

# Principles of security

The most prevalent view of safety and security is public safety and the physical security restricting an individual. However, an initial therapeutic objective is the provision of clients' or patients' personal safety, which is a prerequisite for their personal security. For too many, security is an issue reflected by the height of the wall, number of locks, surveillance and alarm systems. Real security is a human quality, nurtured through trusting interpersonal relationships. Many service users have had damaged, distorted or dysfunctional relationships from childhood. They protect themselves by rejecting and testing their caregivers and find services wanting; as a result of this behaviour, they are moved up the physical security ladder.

Beyond relational security, some individuals, especially those with learning disabilities, require a greater degree of stability in their lives than they can create and maintain independently. For them, clear and simple social guidelines and a predictable routine or pattern of responses from a caring support team are essential for stable functioning. This care planning and the associated guidelines for staff constitute the core of procedural security.

Only a small minority of offenders with learning disabilities require the additional external precautions of physical limitations. These may range from simple confusion locks, safe gardens, location of residence, and perimeter fences, to the range of additional restrictions found in high security. Whatever the style of residential provision, from provisions in the community through open, low-, medium- and high-secure units, the basic principle of security must be relational. Without the fundamentals of relational and procedural security, there is undue reliance on restrictive levels of physical security, and the potential for restrictive and oppressive procedures to develop. Box 16.2 shows the components of security that can be applied to any residential setting with a progression towards heightened structural restriction.

The aim of staff in any physically restrictive environment should be to equip individuals with sufficient skills to allow their safe transfer to a less restrictive environment in which to continue therapeutic intervention designed to address their core deficits, thus reducing the likelihood of recidivism.

---

**Box 16.2**   Dimensions of security

*Core components of security*
Relational
Procedural
Structural

*Residential setting*
Community
Open
Low secure
Medium secure
High secure

# Conclusions

From the earliest part of the 20th century, people with learning disabilities have been identified as 'potential criminals'. However, it is clearly inaccurate to consider the behaviour of a very small percentage of such a heterogeneous population in such a way. It is appropriate to examine why particular characteristics may be more prevalent in offenders with learning disability. Individuals may have poor social skills, with impulse control difficulties. They may have been subjected to physical and sexual abuse, experienced dysfunctional or disjointed social learning and developed maladaptive (although organised) coping strategies. Reduced capacity to resist temptation, inappropriate challenging of others or not considering the consequences of their actions not only places them at greater risk of committing offences, but might also make them less likely to avoid involvement with the criminal justice system and more vulnerable within it. A working knowledge of the civil and criminal legislative frameworks that make special provision for adults with learning disabilities who come into contact with the criminal justice system is necessary for all professions working with this population.

Examination of the predisposing, precipitating and perpetuating factors for criminal behaviours and of the operation of the criminal justice system for adults with learning disabilities will inform the development of more refined and targeted intervention strategies. At the very least, a systematic examination of the pertinent constitutional, developmental, environmental, static and dynamic factors contributing to any alleged offence by a person with a learning disability should inform multidimensional, multi-agency care planning, with sensitive use of the criminal justice system. The basic tenet of a locally available, accessible service provided at the least level of restriction commensurate with the assessed risk remains the starting point for support and service intervention.

# References

Blanchard, R., Watson, M., Choy, A., et al (1999) Paedophiles: mental retardation, marital age and sexual orientation. Archives of Sexual Behaviour, 28, 111–127.

Brooke, D., Taylor, C., Gunn, J., et al (1996) Point prevalence of mental disorder in unconvicted male prisoners in England and Wales. British Medical Journal, 313, 1524–1527.

Clare, I. & Gudjonsson, G. (1995) The vulnerability of suspects with intellectual disabilities during police interviews. Mental Handicap Research, 8, 110–128.

Conley, R. W., Luckasson, R. & Bouthilet, G. N. (1992) The Criminal Justice System and Mental Retardation: Defendants and Victims. New York: PH Brooks.

Craft, M. & Craft, A. (1984) Mentally Abnormal Offenders. London: Baillière Tindall.

Day, K. (1988) A hospital based treatment programme for male mentally handicapped offenders. British Journal of Psychiatry, 153, 635–644.

Department of Health (1957) *Royal Commission on the Law Relating to Mental Illness and Mental Deficiency 1952–1957* (Percy Report). London: HMSO.

Edmondson, C. B. & Conger, J. C. (1996) A review of treatment efficacy for individuals with anger management problems. Conceptual, assessment and methodological issues. *Clinical Psychology Review*, **16**, 251–275.

Everington, C. & Fulero, S. M. (1999) Competence to confess: measuring understanding and suggestibility of defendants with mental retardation. *Mental Retardation*, **37**, 212–220.

Faulk, M. (1976) A psychiatric study of men serving a sentence in Winchester prison. *Medicine, Science and the Law*, **16**, 244–251.

Fedoroff, J. P. & Fedoroff, B. I. (2001) Sexual disorders, developmental disorders, developmental delay, and comorbid conditions. *National Association for the Dually Diagnosed Bulletin*, **4**, 23–28.

Glaser, W. & Deane, K. (1999) Normalisation in an abnormal world: a study of prisoners with an intellectual disability. *International Journal of Offending Therapy Criminology*, **43**, 338–356.

Gudjonsson, G. H., Clare, I. C., Rutters, S., *et al* (1993) *Persons at Risk during Interview in Police Custody: The Identification of Vulnerabilities* (Royal Commission on Criminal Justice Research Study no. 12). London: HMSO.

Hayes, S. (1991) Sex offenders. *Australia and New Zealand Journal of Developmental Disabilities*, **17**, 221–227.

Hodgins, S. (1992) Mental disorder, intellectual disability and crime. *Archives of General Psychiatry*, **49**, 476–483.

Johnston, S. J. & Halstead, S. (2000) Forensic issues in intellectual disability. *Current Opinion*, **13**, 475–480.

Kearns, A. & O'Connor, A. (1988) The mentally handicapped criminal offender: a 10-year study of two hospitals. *British Journal of Psychiatry*, **152**, 848–851.

Kebbell, M. R. & Hatton, C. (1999) People with mental retardation as witnesses in court: a review. *Mental Retardation*, **37**, 201–211.

Kiernan, C. & Dixon, C. (1991) *People with Mental Handicap Who Offend*. Manchester: Hester Adrian Research Centre.

Lindsay, W. R., Olley, S., Baillie, N., *et al* (1999) Treatment of adolescent sex offenders with intellectual disabilities. *Mental Retardation*, **37**, 320–333.

Lund, J. (1990) Mentally retarded criminal offenders in Denmark. *British Journal of Psychiatry*, **156**, 726–731.

Lyall, I., Holland, A. J., Collins, S., *et al* (1995*a*) Incidence of persons with a learning disability detained in police custody: a needs assessment for service development. *Medicine, Science and the Law*, **35**, 61–71.

—, — & — (1995*b*) Offending by adults with learning disabilities and the attitudes of staff to offending behaviour: implications for service development. *Journal of Intellectual Disability Research*, **39**, 501–508.

MacEachron, A. E. (1979) Mentally retarded offenders: prevalence and characteristics. *American Journal of Mental Deficiency*, **84**, 165–176.

Mikkelsen, E. J. & Stelk, W. J. (1999) *Criminal Offenders with Mental Retardation: Risk Assessment and the Continuum of Community Based Programs*. New York: NADD Press.

Murphy, G., Harnett, H. & Holland, A. J. (1995) A survey of intellectual disabilities amongst men on remand in prison. *Mental Handicap Research*, **8**, 81–98.

Murrey, G. J., Briggs, D. & Davis, C. (1992) Psychopathic, disordered, mentally ill and mentally handicapped sex offenders: a comparative study. *Medicine, Science and the Law*, **32**, 331–336.

Pearse, J., Gudjonsson, G. H., Clare, I. C. H., *et al* (1998) Police interviewing and psychological vulnerabilities: predicting the likelihood of a confession. *Journal of Community Applied Social Psychology*, **8**, 1–21.

Singleton, N. & Meltzer, H., Gatwood, R., *et al* (1998) *Psychiatric Morbidity among Prisoners in England and Wales*. London: Stationery Office.

Tredgold, A. F. (1915) Idiocy: imbecility: feeble-mindedness, Chapter XV. In *Early Mental Disease, Lancet* extra numbers (suppl. 2), 66–70.

# Further reading

Ashton, G. & Ward, A. D. (1992) *Mental Handicap and the Law*. London: Sweet & Maxwell.

Clare, I. C. H. & Murphy, G. (1998) Working with offenders or alleged offenders with intellectual disabilities. In *Clinical Psychology and People with Intellectual Disabilities* (ed. E. Emerson), Chichester: John Wiley & Sons.

Day, K. (1990) Mental retardation: clinical aspects and management. In *Principles and Practice of Forensic Psychiatry* (eds R. Bluglass & P. Bowden), pp. 399–418. London: Churchill Livingstone.

Department of Health (1994) *Review of Health and Social Services for Mentally Disordered Offenders and Others Requiring Similar Services. Vol. 7: People with Learning Disabilities (Mental Handicap) or with Autism* (Reed Report). London: HMSO.

Johnston, S. J. (2002) Review of risk assessment in offenders with learning disability: the evidence base. *Journal of Intellectual Disability Research*, **46** (suppl. 1), 47–56.

Reid, A. H. (1990) Mental retardation and crime. In *Principles and Practice of Forensic Psychiatry* (eds R. Bluglass & P. Bowden), pp. 393–397. London: Churchill Livingstone.

# CHAPTER 17

# Consent and decision-making capacity

## Anthony Holland

On 10 December 1948, the General Assembly of the United Nations adopted and proclaimed the Universal Declaration of Human Rights (United Nations, 1948). This Declaration required all countries that were signatories to respect the rights of individuals and to ensure that they were protected from the potentially oppressive powers of the State. The idea enshrined in the Articles of the Declaration is that of self-determination, and it is the duty of the State to care for its citizens, ensuring, for example, the right to life, education, equal protection under the law, privacy, freedom of movement, marriage and a family. The autonomy of the individual is central to the Universal Declaration of Human Rights and to the later European Convention on Human Rights (Council of Europe, 1952) and it applies regardless of 'race, colour, sex, language, religion, political and other opinion, national or social origin, property, birth or other status'. In 1994, the United Nations Standard Rules (United Nations, 1994) on the equalisation of opportunities for people with disabilities reaffirmed that this declaration also applied regardless of the presence or not of a disability. This concept of 'self-determination' underpins legislation in democratic countries. In England, Wales and Scotland, the European Convention on Human Rights has been incorporated into the national laws, requiring that legislation passed by the respective parliaments is compatible with the convention.

An acceptance of the rights of individuals by nation states is required, as history has shown that states tend not to be benign institutions, but can become oppressive. When specific conditions are allowed to develop, members of minority ethnic, religious or tribal groups, for example, become dehumanised and persecuted and, at its most extreme, this can lead to genocide (Glover, 1999). Thus, an appreciation of these general over-arching principles and of the specific laws in the jurisdiction within which we work and live, and their relevance to the health and social care support of people with learning disabilities and of those in other potentially disadvantaged groups, is of great importance.

# Background

People who, for example, have had a traumatic head injury or have learning disabilities, dementia or severe mental illness may develop or already have such serious mental disabilities that their ability to think and reason is adversely affected. Therefore, it is difficult for them independently to make the basic decisions necessary to lead an acceptable and safe life. It is under these circumstances that the concept of decision-making capacity can be particularly relevant. This chapter considers consent and decision-making capacity from both a legal and a clinical viewpoint. I argue that the capacity of individuals with mental disabilities to make decisions for themselves is the pivotal issue that determines whether their autonomy must be respected, or that others can and should take decisions on their behalf in order that they receive the support that is needed.

Case law in England and Wales has established that people who are competent have the right to determine for themselves whether to accept medical treatment or not (*Re T (Adult: Refusal of Treatment)*, 1992). If competent individuals refuse to give consent to treatment for a physical disorder, this must be respected even if it is likely to lead to their death. Similarly, it is unlawful to keep individuals somewhere against their will unless it has come about through an appropriate and recognised legal procedure with due course to appeal, such as a Court of Law sentencing a person to prison, or the Mental Health Act 1983 being used to compulsorily admit a person to hospital (*Collins v Wilcock*, 1984; *R v Rahman*, 1985). In most circumstances, what renders an action that would otherwise be unlawful (for example, surgical treatment) lawful is consent. To give meaningful consent, the person has to be appropriately informed about the decision in question, and has to have the ability (capacity) to be able meaningfully and freely to give or withhold consent.

Historically, there are many examples where these principles of consent have been overridden. For example: information has been withheld; the refusal of treatment by people capable of consent has been ignored, because of some specific characteristic (such as being a member of a particular religious or ethnic group); and individuals presumed to lack the ability to make decisions because of their learning disabilities have had their future determined for them, with little consideration as to what is right and just (Fennell, 1996).

With a greater appreciation of the general principle of individual autonomy and its implications, particularly in health care, the issue of how to resolve the dilemma that arises when an adult, who because of unconsciousness or of some mental disability such as dementia or severe learning disability, is unable to make decisions, or a particular decision, for himself or herself, requires consideration. There needs to be a framework that guides as to when a decision can lawfully be made by another person on behalf of someone unable to make that decision for himself or herself. This framework should also establish the principles that should inform the person making the decision. Clearly, there must be a mechanism whereby health treatment can lawfully proceed when a person is unable to make a health care decision. This is particularly the case when such treatment might relieve suffering and/or prevent death (Fulford, 1989). Although the treatment of a head injury in an unconscious person and the removal of an inflamed appendix in a person with severe learning disabilities unable to consent seem obvious courses of action and good practice, the issue becomes more complex in the case of decisions the benefits of which to the individual are less obvious or even absent (for example, sterilisation or treatment to briefly prolong life in terminal illness). What then is in the person's best interest? Where a person lacks capacity to make these decisions for himself or herself, who should decide? What should the guiding principles be?

In the legal jurisdiction of England and Wales, the issue of autonomy is of central importance. However, in the case of health care decisions, any treatment must be in the incapacitated person's 'best interests'(*Re C (Adult: Refusal of Medical Treatment)*, 1994; *Re F (Mental Patient: Sterilisation)*, 1990. In England and Wales, guidance on health care decisions is still in the form of case law, but in Scotland principles have become part of new statute (Adults with Incapacity (Scotland) Act 2000).

Although these principles apply to the assessment and treatment of physical disorder, they do not apply to the treatment of mental disorder. Mental health legislation in England and Wales enables the compulsory admission and treatment of individuals with mental disorders even if they are capable of making the necessary decision for themselves, provided that particular conditions are met. It has been argued (Department of Health, 1999) that particular ethical principles should apply regardless of whether treatment is for physical or mental disorder (Szmukler & Holloway, 2000; Zigmond & Holland, 2000). However, with respect to the key principle that there should not be a difference between what governs the treatment of physical disorders and mental disorders (i.e. non-discrimination), there is disagreement. It has been rejected by the Government for England and Wales, and modified for Scotland (Department of Health, 2000). This has particularly important implications for people with learning disabilities, because in the proposed new English and Welsh mental health legislation, the definition of 'mental disability' is similar to that proposed in the new mental incapacity legislation (see below). It is so broad that it will clearly encompass all people considered to have learning disabilities, thereby rendering them liable to detention, even if they are capable of making decisions for themselves (Department of Health, 2000). 'Mental disability' is defined as 'any disability or disorder of mind or brain, whether permanent or temporary, which results in an impairment or disturbance of mental functioning'.

The issue of consent and capacity to make decisions has much wider implications than simply in health care. For people with learning disabilities, decisions may be taken as to where they will live and what they will do. Often others manage their financial affairs, and there may well be the assumption that marriage and having a family is not a realistic or an appropriate option for them. Thus, the recognition of the balance between self-determination for those capable of making the necessary decisions and ensuring provision of adequate support for those that lack decision-making capacity becomes crucially important for these people in all aspects of their lives.

A Mental Incapacity Act has been proposed for England and Wales (Lord Chancellor, 1999) that is similar to the Scottish Adults with Incapacity Act 2000, and it is awaiting parliamentary time. At present, in terms of health care decisions, it is for the treating health care professional to decide what is in a person's best interest if that person, by reason of the presence of a mental disability, cannot make that decision for himself or herself (British Medical Association & Law Society, 1995; Wong *et al*, 1999). Although case law does not cover substitute decision-making, it does furnish the treating health care professional with a defence against the potential charge of assault (treating without consent), provided that the professional acted in the individual's best interests in terms of the treatment given. Although in many situations, the course of action that should be taken is obvious and clearly in the person's best interests, the case of *R v Bournewood Community and Mental Health NHS Trust, ex parte L* (1948) highlighted the lack of a direct legal remedy if there is dispute over what is in an 'incompetent' adult's best interest. Although the objection raised by Mr L's paid carers to his initial 'informal' admission to hospital was eventually resolved, leading to his discharge from hospital through the use of the appeal mechanism available when he was eventually detained under the Mental Health Act 1983, this case highlighted the inadequacies of the law in two respects. First, the House of Lords decided that the wording of the Act meant that adults lacking capacity to consent to hospital admission and treatment for their mental disorder could still be admitted informally to hospital. Thus, it was accepted that there was probably a very significant group of people admitted to hospital without their consent (because they lacked the capacity) and without any legal safeguards. Second, there was no easy means whereby a doctor's decision could be challenged in law (other than by judicial review), and therefore no way in which a dispute over what was in the best interests of an incapacitated person could be resolved.

In the House of Lords judgement, Lord Steyn, while noting that 'healthcare professionals will almost always act in the best interests of patients', went on to observe that Parliament had devised the Mental Health Act 1983 partly as a protection against 'misjudgement and lapses by professionals involved in healthcare', saying the following:

'Competence is a pivotal concept in decision-making about medical treatment. Competent patients' decisions about accepting or rejecting proposed treatment are respected. Incompetent patients' choices on the other hand, are put to one side, and alternative mechanisms for deciding about care are sought. Thus, enjoyment of one of the most fundamental rights of a free society – the right to determine what should be done to one's body – turns on the possession of those characteristics that we view as constituting decision-making competent'.

It is recognised in England and Wales that there is a lack of an appropriate legal framework to provide the basis for both substitute decision-making and determining best interest when a person lacks capacity. In addition, there is still only a limited attempt to marry legal principle with clinical practice (for an example, see Wong *et al*, 2000). This may be because there is a tension between the legal concept of capacity and the actual assessment of capacity. From a legal point of view, capacity has to be dichotomous – you have it or you do not have it at a particular point in time for a particular decision. Clinically, it is not as simple as this, and there may well be a grey area between a person's ability passively to assent or not and his or her ability to give informed consent. How capacity in any given situation can be reliably assessed and how a person's capacity can be maximised are key clinical issues.

## Decision-making capacity

Decision-making capacity is a legal concept (Gunn, 1994). Three main approaches to capacity have been considered and are referred to as outcome, status and functional (Wong *et al*, 1999). The outcome approach determines capacity on the basis of the actual decision a person makes. The implication is that if the decision is not in agreement with conventional wisdom, then the person should be considered to lack capacity. This approach goes against the principle of respect for self-determination and autonomy, and has therefore been rejected. The status approach depends on the presence of some specific characteristic, such as being below a certain age or having a clinical diagnosis (e.g. severe learning disability, dementia, schizophrenia) that by itself implies incapacity. Thus, the assumption is made that this particular characteristic will inevitably render the individual incapacitated, regardless of the exact severity and/or nature of the mental disability or the severity

**311**

of the decision in question. This approach has been rejected on empirical grounds (Grisso & Appelbaum, 1995, 1998), although it continues to be a principle underpinning mental health legislation. The functional approach is now widely accepted as the most appropriate (Hoggett, 1994). It is the observed limitations in a person's abilities resulting from the presence of a mental disability, rendering him or her unable to meet the demands of the decision in question that determine whether he or she is incapacitated or not. The key point is that capacity is time- and decision-specific. It is not sufficient to give a diagnosis. It must be determined that the functional abilities required to make a particular decision are impaired. As is discussed below, these abilities might be improved through treatment of the mental disability or individuals may be helped to gain the necessary abilities through the use of different forms of communication or through the use of learning aids.

## Legal standards of capacity

Assessment of capacity, for example for the Court of Protection, has been shown to be very haphazard and most closely to resemble a status approach, i.e. a particular diagnosis is seen as a sufficient criterion (Suto *et al*, 2002). One reason for this may well be that that the legal criteria against which an individual's abilities need to be compared are not widely appreciated. Although there is subtle variation across legal jurisdictions, some key principles have emerged (Lord Chancellor, 1999). The four key requirements of 'capacity' are taken to be: the ability to communicate a choice; to understand and to retain the relevant information; and to balance the information in order to arrive at a choice.

### *Communicating a choice*

Individuals must have the ability to make apparent what they have decided. This is clearly a necessary requirement, but simply having the ability to state a preference is not sufficient to be considered to have capacity, as consideration has to be given to the thinking around the making of that choice (see below). The inability to communicate may arise for many reasons, for example unconsciousness, thought disorder or extreme ambivalence. Some may be unable to communicate a choice through spoken language, but can use other forms of communication. Thus, the use, for example, of sign language, electronic aids or written communication may make individuals, who might otherwise be considered unable to communicate their choices and therefore incapacitated, able to do so. The use of speech and language therapy expertise in this regard may be critical.

## Understanding the relevant information

For health care decisions, the standard of understanding that has to be achieved is low, and is described as understanding in 'broad terms' and 'simple language' (*Chatterton v Gerson Queen's Bench 432*). However, it is also necessary that individuals appreciate that the information directly applies to them. The key issues that individals should be informed about and understand in terms of any proposed health treatment are as follows:

- the nature of the treatment
- the purpose of the treatment
- the risks of having the treatment
- the risks of not having the treatment
- alternative treatments

Individuals therefore need to have a broad idea of what is involved, what the potential outcomes (risks and benefits) are, what the prognosis without treatment is and that there are alternatives. There are therefore two parts: first, making available the information in a manner that maximises the chance that it can be understood, and second, determining whether the individual has understood the relevant information and appreciates that it applies to him or her. With respect to the former, the information may either not have been provided at all or may have been given in a rushed and cursory manner, and therefore the individual cannot have been expected to have understood it. Wong *et al* (2000), in determining the capacity of people with different mental disabilities to consent or not to having a clinically recommended blood test, found that the use of an information sheet was particularly helpful for people with learning disabilities. The five points listed above provide a framework for a structured interview, and the task of the clinician is to explore each of these in the context of the particular decision that an individual is being asked to make.

## Retaining relevant information

There has been some debate as to whether this is a necessary criterion. It was included in the Law Commission's proposals, but may be redundant in that the inability to retain information for an adequate period of time is very likely to result in an inability to understand, and may therefore be covered by the section above.

## Balance the information in order to arrive at a choice

Meeting this criterion requires the ability to consider the information given and its relevance. It is not concerned with the outcome of the decision, but rather the process that the individual has gone through in arriving at a choice. A number of factors might adversely affect this, including, for example, the ability to reason (which might be impaired in severe learning disability, dementia or thought disorder), the impact of delusional experiences consequent to mental illness, and the extreme negative thinking associated with severe depression. If an individual can give no reason for his or her decision, or the reasons given are obviously being affected by a mental disorder or disability, for example, by delusional experiences, then this particular ability is absent.

## Clinical determination of decision-making capacity

The most firmly established method for informing this assessment process is the MacCAT–T Tool for Treatment, which was devised as part of the MacArthur Treatment Competence study (Grisso & Appelbaum, 1998). The conclusion as to whether a person with a mental disability has the capacity to make a particular decision is ultimately a matter of judgement after the necessary assessments have been undertaken in a structured and informed manner. It is decision-specific and requires that the person making the judgement is knowledgeable about the decision in question. With respect to health care decisions, it is therefore usually the treating professional who should be ultimately responsible for determining whether an individual has the capacity to make a given health care decision. However, he or she might wish to seek advice as to whether an individual has a mental disability that might adversely affect decision-making capacity, whether any intervention might improve this capacity (see below) and how capacity might reliably be assessed. In law there is a presumption of capacity, and therefore assessment is undertaken only if there is reason to doubt an individual's ability. Individuals can be considered to lack capacity only if they have a mental disability. As stated earlier, the proposed new Mental Incapacity Act defines 'mental disability' very broadly. Thus, decision-making capacity might be clearly absent (for example, owing to unconsciousness) or it might be in question because an individual is known to have a mental disability or because the treating professional is alerted to that possibility by the nature of the individual's response to particular questions (for example, about his or her symptoms and the nature of his or her suspected illness).

The clinical assessment of decision-making capacity is a process, the four stages of which are outlined below.

First, there is a presumption of capacity, and this can be challenged only if there is evidence of a mental disorder such as a learning disability. Thus, it is important to establish the presence and the nature of any disability. Furthermore, understanding more about the causes of a particular mental disability may aid understanding of the way in which decision-making capacity might be impaired. For example, in the case of a person with early dementia, memory might be a key problem and the use of memory aids might be helpful. Clearly, if the person is unconscious, no further action needs to be taken to establish whether he or she lacks decision-making capacity, and any action can proceed, provided that it is in the patient's best interest and is the least invasive/restrictive option. In emergency and life-threatening situations, treatment in the patient's best interest would follow immediately, but if time allows, further consultation might take place (see below).

Second, using the framework given above, the key facts with respect to the decision in question and what the individual needs to know in order to make an informed decision (e.g. the nature of the treatment, risks and benefits) should be established. Information may need to be repeated or given using aids (such as photographs: see Wong *et al*, 1999) or alternative forms of communication.

Third, the individual is interviewed to determine whether he or she is able to understand and balance the information, and arrive at and communicate a choice. This requires a structured approach, assessing each of the key elements. In an as yet unpublished study (Bellhouse *et al*, further information available from the author upon request) assessing the decision-making capacity of a consecutive series of people admitted to mental health or learning disability services, it was found that the factor that best predicted overall capacity was whether individuals appreciated that they might be unwell. They did not have to accept that they were unwell, but rather that it was a possibility. Similarly, a failure to appreciate the 'purpose of treatment' was a good predictor of overall incapacity. Thus, the assessment takes the form of a semi-structured interview that probes an individual's understanding of why a particular course of action has been recommended (hospital admission, medication, etc.), what form the treatment takes, what the potential risks and benefits of admission/treatment are and the risks and benefits of not following the recommended course of action.

Fourth, if individuals have the relevant knowledge, can they balance it in a manner that informs their decision? Do they appreciate that not receiving a particular treatment could adversely affect their health and that this could lead to death? In the case of people with psychiatric illness, the risks of not coming into hospital may be suicide or harm to others, or a deterioration in their health or social circumstances. This needs to be understood.

At the end of what is, in essence, a semi-structured interview, a judgement is made. What remains unclear is the threshold that should be applied below which an individual should be considered incapacitated. This clearly should not be so stringent that a significant number of those without mental disabilities would be judged incapable, but it should be sufficiently stringent that those with mental disabilities, who are at risk of neglect or harm, can be protected from the consequences of their apparent indecision. Again, there is a balance to be struck between the respect for autonomy that goes with having capacity and the need to ensure that people potentially without capacity do not suffer from benign neglect as neither they or anyone else is willing or able to make a particular decision on their behalf.

## The principle of 'best interest'

The finding of incapacity carries with it continuing responsibilities, whether the decision in question is about health, living circumstances, financial affairs or other matters. The proposed English and Welsh Mental Incapacity Act indicates that the concept of 'best interest' includes trying to identify the discernible wishes of the individual concerned (either now or from earlier in his or her life), and the views of family or other 'significant others', as well as acting in the least invasive/restrictive manner possible. If informed consent is not possible, maximally informed assent should be the objective. For specific situations, such as a request for the sterilisation of a person lacking capacity, it is for a court to decide whether it would 'not be unlawful' to perform the surgery, on the basis of whether, in the court's judgement, such a course of action would be in that person's best interest.

## Conclusions

There are two extremes. One is paternalistic, taking a 'status' approach and arguing that the presence of a mental disability, however minor, is sufficient to consider individuals incapable of taking decisions for themselves and therefore that decisions must be made by others and paternalistically imposed. This view, together with the idea that society must be protected, dominated the early institutional movement and is beginning to appear again with proposed new legislation that lacks clear ethical principles or legal safeguards and enables the detention of those with presumed severe and dangerous personality disorders (Home Office & Department of Health, 1999; Grounds, 2001). The other perspective is that the principle of self-determination should be protected at all costs, and therefore the decisions of individuals should always be respected. In certain settings, this is best illustrated by the statement that it was the individual's 'choice' to do or not to do something, the consequence of which may be at best neglect and at worse suffering or death (Holland & Wong, 1999). The resolution of these two unacceptable extremes comes about through the use of the legal concept of decision-making capacity, and by its valid and reliable assessment. If the legal concept is understood, a framework for its clinical assessment can be established and applied. This requires the structured assessment of the key elements that make up any informed decision. This in turn leads to a judgement about an individual's overall capacity to make a specific decision at a particular time. The key issues are: has the person been informed in a manner that maximises his or her chance of understanding, can he or she understand the relevant information, consider and balance the options, and arrive at and communicate a choice? If capacity is lacking, then the best interests of the person concerned and the least invasive option should be the determining factors in considering the most appropriate course of action. Although the most appropriate option may be obvious and, if there is doubt, the 'duty of care' is to act to save life, there are decisions for which broader issues may be relevant.

# References

British Medical Association & Law Society (1995) *Assessment of Mental Capacity – Guidance for Doctors and Lawyers*. London: BMA.

Council of Europe (1952) *Convention of the Protection of Human Rights and Fundamental Freedoms*. Rome: Council of Europe.

Department of Health (1999) *Reform of the Mental Health Act 1983*. London: Stationery Office.

— (2000) *Reforming the Mental Health Act. Part 1 The New Legal Framework*. London: Stationery Office.

Fennell, P. (1996) *Treatment without Consent. Law, Psychiatry and the Treatment of Mentally Disordered People since 1845*. London: Routledge.

Fulford, K. W. M. (1989) Treatment. In *Moral Theory and Medical Practice* (ed. K. W. M. Fulford), pp. 186–194. Cambridge: Cambridge University Press.

Glover, J. (1999) *Humanity: A Moral History of the 20th Century*. London: Jonathan Cape.

Grisso, T. & Appelbaum, P. S. (1995) Comparison of standards for assessing patients' capacities to make treatment decisions. *American Journal of Psychiatry*, **152**, 1033–1037.

— & — (1998) *Assessing Competence to Consent to Treatment: A Guide for Physicians and Other Health Professionals*. Oxford: Oxford University Press.

Grounds, A. (2001) Reforming the Mental Health Act. *British Journal of Psychiatry*, **179**, 387–389.

Gunn, M. (1994) The meaning of incapacity. *Medical Law Review*, **2**, 8–29.

Hoggett, B. (1994) Mentally incapacitated adults and decision-making. The Law Commission's project. In *Decision-Making and Problems of Incompetence* (ed. A. Grubb), 27–40. Chichester: John Wiley & Sons.

Holland, A. J. & Wong, J. (1999) Genetically determined obesity in Prader–Willi syndrome: the ethics and legality of treatment. *Journal of Medical Ethics*, **25**, 230–236.

Home Office & Department of Health (1999) *Managing Dangerous People with Severe Personality Ddisorder: Proposals for Consultation*. London: Home Office.

Lord Chancellor (1999) *Making Decisions. The Government's Proposal's for Making Decisions on behalf of Mentally Incapacited Adults: A Report Issued in the Light of Responses to the Consultation Paper "Who decides?"*. London: Stationery Office.

Suto, I., Clare, I. C. H. & Holland, A. J. (2002) Substitute financial decision-making in England and Wales: a study of the Court of Protection. *Journal of Social Welfare and Family Law*, **24**, 37–54.

Szmukler, G. & Holloway, F. (2000) Reform of the Mental Health Act: health or safety? *British Journal of Psychiatry*, **177**, 196–200.

United Nations (1948) *Universal Declaration of Human Rights*. New York: United Nations.

— (1994) *Standard Rules on the Equalization of Opportunities for People with Disabilities*. New York: United Nations.

Wong, J., Clare, I. C. H., Gunn, M., *et al* (1999) Capacity to make health care decisions: its importance in clinical practice. *Psychological Medicine*, **29**, 437–446.

—, —, Holland, A. J., *et al* (2000) The capacity of people with a 'mental disability' to make a health care decision. *Psychological Medicine*, **30**, 295–306.

Zigmond, A. & Holland, A. J. (2000) Unethical mental health law; history repeats itself. *Journal of Mental Health Law*, **3**, 49–56.

*Chatterton v Gerson (1981) Queen's Bench 432*
*Collins v Wilcock* [1984] 3 AllER 374.
*Re C (Adult: Refusal of Medical Treatment)* [1994] 1 AllER 819.
*Re F (Mental Patient: Sterilisation)* [1990] 2 AC 1.
*Re T (Adult: Refusal of Treatment)* [1992] AllER 649.
*R v Bournewood Community and Mental Health NHS Trust, ex parte L* [1948] 1 AllER 634.
*R v Rahman* [1985] 81 Criminal Appeal Reports 349.

# Selective glossary of terms used in molecular genetics

**Allele**

The name used for any one particular form of a specific gene or stretch of DNA. There may be several alternative alleles – in which case the gene is said to be polymorphic.

**Aneuploid**

Where a cell contains other than the normal number of chromosomes, usually due to loss or gain of a chromosome. It excludes those whose number is a whole multiple of the haploid count (i.e. normal diploid count, triploidy, tetraploidy, etc.).

**Anticipation**

Originally meant that a condition had an earlier age of onset in subsequent family generations; nowadays it may also mean an increasing severity.

**Autosome**

A chromosome other than a sex chromosome, 22 pairs in humans.

**Bacterial artificial chromosome (BAC)**

A large specific stretch of foreign DNA can be inserted into this bacterial construct to allow further copies to be made (a clone). They have become almost ubiquitous tools for sequencing of chromosomes.

**Biallelic**

Where only two forms of a gene or stretch of DNA exist in a population.

**Centromere**

A specialised region near the middle of a chromosome where the spindle apparatus attaches during cell division.

**Chiasma**

During meisois, this is the point on two homologous chromosomes where material is exchanged between them (recombination).

## Chromatid

The copy of a chromosome produced during its replication.

## Complementary DNA (cDNA)

This is a synthetic single-stranded form of DNA made complementary to mRNA, using a reverse transcriptase enzyme. More chemically stable than mRNA, it is an easier tool to manipulate.

## Contig

A construct of overlapping pieces of DNA that provides complete coverage of a given region of a chromosome to facilitate mapping and sequencing.

## CpG island

A stretch of DNA that contains a great excess of cytosine–guanine nucleotide pairs. It usually resides near a gene and hypermethylation of the island and gene is a method of control of gene expression.

## Cytogenetics

The study of chromosomes and their aberrations.

## Diploid

A cell that has two of each of the autosomes and two sex chromosomes as its complement (in humans, a total of 23 pairs, or 46 chromosomes).

## Dominant negative

Where a mutant protein from one chromosome forms an inactive complex with, or acts competitively on a target with, the normal protein from the other chromosome to produce an apparent reduction or complete silencing of gene activity. The opposite, whereby activity is increased, is termed 'dominant positive' and is one form of gain-of-function mutation.

## Dynamic mutations

Mutations that change in form across generations, classically the expansion of triplet repeat DNA.

## Epigenetic

Those changes in a cell that are inherited but are not coded for directly by DNA.

## Fluorescent in situ hybridisation (FISH)

An important method of cytogenetics where fluorescently tagged DNA probes are used to study specific regions of chromosomes, usually with a resolution greater than that available under a light microscope.

## Fragile site

A region of a chromosome that does not stain, resulting in an apparent gap. Nearly all are seen only under certain culture conditions. Divided into heritable ('rare') forms such as that produced in a folate deficient medium in carriers of fragile-X, and non-heritable ('common') forms.

## Functional polymorphism

A site on a chromosome that exhibits various forms in the population, some (or all) of which are associated with altered expression levels of a related gene.

## Gamete

A germ cell, sperm or ovum, with a haploid number of chromosomes.

## Gene

Stretch(es) of DNA (exons) that code for a given polypeptide and now usually also meaning the intervening non-coding sequences (introns), the promoter region and the tailing sequences.

## Gene rescue

Essentially an experimental form of gene therapy by which the phenotypic consequences of a specifically created gene mutation are reversed by insertion of an active copy of the gene into the genome.

## Gene therapy

The correction for lack of a gene product by the insertion of an extraneous active copy of a gene into a genome. Divided into somatic cell gene therapy, where non-germ cells are altered (e.g. by DNA insertion using a virus into lung epithelial cells in patients with cystic fibrosis) and the much more controversial germ cell gene therapy.

## Green fluorescent protein (GFP)

A jellyfish protein that glows green under fluorescent light. It can be fused to another protein, with the complex remaining fully functional. Increasingly used as a reporter in dynamic studies of protein functions.

## Haploid

A cell that contains only one of each pair of autosomes and one out of the pair of sex chromosomes (23 chromosomes in total in humans).

## Haplo-insufficiency

Is used to describe the situation when inactivation of a gene on one chromosome results in a decrease, not absence, of product genes; probably common, as most genes are expressed from both chromosomes.

## Heterozygote

Refers to the presence of different alleles of a given locus on the individual chromosome of a pair.

**High-resolution banding**
A cytogenetic method which reveals much finer detail in the banding pattern of chromosomes than classical staining.

**Homoeobox**
A specific 180 base pair DNA motif contained within a HOX gene; it codes for the homoeodomain part of a transcription factor.

**Homozygote**
The situation where both alleles at a given locus of a chromosome pair are identical.

**HOX genes (or homoeotic genes)**
A family of genes that are crucial to normal development, all containing a homoeodomain DNA motif.

**Hypermethylation**
A stretch of DNA with an excess of methylated nucleotides over other regions. Such methylation takes place after DNA synthesis and is important, for example, in imprinting.

**Imprinting**
Occurs when a gene is expressed on only one chromosome of a pair that originates from a specific parent, the parent-of-origin effect.

**Intrasyndromic variation**
The variation in phenotype seen between individuals who have the same genetic syndrome.

**Karyotype**
The complete chromosomal complement of an individual cell defined according to standard notation.

**Kinetochores**
An architectural feature of the chromosome where the microtubules of the spindle apparatus attach.

**LINES (long period interspersed sequences)**
Repeated blocks of DNA that are thought to be due to retroposon activity.

**Linkage analysis**
A set of tests that determine whether the segregation of chromosomal markers, or markers and a disease, within a pedigree has occurred by chance. The LOD score is a statistical measure of this likelihood.

**Linkage disequilibrium**
The situation where genetic markers in a population occur together at a frequency different from that predicted by their known separation on a

chromosome. Its interpretation is complex and can be due to founder effects or inhibition of recombination.

**Locus**
The exact location of a stretch of DNA on a chromosome.

**Lyonisation**
The compaction of any X chromosomes in a cell above a numerical count of one. 'Barr bodies' were an early detection of this in saliva.

**Megabase**
A million base pairs of DNA (or RNA); one of the standard units of measure in the genome.

**Meiosis**
The type of cell division that results in germ cells whereby the number of chromosomes in each gamete is half that in somatic cells.

**Mendelian**
Inheritance that follows the classical rules first identified by Gregor Mendel – autosomal dominant and negative and the sex-linked equivalents.

**Message**
Geneticist's shorthand for mRNA.

**Messenger RNA (mRNA)**
The ribonucleoprotein intermediate transcribed from coding DNA (genes) and usually passed out of the nucleus to be translated into a polypeptide or protein.

**Metaphase**
The highly condensed phase of chromosomes during cell division, this allows easy visualisation under the light microscope.

**Microarrays**
Grids (often termed chips) containing a large number of tiny biochemical reaction sites that can be used to analyse small amounts of DNA, RNA or proteins in a highly parallel fashion.

**Microdeletions**
Deletions of parts of a chromosome that are too small to be visible using classical staining techniques.

**Mitosis**
Cell division in somatic tissues that generates cells with the full normal chromosome count.

**Molecular probe**

A piece of cDNA that has been labelled using radioactivity or a fluorescent tag that is then used to bind and identify the complementary underlying DNA from a chromosome.

**Monogenic**

A phenotype (often we mean here a clinical disorder) that is caused by the action of one gene.

**MRX**

Non-syndromal X-linked mental retardation; inherited learning disability is the only clear phenotypic feature.

**MRXS**

Syndromal X-linked mental retardation; learning disability is present, along with other clinical features such as dysmorphisms.

**Mutations**

Alteration in the DNA of a gene from the population common form (wild type). The alteration may be beneficial, deleterious or have no apparent effect (null mutation).

**Oligogenic**

A phenotype that is caused by the synergistic, additive or interactive effects of only a few genes. The exact number is not defined clearly in the literature.

**Oligonucleotide primers**

The synthetic molecules used to bracket and define stretches of DNA for amplification by polymerase chain reaction.

**P chromosome arm**

The shorter arm of a chromosome, defined from centromere to telomere.

**Partial penetrance**

The situation in which the carriage of a mutant gene does not always lead to a clinical disorder. This is the normal situation for a very large number of clinical conditions.

**Penetrance**

How frequently a given outcome (e.g. clinical disorder) is seen when a mutant gene is present.

**Phenotype**

The detectable or observable effects of the interaction of genes with environment. In medicine it is often narrowed to mean a specific clinical outcome.

**Polygenic**

A phenotype that is the result of a large number of genes taken together.

**Polymerase chain reaction (PCR)**

One of the most important tools available to molecular science, which allows the specific and very sensitive amplification of small stretches of DNA.

**Polymorphism**

A site on a chromosome (allele) that exists in different forms in the population, in most cases without clinical effect (but see functional polymorphism).

**Position effect**

Where the phenotype resulting from a gene depends on the chromosomal environment and architecture in which the gene is embedded; an example would be a different expression of a gene due to a nearby structural chromosomal abnormality.

**Proteome**

All the proteins expressed by a cell or organ at one particular time under a given set of conditions.

**Pseudoautosomal**

Special regions of the X and Y chromosomes that recombine with each other at meiosis and thus are inherited in a fashion that does not show apparent sex-linkage.

**Q chromosome arm**

The longer arm of a chromosome defined from centromere to telomere.

**Quantitative trait locus (QTL)**

Variation can be quantitative (e.g. height) rather than form discrete categories (e.g. biological sex). QTLs are genetic loci that make a contribution to the overall trait. The term is often applied to genes assumed to make small, summed contributions to a polygenic multifactorial condition.

**Recombination**

In humans this is the process by which chromosomal material is exchanged (by crossing over) between chromosomes of a pair during meiosis.

**Restriction endonuclease**

An enzyme that cuts ('digests') DNA at a specific site defined by the sequence of underlying DNA base pairs.

## Restriction fragment length polymorphisms (RFLPs)

Stably inherited differences in the sites for DNA-digesting enzymes (restriction endonucleases) yielding different fragment sizes between individuals.

## RNA interference

A method where short strands of RNA are used specifically to induce the degradation of the targeted gene's mRNA.

## Sex chromosomes

The differently shaped (heteromorphic) chromosome pair that determines the biological sex of an individual, termed X and Y in humans.

## Simple tandem repeats (STRs)

Collective name for stretches of DNA of differing lengths and underlying DNA sequence that repeat themselves and where the number of repeat units is variable in a population.

## Single-nucleotide polymorphisms (SNPs)

A simple polymorphism that takes the form of one nucleotide replacing another at a given site in different subsets of a population. At present, the focus of much research as a tool to study genomic variation.

## Single-stranded DNA (ssDNA)

This is formed experimentally from normal DNA by gentle heating ('melting') and *in vivo* as an intermediate during transcription.

## Subtelomeric rearrangements

Chromosomal abnormalities occurring in the (usually) gene-rich regions immediately centromeric to the telomere. They are difficult to detect by routine karyotyping methods.

## Telomere

A specialised DNA–protein structure at the end of the chromosomal arms formed of repeat DNA sequences and single-strand loop, maintained by a key cell enzyme called telomerase. They are essential to prevent chromosomes from fusing with each other and to avoid DNA loss.

## Transcriptosome

All the mRNA expressed by a cell or organ at one particular time under a given set of conditions.

## Transgenic

An organism created by the insertion of externally derived DNA sequences into the germ cells.

**Translation**

The synthesis of polypeptides and proteins by the ribosomal machinery in the cytoplasm under the direction of mRNA coding sequence.

**Transposable elements**

A group of mobile genetic units that includes transposons, retroviruses, etc. that can insert into, exit from and relocate between chromosomes.

**Trisomy**

Three copies of an autosome or sex chromosome present in a normally diploid cell.

**Uniparental disomy (UPD)**

Occurs when both chromosomes of a pair arise from a single parent.

**Yeast artificial chromosome (YAC)**

A bacterial–yeast construct that can be used to clone and manipulate very large stretches of DNA.

# Index

Compiled by Linda English